PRAISE FOR THE FIRST EDITION OF "HAVING CHILDREN"

". . . provides a clear pathway through the forest of alternatives available to couples who want information before they make important decisions about pregnancy, childbirth, and their first year of parenting. Parents can quickly and easily find the best resource to help them gain the understanding they seek . . ."
Connecticut Family Newspaper
New Haven, Connecticut

"[the editors] realize you can't glean all the necessary child-care information from one source and have done all the hunting and gathering for you."
Chicago Tribune

"What a wonderful resource! It will lead the reader to multiple sources of information for any subject they need. Book titles, Internet sites, videos . . . This book has it all."
Deborah Wage, MSN, FNP, CNM, Certified Family Nurse Practitioner
Nashville, Tennessee

"First-time parents are often overwhelmed with the challenges of pregnancy, birthing, and preparing for that vital first year. . . . this easy-to-use guidebook provides a shortcut to the information and answers that concerned parents seek."
Northwest Family Magazine

"The resources identified are terrific and very inclusive. The rating system is great!"
Joseph Shaeffer, ARNP/CNM, Certified Ob/Gyn Nurse Practitioner
Spokane, WA

"Helping expectant and new parents sort through the maze of available information . . ."
Seattle's Child

". . . the margins with ratings and brief descriptions are a good idea . . . Organizing the book by topic is especially helpful . . ."
Anne Barash, MSW, MD, State University of New York Health Science Center
Syracuse, New York

"The format of the book and the multiple indexes are great, especially the Subject Index which is an excellent way to reference topics."
Karen Stern, OTR/ICCE-CPE, ICEA Certified Childbirth Educator
Philadelphia, Pennsylvania

"This guidebook is a comprehensive and valuable source of information."
Shirley Wingate, RNC, CD, Childbirth Educator, Certified Doula
Urbana, Illinois

"Without exception I thought it was a wonderful and important resource, and applaud your efforts. The book is thorough, interesting, and easy to use. The collection of 'recommended resources' was very good, and I agree with your 'best' and 'worst' recommendations."
Janice Anderson, MD, Family Physician
Monroeville, PA

HAVING CHILDREN

The Best Resources To Help You Prepare

Second Edition

Anne Montgomery, MD, IBCLC, FAAFP

Editor

A Resource Pathways Guidebook

Seattle, Washington

Published by Resource Pathways, Inc.
22525 S.E. 64th Place, Suite 253
Issaquah, WA 98027

Editor: Anne M. Montgomery, MD, IBCLC, FAAFP

Managing Editor:
    Lisle Steelsmith, MA

Researchers:
    Kathie Jackson Anderson, Lucy Campos,
    Joan Elmenhurst, Julie Glassmoyer, Jill K. Nixon

Book Design and Production:
    Sandra Harner and Kelly Rush,
    Laing Communications Inc., Redmond, WA

Printing: Hignell Book Printing, Winnipeg, Manitoba, Canada

Publisher's Cataloging-in-Publication

Having children : the best resources to help you
        prepare / Anne Montgomery, editor. -- 2nd ed.
        p. cm.
        Includes bibliographical references and
    indexes.
        LCCN: 99-60549
        ISBN: 1-892148-06-4

        1. Parenting--Bibliography. 2. Childbirth--
    Bibliography. 3. Prenatal care--Bibliography. 4.
    Fertility, Human--Bibliography.   I. Montgomery,
    Anne M. II. Resource Pathways (Firm)

    Z7164.M2H46 1999   016.649'1
                    QBI99-306

Printed in Canada.

CONTENTS

INTRODUCTION

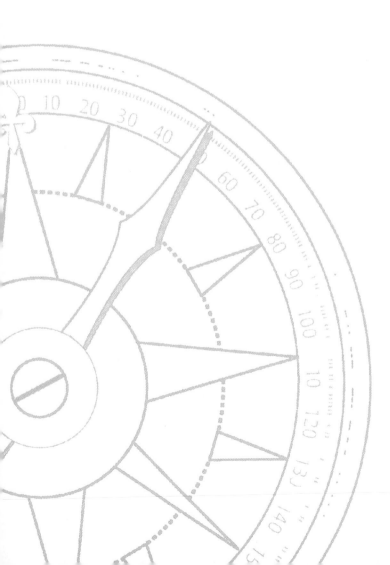

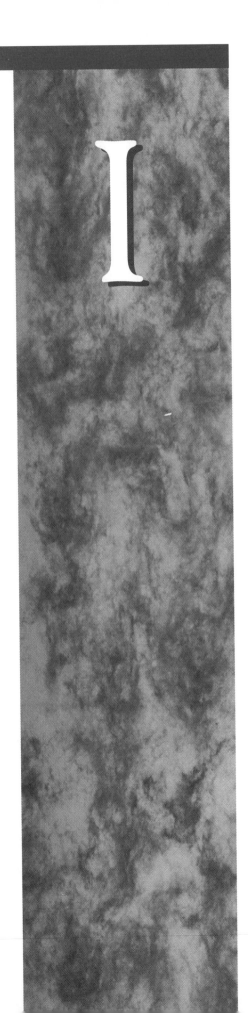

INTRODUCTION

Congratulations on your decision to have a child. Your life will never be the same! You can look forward to new joys, new fears, and many changes in yourself and your relationships. Parenthood is an amazing adventure, and we hope to help you get the best start along that new path.

We've designed *Having Children* to help you in four crucial ways:

- By laying out the broad issues you'll face as you prepare to become a parent and once you have a baby—from pregnancy through childbirth and during the first few months of your newborn's life, as well as how to handle possible infertility concerns that may arise.

- By creating clear "pathways" to the most useful resources at each stage of your journey—a unique feature of this guide. We tell you who has worthwhile information, and where to find it.

- By providing detailed and candid full-page reviews of all the resources we cover—215 of them, over 40 of which are sites on the World Wide Web—so you'll know what's available for free on the Internet, and what's worth buying.

- By building "search engines" to make it easy for you to find and sort reviews, as well as where to go to find additional information—that's why there are multiple indices and a comprehensive chapter which lists support organizations.

People have been having babies throughout human history, of course, and the basic biology of it all hasn't changed. Babies are the same as babies have always been. However, human culture has evolved and changed, and with it our approach to birth and parenting. Most of us in the United States have not grown up in the large, extended families typically found in other cultures and throughout our history. As a result, we have not learned much about bearing babies and parenting children while we were growing up, so we have to read and question and observe as adults. Consequently we get our experiential learning of how to give birth and parent when we have our first child. In addition, changes in the roles played by men and women in our society, as well as newer research about health and development, have profoundly affected our approach to parenting.

Most women in history and throughout the world have given birth in the comfort of their homes in the company of their families. However, in the 20th century, birth has shifted from the home to the hospital. Birth, breastfeeding, and child rearing became "scientific" and medicalized, by mutual agreement of physicians and parents. Over the past few decades, however, women have chosen to regain control of the birth process, and the process of having a baby has returned to a more "natural" approach. Mothers and fathers participate in decision-making about birth, breastfeeding, and parenting. And fathers are often present for the birth and participate fully in parenting their new baby.

Hopeful and expectant parents try to tailor their lifestyles to provide the best start for their baby-to-be, making healthful choices about nutrition and lifestyle. They choose their maternity care provider carefully, consider their preferences for an obstetrician, family physician, or midwife. They choose the setting for their birth—hospital, birth center, or home. They educate themselves about childbirth so that they can participate with their provider in decision-making.

Extended families can provide support, but often, young couples make choices about birth, child care, employment, and lifestyle that don't reflect their parents' experiences or preferences. They will need to sort through conflicting information to find out what fits best for them. Also, couples having difficulty getting pregnant face additional decisions about infertility evaluation and treatment, as well as whether or not they should consider adoption. Couples who have lost a pregnancy through miscarriage or stillbirth will need to grieve, and will wonder about their chances to have a baby in the future.

Parenting today is, in many ways, characterized by the same challenges parents have always faced. Yet, in some ways, parenting today is dramatically different than it was just a generation ago. New findings in infant and child development, medical research in obstetrics, gynecology, urology, and pediatric care, and progress in assisted reproductive technology all contribute to new decisions that prospective parents must make. This new body of knowledge, coupled with societal changes, lifestyle trends, and the evolving roles of men and women all potentially make some issues facing new families more complex than they've been before.

This book contains advice and information relating to health care for women and babies. It is not intended to replace medical advice, and should be used to supplement rather than replace regular care by your health care providers. Since every obstetrical and pediatric situation is unique, always consult with your doctors for your specific health care and decisions.

HOW THIS BOOK IS ORGANIZED

As part of our ongoing research and analysis, we've identified books, websites, videotapes, CD-ROMs, and other resources that are widely available to both men and women as they learn about pregnancy, childbirth, and becoming a parent.

We've organized these resources into seven broad categories, found in **Chapters II through VIII**:

- Pregnancy and Fetal Development

- Childbirth

- Postpartum Maternal Care

- Specifically for Fathers

- Your Newborn

- Solutions for Infertility

- Gaining an Overview

Each chapter begins with background information and advice on the topic. Reviews of resources covering each topic then form the heart of each chapter. These full-page, fact-filled, candid reviews offer an appraisal of each resource. And each follows the same format making it easy for you to do cross-comparisons as you find the resource that best meets your individual needs.

We separate evaluations from descriptions, so you can focus either on what a resource contains or what we think of it—and why. Facts of publication (author, author background, publisher, edition's latest copyright date, ISBN, and price) appear in a sidebar. Here, you will also find a phrase that sums up our evaluation of each resource's "ease of use" along with our "overall rating," and we give each resource 1–4 stars. We always place the highest-rated resources first in each chapter. If there are more than one resource with the same Star Rating, we list them alphabetically by title.

Recommended resources can be found directly following each chapter's introduction and are noted by the following icon:

 "Recommended For:"

Our Star Rating system is defined as follows:

Four Star Rating System

★★★★   Highly recommended—top quality at a fair price!

★★★   Well done; a good resource but not outstanding.

★★   Worth considering; check the description.

★   Your time and money would be better spent elsewhere.

Chapter IX lists resources that we not only recommend for our book's general chapter topics, but are "terrific" resources in how they address a *specific* situation, such as: exercising for an easier labor and faster recovery; dealing with a teen's unplanned pregnancy; handling the pregnancy, childbirth, and parenting of twins or multiples; choosing alternative childbirth practices; breastfeeding and returning to work; facing the emotional aspects of infertility; and more. These resources are designated in this section and throughout our book with the following icon:

 "A Terrific Resource for a Selected Topic"

Chapter X includes a helpful listing of over 80 organizations and other groups you may want to contact for additional information and parent support. Finally, in **Chapter XI**, we've also provided several useful indices which list *all* the resources reviewed in this guidebook, arranged alphabetically by Title, by Author, by Publisher, by Media, and by Subject.

MEET RESOURCE PATHWAYS

As consumers in this Information Age, we all want to take advantage of the many sources of information available to help us make important decisions or deal with major events we experience. Unfortunately, we don't always know where to find these sources of information. Often, we don't know very much about their quality, value, or relevance. In addition, many times we don't know much about the issue we're facing, and as a result don't really know where to begin our learning process.

Resource Pathways guidebooks solve the problem of "information overload" faced by those who want to learn about a topic of critical importance in their life. Those interested in doing such research typically:

- Don't know what resources are available, particularly those outside traditional print media.

- Don't know where to find most of those resources, particularly since most bookstores stock only a limited selection.

- Can't assess the quality or focus of those resources **before** spending time and money first finding, then evaluating, and perhaps buying them.

- Don't understand which resources will be particularly useful for each dimension of a multi-dimensional issue. For **each** aspect of the challenge we're trying to deal with, certain resources will be very helpful, while others may be completely worthless.

This guidebook, focused on the best resources for helping you as you become a parent, will help you overcome these hurdles. In this guidebook, you will find that:

- Virtually all available quality resources are reviewed, including those from "high-technology" media like the Internet or CD-ROMs.

- We make a reasoned judgment about the quality of each resource, and decide whether or not a resource should be recommended (only 25% are recommended).

- We define and explain the different issues typically encountered during your pregnancy through childbirth and after your baby is born. We classify each resource we review according to its primary focus. This helps ensure that you buy or access only the **best** resource for each step.

- We provide information on where to buy or access each resource, including ISBN numbers for obscure print media, direct order numbers for publishers, and URL "addresses" for sites on the Internet's World Wide Web.

After you have used this guidebook to learn which sources of information are best suited to you, you can then acquire or access those resources knowing that your time and money will be well spent.

Our Quality Standards

Those who turn to Resource Pathways guidebooks find the **best** sources of information on critical issues having an important impact on their lives. To ensure that we merit the trust placed in our recommendations, we've developed a proven set of quality standards:

- We are independent from the publishers of products we review; we do not accept advertising or compensation of any kind from those companies.

- Our Editors and Advisory Councils are independent professionals with many years of experience in each area we cover. These professionals help ensure that we keep abreast of developments in the field, and that our evaluations meet their standards for relevance and accuracy.

- We review new products and editions as they become available, so that our guidebooks include the most up-to-date information. We revisit websites on the Internet and the online services frequently to keep up with changes.

How We Develop Our Reviews and Recommendations

This guidebook includes our reviews of over 200 resources that can help you and your partner before you become pregnant and after your baby is born.

Our Editors and Researchers have found virtually all available sources of information focused on having a baby and becoming a parent, including books, the Internet, CD-ROMS, videotapes, and commercial online services. We've created a concise, one-page review of each resource. Each review contains information about the resource (author, publisher, edition, etc.), describes its content and focus, evaluates the comprehensiveness, quality, style, and effectiveness of the resource, and summarizes these findings in one rating for overall quality and one for design (a "1–4 Star" rating system is used). We expand these ratings with written evaluations explaining the rationale behind our ratings and providing guidance on how each source can be best applied. We also provide prices and "where to buy" information for each product.

We put a great deal of time and effort into reviewing and evaluating each resource carefully. Here's what that process includes:

- **Printed Guidebooks:** For these resources, we read the book from cover to cover, identify the particular focus taken by each author, and make a judgment about how the book's contents could be best applied. Our judgment about the relative quality of each source is based upon useful content, breadth, depth, readability, organization, and style. We make every effort to ensure that the latest editions of books are reviewed, and that no out-of-print resources are included.

- **Internet Websites & Online Services:** We review all websites and online services that have any significant amount of original material related to the subject of having a baby and becoming a parent. Our reviews include judgments about the site's graphic and navigation design, as well as the usefulness of material provided relative to that available in other media. We revisit sites frequently to stay abreast of changes and improvements.

  Our criteria for including a site or online service:

  - Content must deal substantially with pregnancy, childbirth, parenting a newborn, or infertility. This is the part we evaluate. We don't evaluate the site as a whole if that site also covers other topics.

  - It must be substantially complete, not substantially under construction.

  - A commercial site must have some relevant content that's free to users.

  - We do not review the websites of parenting organizations unless they contain substantial information for prospective and new parents.

- **CD-ROM & Software:** We carefully review each facet of each CD, including all branches and multimedia options, and thoroughly test software applications available on disk. Our reviews include judgments about the "cost/benefit" of multimedia additions, as well as the usefulness of the content provided relative to the same offering in other media. We note technical problems in loading or using programs provided.

- **▣ Videotapes:** We listen to and view each tape from beginning to end. We then make our judgment based on how well the tape covers its topic (breadth and depth), its organization, and production quality.

Note: We do not review high-cost CD-ROM based products or videotapes sold primarily to professionals with costs that are out of reach for most families.

Because our mission is to help you find your way through this "forest" of information, we also provide you with our recommendations on which resources are best to help you each step of the way (only 25% of the resources we review are recommended). In making these recommendations, we have attempted to err on the side of providing too many choices rather than too few. Our recommendations are based upon our judgment of value, not only relative to alternatives in the same media, but against **all** available resources regardless of media.

Publisher's Note:

In our reviews of websites, we include the current "address" of the website homepage or specific page within a website, to facilitate direct access on the Internet. The nature of the Internet's World Wide Web is, of course, dynamic; this means that many website/page "addresses" change over time. If you find that an address is outdated, the recommended solution is simple—just delete the last expression within the address and hit the "Enter" or "Return" key again.

This will simply point your browser to a file "further up" in the website's file directory. In most cases, you can follow this procedure until you find yourself at the website's homepage (indicated by the phrase ending in ".com" or ".edu" or ".gov," etc.). Usually, you can then find your way back to the specific information (or page) that you were interested in.

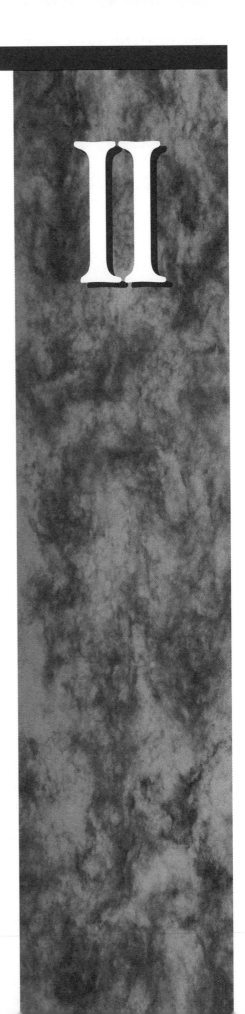

PREGNANCY AND FETAL DEVELOPMENT

II

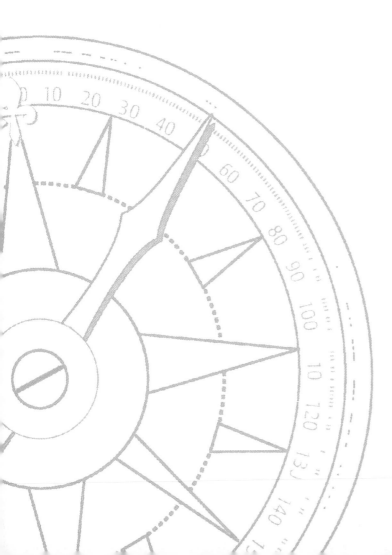

INTRODUCTION

Pregnancy offers a time to focus on the growth and development of your baby, and to plan for your future as parents. Many pregnant women find these nine months offer a chance to examine their ideas about themselves, to improve their own self-care, and to ready themselves for motherhood. Dramatic physical and emotional changes occur during pregnancy. Relationships evolve and grow. Some days, the pregnancy will seem endless; other days it will seem to be moving much too fast.

If your pregnancy was unplanned, you may be struggling with choices about whether or not to parent. Well-meaning people and health care providers may assume you are happy about your pregnancy, when you are instead ambivalent. Facing pregnancy and parenting without a supportive partner can also be difficult. If you are in these kinds of situations, preparing yourself and finding support for your choices and needs will be even more important.

Even before conception, a mother's choices can affect her future baby. Mothers with chronic medical problems such as hypertension or diabetes need to carefully discuss pregnancy with their physicians. All women who are trying to get pregnant should watch their nutrition, get a source of folic acid in their diets, cut down or preferably eliminate smoking, and minimize alcohol use. The most critical phase of fetal development occurs in the first eight weeks after conception, a time when many women don't yet know they are pregnant. By 16 weeks, a baby is essentially fully formed and just needs to grow and mature enough to be able to live outside the mother's womb.

One of the first decisions you need to make is which care provider to choose, and where you wish to give birth. Choices may range from home birth with a direct-entry midwife, to a birth center or hospital birth attended by a Certified Nurse Midwife or Family Practice physician, to a birth in a higher-risk setting attended by an obstetrician, or many other combinations of these options! If you are contemplating pregnancy or are early in your pregnancy and haven't yet chosen a caregiver, ask around for recommendations and then interview several caregivers. You will also want to check with your insurance carrier first about the coverage you will have, but you should make your ultimate decision thoughtfully. Does the caregiver attend births of his or her own patients or might another provider be covering births at the time when your baby is born? How supportive is the care provider of breastfeeding? If the waiting room is full of formula samples, coupons, or commercial literature from only certain companies, you may want to check this out. Consider other factors that might be important to you personally. It is important that you are able to work with your provider and trust his or her recommendations.

During pregnancy, mothers-to-be may experience common conditions such as nausea, backaches, and other physical discomforts. They will need to choose how and how much to exercise, what and how much to eat, and how to get comfortable so they can sleep and feel rested. Prospective mothers will also begin to learn about breastfeeding and infant care, and contemplate their future parenting philosophy.

Most commonly, a pregnant woman will see her maternity care provider as soon as she knows she is pregnant. The first visit is a comprehensive examination and includes a pap smear and pelvic exam, cultures for urinary and vaginal infections, and blood tests. These blood tests generally include blood type, blood counts for anemia, tests to see if the woman has been exposed to hepatitis B or syphilis, and a test to see if the woman is immune to rubella (German measles). The woman will be offered an HIV test. Evaluation for risk of Down's syndrome and/or spina bifida in a low-risk woman may include a "Triple Screen" test at about 16 weeks gestation. Screening for diabetes may be done at about 26 weeks gestation. Finally, urine may be tested at each prenatal visit for evidence of protein and/or sugar. Prenatal visits commonly occur about once a month for the first seven months, then every two weeks until the ninth month, then weekly until the baby is delivered.

A "due date" will be assigned based on the woman's last menstrual period, or on the date of conception if known. It is important to remember, however, that a "due date" is an estimate. About 75 percent of babies are born within one week either side of their due date. Only about 5 percent of babies actually come on that assigned day. A full-term pregnancy averages 38 weeks from the date of conception, or 40 weeks from the first day of the last menstrual period, but first pregnancies tend to be about three days longer on average.

Although most pregnancies progress normally, there are sometimes complications. Some pregnancies sadly end in miscarriage or fetal death. Others are complicated by pregnancy-related conditions. And women over 35 have an increased risk of chromosomal abnormalities and may consequently be offered genetic testing with an amniocentesis or chorionic villus sampling.

Some maternity care providers do ultrasounds for every pregnancy, others only do them when they are medically indicated.

There are no known risks of ultrasound to the fetus. The best time to do a single ultrasound is between 18–20 weeks gestation, because the baby is large enough for any significant abnormalities to be seen, and dating is reasonably accurate (plus or minus 10 days). After 20 weeks however, growth rates vary so due dates won't be changed based on a late ultrasound. Keep in mind that a due date from an ultrasound is never better than a known conception date or a reliable menstrual period date. Ultrasounds may be done at other times to follow fetal growth, assess the quantity of amniotic fluid, or to evaluate the position of the baby or the placenta. Many parents want to know the gender of their baby, but this is not a sufficient medical reason to do an ultrasound and may add unnecessary expense and even worry, since all medical tests have the possibility of error.

Exercise And Nutrition

Pregnancy is a great time to continue or improve important self-care activities. "Eating for two" doesn't mean eating twice as much, though! Normal-weight women should gain between 20 and 30 pounds during pregnancy to assure adequate nutrition for themselves and their babies. A good, balanced diet with about 300 extra calories per day will generally be adequate. If you have severe nausea and vomiting, be sure to keep yourself hydrated and don't worry too much about calories in the first trimester; you'll want to just eat whatever will stay down! However, unless you are severely underweight, it's best to avoid excessive "junk food" with empty calories.

Your health care provider will likely prescribe a prenatal vitamin to assure that you take in enough essential vitamins. Folic acid, found in green leafy vegetables and fortified breads and cereals, is critical in the first trimester to reduce your baby's risk of having spina bifida. Adequate iron and calcium are important as well, but if you don't like milk, don't worry! There are many other sources of calcium, and supplements are available that can be used as well. Vegetarian mothers will want to pay particular attention to getting adequate iron and protein intake.

Exercise can contribute significantly to your sense of well-being in pregnancy, as well as prepare you for the physical demands of labor and birth and, later on, chasing a toddler. Exercise can continue at the same level as before pregnancy, as long as you stay well-hydrated and avoid over-exertion. Pregnant women have even competed in the Olympics! For women who haven't been active before pregnancy, starting gradually and gently works best. Walking and swimming both provide excellent general conditioning. Pelvic tilts and back arches can help with back pain during pregnancy. If you are starting to exercise for the first time, be sure to consult your provider for a recommendation first.

Loss Of Pregnancy

Losing a pregnancy through miscarriage, stillbirth, or infant death can be devastating. Miscarriage is very common—up to 25 percent of pregnancies may end in miscarriage, generally before the 16th week. When one considers everything that has to go right for a pregnancy to proceed to a normal outcome, it's not surprising that many pregnancies do not. However, from the time of conception or soon thereafter, most pregnant women are very aware of their pregnancies and already forming ideas, hopes, and dreams about their baby-to-be. Even in unplanned or undesired pregnancies, miscarriage frequently brings a sense of grief and guilt. Although a sense of responsibility is quite understandable, usually there is nothing the mother could have done or not done to prevent a miscarriage. The risk of miscarriage rises with maternal age, so unfortunately it is also more common for those very women who are often struggling to become pregnant in the first place.

If you tell people about your miscarriage, you will undoubtedly begin to hear stories about their miscarriages, be given consolation, or be offered advice. For some, this will be helpful. However, couples need to grieve in their own ways. And men and women often differ in their response to losing a baby. Many couples find it helpful to name the baby and hold a memorial service, particularly if the pregnancy had already been announced. For pregnancies that end later in stillbirth or early neonatal death, be sure to hold the baby and get pictures to save. These may be very treasured in the future, even if they must be put away for a time to allow for grief.

Fortunately, miscarriage or other pregnancy losses rarely mean the woman cannot have children. Unless there have been three or more consecutive miscarriages, no medical evaluation is usually necessary in terms of finding the cause of the miscarriage. However, a stillbirth or other infant death will likely be investigated to see if there is a cause that could be repeated and possibly prevented in a future pregnancy, but usually the couple will be able to conceive again and carry the next pregnancy to term. Couples should allow themselves enough time to grieve the loss of the pregnancy and address any medical concerns before conceiving again. Although a woman's body is able to conceive again right away, it is also best to wait until at least one normal period has occurred after the pregnancy loss. This will also allow for accurate dating of the next pregnancy. Generally, a woman's body will be ready when her emotions are.

During pregnancy, as your baby grows and develops inside you, you may find that you have different concerns than you did the month before. The resources we have recommended in the following pages should help ease your mind and your body as they change during pregnancy, and as your baby develops. To help focus your search for answers, we've divided these resources into three categories:

General Overview	17
Nutrition and Exercise	31
Loss of Pregnancy	35

We also highly recommend that prospective parents read the reviews of resources we recommend in **Section III—"Childbirth"**—and **Section VIII—"Gaining an Overview: All-Inclusive Resources."** Within these sections, some resources specifically address both pregnancy and childbirth, while others address pregnancy, childbirth, and newborn care. Resources we recommend can help answer questions you have pertaining to pregnancy.

As you look at these resources, begin to consider your own approach to your pregnancy. You might ask yourself questions such as, "What birth setting do I want?" "How will I care for myself during pregnancy?" "How do I find a caregiver who will help me have the experience I want?" By empowering yourself with knowledge about normal pregnancy and common complications, you will be able to act in partnership with your physician or midwife to assure the best possible outcome for you and your family.

General Overview

THE PREGNANCY BOOK
A Month-By-Month Guide

 Recommended For:
Pregnancy & Fetal Development

Description:

This 430-page book is a compendium of pregnancy and childbirth information organized in a month-by-month workbook format. Each of the first nine chapters corresponds to a month of pregnancy. The authors have designed the book so that a central design theme is consistent throughout. Each chapter suggests questions a prospective parent may have for a health care provider at that stage of pregnancy; each chapter has a designated place for a monthly photograph to provide a record of the pregnancy's progression. Each chapter also gives guidance on the same set of topics: "How You May Feel Emotionally," "How You May Feel Physically," "How Your Baby Is Growing," "Concerns You May Have" and a monthly diary. Other topics then are added each month. Chapter 9 includes labor and delivery; Chapter 10 covers the postpartum period. Included as appendices are "If You Get Sick," "Additional Resources," and "Emergency Delivery." A glossary of obstetrical terms and an index close out the volume.

Evaluation:

Sometimes prospective parents just need some basic information about what's normal and what's not. This is a gentle book that compels the reader to take out a pencil with which to make notes in the margins; spaces are provided for thoughts, dreams, goals, room to record one's pre-birth conversation with one's child, and more. Included are checklists on dozens of topics, from "Discovering Your Personal Bests" (designed to make sure your baby has a happy mother) to "What The Laws Allow" (an overview of employment law as it relates to pregnancy). This book ducks no tough questions. Included in Chapter 8 is a common sense discussion of the sometimes controversial issue of Cesarean/surgical birth. While the authors are thorough and straightforward in their approach, their goal is to be supportive to pregnant couples. Example: "To avoid cluttering . . . the already overwhelmed minds of pregnant women, we have placed the rare conditions in the glossary . . . we don't want to worry the 99 percent of mothers-to-be needlessly with unusual problems that may occur in the other 1 percent." There undoubtedly are flashier books on pregnancy and childbirth than this one, but there are few that accomplish so much in such a practical manner.

Where To Find/Buy:

Bookstores and libraries.

★★★★

Overall Rating
★★★★
Good, overall source of general information, written in a helpful, supportive tone

Design, Ease Of Use
★★★★
Excellent monthly format, helpful lists and ample room for notes and photos

1–4 Stars

Author:
William Sears, MD; Martha Sears, RN; and Linda Hughey Holt, MD, FACOG

William Sears teaches at the University of Southern California School of Medicine and hosts America Online's "Parent Soup" forum. Martha Sears is a certified childbirth educator; the Sears, who have eight children, have authored 15 books. Linda Hughey Holt is medical director of the Evanston Hospital Institute for Women's Health.

Publisher:
Little, Brown and Company

Edition:
1997

Price:
$22.00

Pages:
430

ISBN:
0316779148

Media:
Book

Principal Subject:
Pregnancy & Fetal Development

Pregnancy Subject:
General Overview

★★★★

Overall Rating
★★★★
Objective overview of childbirth choices, tips on how to be proactive while pregnant

Design, Ease Of Use
★★★★
Good layout, well-illustrated

1–4 Stars

Author:
Sheila Kitzinger

Sheila Kitzinger is a social anthropologist and a childbirth educator. She studied at Oxford University and has conducted research on birth, breastfeeding, and motherhood in cultures around the world. She lectures widely on the issues of birth and parenthood.

Publisher:
Pantheon Books

Edition:
1987

Price:
$11.95

Pages:
352

ISBN:
039475249X

Media:
Book

Principal Subject:
Pregnancy & Fetal Development

Pregnancy Subject:
General Overview

General Overview

YOUR BABY, YOUR WAY
Making Pregnancy Decisions And Birth Plans

 Recommended For:
Pregnancy & Fetal Development

Description:

This 352 page book contains five parts (19 chapters) focusing on the range of choices available in pregnancy care and childbirth, and the changes and challenges a woman experiences during pregnancy. This book states and supports the concept that the care a woman gives herself (and that she receives from her partner and other family members) has more affect on her and her baby's well-being than any provided by doctors. In order to create the best care, a woman must assess the options available to her so she can be responsibly proactive. By including chapters on emotional changes, drugs and health, diet, exercise, and medical tests as related to pregnancy, this book guides women to master this life-transforming process. Chapter 18 offers the author's final opinion by comparing "obstetrically managed birth" and "autonomous birth." The last chapter then imparts the author's strategy of how to take a proactive role by offering tips on creating your birth plan. Six plans are given ranging from simple plans (half a page) to more complex and detailed plans; a C-section plan is also included.

Evaluation:

This book was written from an international perspective on what women's options are when pregnant. It provides, for the most part, an objective dialogue of their choices for childbirth (the book frequently portrays a negative view of the medical profession and hospitals, however). It takes the reader through the experience with a voice that is supportive and also full of good common sense advise. It does not tout a particular birthing method, but supports the reader in making her own inventory of what she needs, what she expects, and how to be responsible for achieving this. Her section on "Ripe with Child" leads readers to an awareness of their baby, its growth, its response to stimuli, and ways to feel connected. This book mirrors other books that stress personal responsibility and autonomy. Although it is ten years old, it is as fresh and useful today as the day it was printed. While not comprehensive on the subject of childbirth, this book is a useful one for a woman who would like some guidance through her own decision-making process.

Where To Find/Buy:
Bookstores and libraries.

General Overview

I'M PREGNANT, NOW WHAT DO I DO?

Terrific Resource For:
Pregnant teenagers considering their options for handling an unplanned teenage pregnancy

Recommended For:
Pregnancy & Fetal Development

Description:

The authors present three options for teenagers finding themselves in an unplanned pregnancy: giving the child up for adoption, terminating the pregnancy (abortion), or continuing with the pregnancy. The book's intent is to provide up-to-date information so you will be "getting as many facts as you can about your options (that) will help you choose what's best for you." The 11 chapters of this 228 page book include discussions on the following: facts about the reproductive system, brief description of pregnancy (1/2 page plus per trimester), developing support systems, tips on the decision-making process, and the role of your partner in your decisions. The bulk of the book focuses on separate chapters dealing with becoming a parent, considering adoption, and choosing abortion. Each of these chapters present the facts, the pros and cons, how to deal with the changes and associated losses, and "things to consider." Also given are additional chapters that describe case studies of three women who have chosen one of these options and examples of how their lives were impacted. A glossary and list of resources is also given.

Evaluation:

Lack of knowledge about sex, accompanied by conflicting messages teens get about their sexuality through the media, can result in unplanned teen pregnancies. The U.S. still has the highest rate of adolescent pregnancies in the developed world. Societal avoidance only adds to the denial many teens exercise when they find out they are pregnant. This book presents a fair, unbiased, and factual account of alternatives available to teens. It contains numerous stories from teens that describe their situations, the way they made decisions about what to do, and the effect those decisions made on their lives. These accounts are personal, engaging and supportive. This is a book that not just pregnant teenagers need to read; it would also be of great use for any teen who is considering sexual intercourse. Knowing the consequences and the ensuing decisions that may need to be made would better enable them to make informed decisions.

Where To Find/Buy:

Bookstores and libraries.

Overall Rating
★★★★
Sensitive, factual account of decision-making involved with an unplanned pregnancy

Design, Ease Of Use
★★★
Straightforward headings in table of contents; chapter organization sometimes unclear

1–4 Stars

Author:
Dr. Robert W. Buckingham, PH & Mary P. Derby, RN, MPH

Buckingham is a professor of public health at New Mexico State University in Las Cruces and author of ten other books. Derby is a maternal child health clinical nurse specialist at Harvard Pilgrim Health Care in Boston and has worked extensively with adolescents.

Publisher:
Prometheus Books

Edition:
1997

Pages:
228

ISBN:
1573921173

Media:
Book

Principal Subject:
Pregnancy & Fetal Development

Pregnancy Subject:
General Overview

★★★

Overall Rating
★★★
Handy reference book that defines 850+ terms from preconception through postpartum

Design, Ease Of Use
★★★
Alphabetical with subject index for cross-references; cross-related bibliography needed

1–4 Stars

Author:
Nancy Evans
Evans has developed major medical and nursing textbooks and references for leading medical publishers and has served as a consultant to physicians, nurses and schools of nursing. She is president of Breast Cancer Action working toward the prevention and cure of breast cancer.

Publisher:
Hunter House

Edition:
1994

Price:
$16.95

Pages:
336

ISBN:
0897931297

Media:
Book

Principal Subject:
Pregnancy & Fetal Development

Pregnancy Subject:
General Overview

General Overview

THE A TO Z OF PREGNANCY AND CHILDBIRTH: A CONCISE ENCYCLOPEDIA
Over 850 Easy-To-Find Answers To The Questions And Needs Of Expectant Parents

Description:
The purpose of this book is to provide a concise explanation of terms that the reader will encounter in preconception through postpartum. Oftentimes these terms are used freely by care givers and within the literature with resulting confusion for the reader. By presenting these terms with conciseness and reflective of current research findings, the author intends to empower the reader to meet her/his individual needs and to make informed decisions regarding the pregnancy and birthing process. In this 336 page reference book, then, she has organized 850+ terms which are arranged alphabetically in a dictionary-like fashion. Terms within entries are capitalized to show that they are cross-related and defined elsewhere in the text. A subject index is located at the back of the book listing all relevant terms by major category, such as labor and delivery, diagnostic tests and procedures, etc. Also provided is a bibliography listing current references along with a resource section listing organizations and contact information by subject matter (infertility, grief and loss, etc.).

Evaluation:
This book is a handy reference tool. The entries are void of clinical jargon that would tend to put off those not directly involved with the medical field. Each definition is exactly what the author claims—clear and concise. Sometimes these definitions are too concise and one looks for more information which is not provided. On the other hand, pregnancy is a time when unfamiliar terms are thrown at one during birthing classes, doctor's visits, and one's own reading. Consequently, there is a need to become familiar with these terms in a relatively short period of time. This guide can be quite helpful in doing so, for it contains over eight hundred defined terms. Because of this broad scope, however, other resources will be needed to get more in-depth backgrounds on given subjects, e.g. "miscarriage." It would be helpful in these cases to organize the bibliography section according to subject categories so that one could be directed to other resources, e.g. "for further reading on miscarriage see . . ." Perhaps this will happen in a future edition.

Where To Find/Buy:
Bookstores and libraries, or order direct by calling (510) 865-5282.

General Overview

THE ESSENTIAL OVER 35 PREGNANCY GUIDE
Everything You Need To Know About Becoming A Mother Later In Life

★★★

Description:

This two part, six chapter book contains chapters on preconception, prenatal testing, fertility treatment, miscarriage and becoming pregnant again, and a month-by-month look at the stages during pregnancy. In the Preface, Lavin shares her own experience with becoming a mother for the first time at age 41. About a fourth of the book concentrates on preconception: learning when your body is most fertile; preconception physical and reproductive health exam; diet, weight, health, and exercise; fertility treatment; preconception genetic testing; pregnancy risks, and more. Chapter 3, "Prenatal Testing," covers the various tests available: amniocentesis and early amniocentesis, chorionic villus sampling, alpha fetoprotein screening, multiple marker screening, and ultrasound. Chapter 6, "Pregnancy Month by Month" tracks the growth and changes in mother and baby each month, as well as things to expect and plan for during the months. Two appendices are provided. Appendix A gives a summary of potential danger signs during pregnancy. Appendix B is a "Basic Food Guide" for preconception, pregnancy, and nursing. References and an index conclude the book.

Evaluation:

This is a good resource for women 35 and older who want to become mothers. Lavin, who miscarried twice at age 40 before having a child at 41, writes with encouragement to her readers. Her firsthand experience with miscarriage as well as a successful delivery in "midlife," as she calls it, is reflected in this book. Lavin combines her knowledge along with medical studies and facts in an attempt to ease worries and dispel myths about pregnancy and childbirth for those in their mid-30s and older. For example, she states that "a healthy 35-plus woman without pregnancy complications is as likely as a younger woman to have a baby without medical problems." Many of the questions that women in this age category may have are addressed. There is good coverage on preparing for pregnancy, how to determine ovulation and peak fertility times, and other alternatives to achieving pregnancy. Chapter 6, "Pregnancy Month by Month" is a nice introduction to what to expect. Presenting excellent preconception information, any expectant parents will want more complete resources to obtain details about the stages of pregnancy, labor, and birth.

Where To Find/Buy:
Bookstores and libraries.

Overall Rating
★★★
Helpful information for those women over 35 years old who want to become pregnant

Design, Ease Of Use
★★★
Easy to read; information presented in a logical order from preconception through pregnancy

1–4 Stars

Author:
Ellen Rose Lavin, PhD and Samuel H. Wood, MD, PhD

Lavin has a Ph.D. in Psychology, has been a practicing licensed Marriage, Family and Child Counselor for 13 years, and specializes in pregnancy issues. Wood, M.D., Ph.D., is a board-certified reproductive endocrinologist.

Publisher:
Avon Books

Edition:
1998

Price:
$11.00

Pages:
196

ISBN:
0380788195

Media:
Book

Principal Subject:
Pregnancy & Fetal Development

Pregnancy Subject:
General Overview

★★★

Overall Rating
★★★
Fascinating, scientific account of fetal activity

Design, Ease Of Use
★★
Text is heavy and difficult reading for most

1–4 Stars

Author:
Peter W. Nathanielsz, MD, PhD

Since 1982 Peter Nathanielsz M.D. has taught at Cornell University where he is the Director of the Laboratory for Pregnancy and Newborn Research. He is also the chairperson of the Maternal Child Health Research Committee of the National Institute of Child Health and Human Development.

Publisher:
Promethean Books

Edition:
1992

Price:
$31.25

Pages:
237

ISBN:
091685955X

Media:
Book

Principal Subject:
Pregnancy & Fetal Development

Pregnancy Subject:
General Overview

General Overview

LIFE BEFORE BIRTH
A Time To Be Born

Description:

This 237 page book, written by a researcher/scientist summarizes the current understanding of the life and birth of the fetus. Such information exploded in this hi-tech age with ultrasonic methods of visualizing the interior of human fetuses and its electronic methods of continuously observing every conceivable function. The bulk of the book consists of sixteen chapters which report of what has been found. Topics those chapters address range from "The Placenta," to "Fetal Circulation," to "A Time to be Born." The information presented in all of these chapters play and replay the overture of this work: that the fetus is not a passive passenger in the uterus, but rather that he/she is a being developing the ability to respond and react very purposefully to all manner of challenges and that he/she is very much in control of what goes on in the womb. The book also contains an extensive glossary and index.

Evaluation:

This book is not an easy read, because it is filled with scientific data relative to the development of the fetus in the womb. But if the reader has at least an elementary scientific background, a large vocabulary, an endurance to work one's way through a heavy text, this is a fascinating book. Ultrasound and other scientific advancements have given us a window to the fetus which has been shrouded in darkness and mystery until a relatively short time ago. We now know, for example, that the fetus starts the birth process (not the mother); that the placenta (our only truly throw-away organ) has all the properties of a lung, a digestive system, a kidney, and a food store; that prenatal events do predispose the child to SIDS. This is not a "how to" book (although it emphatically points out how maternal behavior—or misbehavior—can affect the fetus); it is, rather, an informational sharing concerning what is presently known about fetal development. With all the caveats that have been listed, it certainly enables one to understand what the fetus is up to.

Where To Find/Buy:

Bookstores and libraries.

General Overview

WHAT TO EXPECT WHEN YOU'RE EXPECTING

Description:

In its second edition, this 477 page guidebook for prospective parents offers four parts entitled "In the Beginning," "Nine Months and Counting," "Of Special Concern," and "Last But Not Least: Postpartum, Fathers, and the Next Baby." The first part offers information regarding pregnancy signs, choosing and working with a practitioner, special concerns (over 35, physical history, smoking, etc.), prenatal diagnosis (amniocentesis, ultrasounds, etc.), and diet. Part 2 offers month-by-month narratives of what to expect at your check-up, what you may be feeling, what you may be concerned with, and important things to know. "Of Special Concern" includes major revisions from the book's first edition. Here you will find questions and answers focusing on what happens if you get sick, are coping with a chronic condition (asthma, MS, etc.), or if something goes wrong (miscarriage, preterm labor, etc.). The last part includes sections on breastfeeding, the postpartum period, and effects on the father; this second edition also includes more information on preparing for the next baby. An appendix lists treatments and tests occurring during pregnancy.

Evaluation:

This book's linear format makes it definitely one of the more "user friendly" resources in the field. It is well-organized, offers medical information in an easily digested fashion (no jargon), and highlights important questions that pregnant women want answers to—"I get tired when I am exercising or doing heavy cleaning; should I stop?" Continuing the same format into each month makes this book an easy read; one is able to glean the facts at a glimpse. While many resources neglect men's adjustment as a baby is introduced into the family, this book briefly addresses some of the feelings, fears, and hopes of new fathers. One major drawback to this book is that readers may be scared away by the book's heavy descriptions of possible complications during pregnancy and childbirth. Others may object to the book's limited focus—it presents a standard hospital birth, but does little in presenting other childbirth alternatives. Still others, seeking an assertive stance during their pregnancy, may find the book's overall patronizing tone (in which the doctor is put in charge guiding the woman) objectionable. This resource is better used with other broader-based and proactive resources.

Where To Find/Buy:

Bookstores and libraries.

Overall Rating
★★
Information presented in a month-by-month format highlighting concerns at that stage

Design, Ease Of Use
★★★★
User-friendly format using Qs & As, with major headings; visually appealing

1–4 Stars

Author:
Arlene Eisenberg, Heidi E. Murkoff, Sandee E. Hathaway, BSN

Publisher:
Workman Publishing

Edition:
2nd (1996)

Price:
$10.95

Pages:
477

ISBN:
089480829X

Media:
Book

Principal Subject:
Pregnancy & Fetal Development

Pregnancy Subject:
General Overview

★★

Overall Rating
★★

Lengthy, repetitive explanations of how a woman's responses affect her unborn child

Design, Ease Of Use
★★

Good basic design, but not easily thumbed for pertinent points

I–4 Stars

Author:
Thomas Verny, MD, with John Kelly

Verny, a psychiatrist in private practice, earned his doctorate at the University of Toronto. He has taught at Harvard and York Universities and is the founder of Toronto's Center for Psychotherapy and Education. Kelly is a freelance writer specializing in medical subjects.

Publisher:
Dell Publishing (Bantam Doubleday Dell)

Edition:
2nd (1981)

Price:
$12.95

Pages:
253

ISBN:
0440505658

Media:
Book

Principal Subject:
Pregnancy & Fetal Development

Pregnancy Subject:
General Overview

THE SECRET LIFE OF THE UNBORN CHILD
How You Can Prepare Your Unborn Baby For A Happy, Healthy Life

Description:

Do a woman's actions, thoughts and feelings influence her unborn child? This 253 page book is basically a thesis addressing this topic. Dr. Verny takes a psychiatrist's view of the life of the unborn child. This essential difference is revealed in this book by noting scientific studies focusing on neurobiological processes and their effects on mother and child. This book explains how a mother's emotional response is communicated to her child through changes in her body chemistry—neurohormones which are shared with the fetus. Beyond genetic predisposition, this book explains how a physical predisposition is imprinted on a child's emotional processing centers of the brain. Chapter titles highlight topics covered in this book: "The Secret Life of the Unborn Child," "The New Knowledge," "The Prenatal Self," "Intrauterine Bonding," "The Birth Experience," "The Shaping of Character," "Celebrating Motherhood," "The Vital Bond," "The First Year," "Retrieving Early Memories," and "Society and the Unborn Child."

Evaluation:

The most positive note in this book, and one that many have expanded on since it was published in 1981 is the idea that a women can make her thoughts, feelings, and prenatal environment into a positive force (or negative force) in her child's life. The obvious use of this information is one seen in most arguments for natural childbirth, for emotional support of the mother, and for a gentle entry into the world for the child. And so, this book was a landmark book in the field. But since it was published, most of its information has been condensed by others and, while some readers may be interested in the details of how the investigation began and what ideas and insights led the way, the book seems to drag and become repetitive. Also, in the very fast world of scientific research and medical practices, this resource feels outdated despite its scientific foundations. Reading the sections on artificial insemination, for example, makes one uniquely aware of just how far we've come since this book was written.

Where To Find/Buy:
Bookstores and libraries.

General Overview

★★

YOUR PREGNANCY WEEK BY WEEK

Description:

This book begins by explaining the importance of the three months prior to becoming pregnant as a time for the mother-to-be to evaluate and prepare so that her baby is offered the best start possible. Curtis's goal is to provide patients with "information about gynecological and obstetrical conditions they may have, problems they may encounter and procedures they may undergo." As indicated by the title, the book is presented in a week-by-week format. The following topics are highlighted for each of the 38 weeks of fetal development: "How Big Is Your Baby?," "How Big Are You?," "How Your Baby Is Growing and Developing," "Changes In You," "How Your Actions Affect Your Baby's Development," and "You Should Also Know." This last topic presents warnings or concerns for the reader to consider. In addition, a boxed "tip" is offered for each week. Illustrations of the baby's development are included for each week, and occasionally a corresponding visual of a sonogram or a separate illustration is provided which depicts fetal development within the mother. This book contains a 10 page glossary and an index.

Evaluation:

Curtis advises readers to read this book through, and then read it over a week at the time; that is good advice given the fact that information contained within a particular week may not be unique to that time period. When describing "How Big" for fetus and mother, typical ranges are indicated and there is not much elaboration. Greater detail about development is found under the headings for fetal development and changes in the mother. While this detail may be pertinent to the week within which it is printed, elaboration often ties the information to periods of time beyond the specified week (before and/or after). A broad range of issues are discussed that would not apply to the experience of all readers (for example, in Week 23—Urinary-Tract Infections, and in Week 29—Treatment of Premature Labor). Although the comprehensive scope of this 371 page book may not be best suited to the week-by-week format, the index and glossary are always available to help the reader who is seeking specific information at any point during her pregnancy.

Where To Find/Buy:

Bookstores and libraries.

Overall Rating

★★

Week-by-week account of pregnancy isn't as easily delivered as the title indicates

Design, Ease Of Use

★★

Easily referenced with consistent format, but is repetitive and is best read cover to cover

---

1–4 Stars

Author:

Glade B. Curtis, MD

Curtis is in private practice in obstetrics, gynecology, and infertility. He has also written *Your Pregnancy Questions & Answers* and *Your Pregnancy After 30.*

Publisher:

Fisher Books

Edition:

3rd (1997)

Price:

$12.95

Pages:

371

ISBN:

1555611435

Media:

Book

Principal Subject:

Pregnancy & Fetal Development

Pregnancy Subject:

General Overview

Overall Rating

★★

Much help for women experiencing unpleasant and painful symptoms during pregnancy

Design, Ease Of Use

★

Confusing lack of focus; dense writing style with no graphics

1–4 Stars

Author:

Virginia Hege Tobiassen

The author is an experienced mother who underwent her own "miserable but uncomplicated pregnancy" before the birth of her son.

Publisher:

Chicago Review Press

Edition:

1995

Price:

$14.95

Pages:

204

ISBN:

1556522444

Media:

Book

Principal Subject:

Pregnancy & Fetal Development

Pregnancy Subject:

General Overview

General Overview

AM I GLOWING YET?

Understanding And Coping With The Common & Not-So-Common Miseries Of Pregnancy

Description:

The author, a "survivor" of a difficult pregnancy, wrote this book to dismantle the myth of pregnancy as a trouble-free period of time in which a mother-to-be "glows" with good health and well-being. Written primarily for pregnant women, this book is also intended as a "wake-up call" to medical practitioners who often dismiss women's real pain and suffering as minor "discomforts" of pregnancy. By describing symptoms and treatment for the very real ailments of pregnancy, the author hopes to prevent women from blaming themselves if they feel miserable, to help them understand "they are not alone," and that it is not "all in your head." The fifteen chapters run the gamut of common and less common afflictions during pregnancy, from nausea and vomiting, headache, and breast pain to Bell's palsy, ear, nose, and mouth problems, and carpal tunnel syndrome. In each chapter, the author discusses both effective and ineffective medical treatments and current research, first-hand accounts of women who have experienced these symptoms, and non-standard treatments such as dietary changes, herbs, acupressure, and exercises.

Evaluation:

As the author says at one point, "There may be days when you feel that being pregnant is about on par with receiving a punch in the mouth. . . ." This book is extremely effective in overturning many of the cherished myths of a "normal" pregnancy, showing a realistic side of it that is so often not written about and/or discussed. It presents an interesting, but at times unclear, hodgepodge of themes: part social activism, part medical research, part psychology, with a historical perspective of pregnancy ailments and treatments coupled with medical research's future outlook. However, this resource offers support and information to those women whose pregnancies leave them far from "glowing," who may have been let down by medical practitioners and others who minimize their symptoms. The real challenge is that "most causes of pregnancy symptoms are largely unknown, and the only real cure is the end of the pregnancy." Readers may find some solace in this book as it provides information, support, and suggestions for those misunderstood "miseries of pregnancy."

Where To Find/Buy:

Bookstores and libraries.

General Overview

SEASONS OF CHANGE
Growing Through Pregnancy And Birth

★★

Description:

This 184 page book is a journal following one woman's experience through her pregnancy. Illustrated with photographs of pregnant woman, their mates and their babies, pictures were taken by the author to illuminate her recorded impressions. This book was written to directly support the decision to have a home birthing experience. The decision process is detailed and includes events and thoughts leading up to the author's departure from the current medical establishment, through her search for information about birth mid-wives, and her actual experience of having the baby at home. Personal impressions, insights, and discussions with family and friends are included. The entire experience from the moment of realization through a month after delivery is conveyed from the first person perspective.

Evaluation:

This book's intent is to share the deeply personal experience of pregnancy, giving birth, and adjusting to the presence of a new baby in one's life. The photographs give the impression that the people depicted are the same as the ones speaking, but we find some confusion here that is not clarified. Obviously, some of the pictures are of other women, not the speaker, yet no element of their stories, or even their names are mentioned. This detracts from the overall impression of the book. Most of the photographs are of the home snapshot variety, which lends itself well to the the first person perspective of the book. This book might interest a first time mother who wants to hear about and view her upcoming experience from another first-time mother. A major flaw in this book is the lack of dates. One would assume that using a journal approach would also include noting the time period, the month of pregnancy, or the trimester. However, omission of any actual or implied time reference makes this book awkward to navigate.

Where To Find/Buy:

Bookstores and libraries.

Overall Rating
★★
This personal journal detailing pregnancy and childbirth will appeal to some

Design, Ease Of Use
★
Difficult to note months of pregnancy (undated entries), no table of contents or index

1–4 Stars

Author:
Suzanne Arms

Suzanne Arms is an internationally-recognized writer, photojournalist, and public speaker. She is dedicated to seeing that women and birthing families have all the information and support they deserve. Her images and words have inspired two generations of women.

Publisher:
Kivaki Press

Edition:
1994

Price:
$14.95

Pages:
184

ISBN:
1882308581

Media:
Book

Principal Subject:
Pregnancy & Fetal Development

Pregnancy Subject:
General Overview

Overall Rating

★

Chatty, overly personal opinions conveyed as reality

Design, Ease Of Use

★★

Well organized under topic headings, uses primarily a text style with little graphics

1–4 Stars

Author:

Vicki Iovine

Formerly a *Playboy* centerfold, with careers in TV and radio, and law degrees, Iovine is now the mother of four children. This book reflects the "combined point of view" of Iovine, her agent, and her editor.

Publisher:

Pocket Books
(Simon & Schuster)

Edition:

1995

Price:

$14.00

Pages:

262

ISBN:

0671524313

Media:

Book

Principal Subject:

Pregnancy & Fetal Development

Pregnancy Subject:

General Overview

General Overview

THE GIRLFRIENDS' GUIDE TO PREGNANCY
Or Everything Your Doctor Won't Tell You

Description:

Iovine says that this book "is the compilation of the experiences, opinions, concerns, complaints and remedies that my Girlfriends and I had when we were pregnant." She begins the book by talking about typical symptoms of pregnancy: "Breasts," "Peeing," "Exhaustion," "Crampiness," "Dizziness," "Nausea," "Sensitivity to Odors," "Insanity," "No Period," and "Intuition." In this first chapter and the 17 chapters that follow, topics are discussed from her personal point of view. There is an emphasis on the mother-to-be's appearance, emotions, and experiences (such as announcing a pregnancy, sex, exercise, etc.). While continuing to express a non-medical perspective, some medical issues are considered under the following chapter titles: "You and Your Doctor," "Prenatal Tests," "Labor Begins (Finally!)." Chapters entitled "What to Take to the Hospital" and "Baby 'Stuff'" offer advice on what to take or buy to be adequately prepared for giving birth and coming home with your baby. The book wraps up with labor, delivery, and the long-term effects of giving birth ("Losing the Weight," and "The Legacy of Pregnancy.")

Evaluation:

The detailed "Acknowledgments," "Foreword," "Why I Wrote This Book," and "Postscript" convey much about Iovine's personality as does the writing contained within each of her 18 chapters. She believes that the advice shared by girlfriends and other mothers in your life are what get you through pregnancy. This book, then, is Iovine's attempt to fill the gap for any mother-to-be who does not have a full supply of her own consultants, i.e., girlfriends. Although parts of the book offer good advice, the level of personal orientation narrowly define many issues (as exhibited in "Sharing the Wonderful News," "You and Your Doctor," "Exercise and Pregnancy"). In effect, the book's tone reads just like a one-way sounding board from someone who enjoys gossiping or chatting on topics personally relevant mainly to themselves. While Iovine explains in the introductory portion of the book that all mothers share a bond due to their shared experience of pregnancy and delivery, the book does not convey this common ground. This book is worthwhile reading for some personalities, but it does not speak truly for the majority of mothers-to-be.

Where To Find/Buy:

Bookstores, libraries, or order direct by contacting Mail Order Department, Simon & Schuster, Inc., 200 Old Tappan Road, Old Tappan, NJ 07675.

General Overview

SABRINA'S PREGNANCY PAGE

Description:

This website, created and maintained by Sabrina Cuddy, a childbirth educator and breastfeeding counselor, offers 13 main options at its homepage. Three choices focus on discussion and support via email or a "Pregnancy Chat" manned by Cuddy or another "birth professional," and "bulletin boards." Three options list links for: "pregnancy, birth and breastfeeding resources," "parenting resources," and "women's health." FAQs comprise another option focusing on pregnancy, birth, and labor concerns. One other option at this site provides access to informational archives for pregnancy, labor, and birth topics from midwives, labor assistants, childbirth educators, and parents. Cuddy's background, her book reviews and recommendations, her childbirth classes and services, and awards her site has won make up the final three options. In addition, there are FAQs regarding various medical procedures and methods, such as the Bradley® Method, Pregnancy Nutrition, Birth Planning, Epidural Anesthesia, and General Pregnancy. "For high-quality sites with an emphasis on information rather than the selling of a product or service . . . " a visitor can travel through a series of connected, related websites called the Pregnancy Ring.

Evaluation:

This site hosts nothing more than a forum for one person's point of view (with numerous disclaimers). The creator's background in childbirth education consists primarily of her three year stint as a Bradley® Method Childbirth Educator; her homepage suggests she is "not qualified to give medical advice . . . and all material is her opinion only." Consequently, this site lacks credibility, infrastructure and can be a possibly dangerous venture for the user who is looking for medical advice. The one positive element of this site are all the links it contains. But the links are usually vague, e.g. "Another site with resources for women is Here." Some summaries would have been helpful. If one is looking for serious answers to questions about pregnancy, birth, labor, or any health issue related to women, she/he needs to look elsewhere.

Where To Find/Buy:

On the Internet at the URL: http://www.fensende.com/Users/swnymph/index.html

---

Overall Rating

★

Only useful for various links and one woman's opinions on various pregnancy issues

Design, Ease Of Use

★

Links need better descriptions; subjects ramble without structure

---

I–4 Stars

Author:
Sabrina Cuddy

Media:
Internet

Principal Subject:
Pregnancy & Fetal Development

Pregnancy Subject:
General Overview

Overall Rating

★

An intellectual discussion of the issues around prenatal testing; strong anti-male flavor

Design, Ease Of Use

★

Heavy style sprinkled with anecdotes; many chapter titles vague

1–4 Stars

Author:

Barbara Katz Rothman

Barbara Katz Rothman is the author of *Recreating Motherhood: Ideology and Technology in a Patriarchal Society* and *In Labor: Women and Power in the Birthplace*. She is a professional writer who drew on the experiences of over 120 women for this book.

Publisher:

W. W. Norton & Company

Edition:

2nd (1993)

Price:

$9.95

Pages:

281

ISBN:

0393309983

Media:

Book

Principal Subject:
Pregnancy & Fetal Development

Pregnancy Subject:
General Overview

General Overview

THE TENTATIVE PREGNANCY
How Amniocentesis Changes The Experience Of Motherhood

Description:

This 281 page book is an intellectual discussion of the issues surrounding amniocentesis and its effect on women's pregnancies. Chapter 1, "The Products of Conception," question society's values in terms of treating people and their body parts as "commodities" (organs, blood, sperm, etc.). Chapter 2, "Prenatal Diagnosis in Context," reviews the social and technological changes that have made "amnios" possible. Chapter 3, "Making Choices," focuses on how women decide whether or not to take advantage of current technology. Chapter 4, "The Tentative Pregnancy," and Chapter 5, "On Fetal Sons and Daughters," share the experiences and decisions of women who have had an amniocentesis. Chapter 6, "Ambiguous Diagnoses," addresses bad or inconclusive news about a pregnancy. Chapter 7, "Grieving the Genetic Defect," points out that in some cases of amniocentesis, the child was wanted but a decision was made to "start over," which for most women includes grieving the loss of a child which was very real to her. Chapter 8 closes with a review of the issues, focusing on the social impact as well as the personal impact of each parental decision.

Evaluation:

The 1993 edition of this work contains a new introduction and two new appendixes. The bulk of the book, however, was published in 1986 and leaves one with a sense of its being out of date, even though the issues raised are by no means resolved. Since this book was published, many of the issues raised here have been hashed out in the American public forum. But it leaves her work caught in the rhetoric of that period in time. Aside from giving her views on the consequences stemming from an amnio, the author harbors an anti-male sentiment that distracts from an objective discussion of these issues. Also, the author is offended over the issue of body parts becoming commodities, likened to slavery in a subtle way. This slants the discussion in such a way that it becomes more difficult to grasp the heart of the matter—how women feel about their pregnancies. So, while the work is valuable in raising important social issues, one must be in a certain frame of mind to be interested in it. This book is recommended only for those interested in the political, bioethics and sociological issues raised by the author.

Where To Find/Buy:

Bookstores and libraries.

Nutrition And Exercise

MATERNAL FITNESS
Preparing For A Healthy Pregnancy, An Easier Labor, And A Quick Recovery

Terrific Resource For:
An exercise program to help prepare for a fit pregnancy, easier labor, and fast recovery

Recommended For:
Pregnancy & Fetal Development

Description:
In her 160 page book, Tupler, a personal trainer and fitness instructor, details an exercise program called "Maternal Fitness" (MF). Her routine is based upon three goals: prevention, preparation, and restoration. Through her fitness program she believes that certain discomforts (backaches, urinary incontinence, etc.) will be prevented as you learn to align and balance different parts of your body as it changes. She equates having a child to "the marathon of labor" and suggests ways to prepare yourself by strengthening your transverse muscle (the innermost abdominal muscle), thigh muscles, and pelvic floor muscles. Restoration includes helping your body during the postpartum period as it readjusts to taking care of yourself and your baby. The first third of the book explains the rationale for these exercises by outlining the anatomy of the human body; the nature of pregnancy, childbirth and breathing. The next section describes the BAKS Basics (breathing, abdominal work, kegels, squatting). The bulk of the book offers narrative and illustrations for Maternal Fitness.

Evaluation:
Tuppler's knowledge of body structure and mechanics coupled with "Dos and Don'ts, and Other Stuff to Know About Pregnancy and Exercise," make this a necessary book for anyone continuing in a work-out program during pregnancy. The exercises are detailed, movement by movement, in both picture and narrative form. This makes this resource a "user friendly" one, especially in the early stages of becoming accustomed to the exercises. Also, the author/ physical trainer starts you off slowly in her BAKS Basics program, and then helps you progress into her Maternal Fitness. Because bodies change during pregnancy (often without our knowledge until we unfortunately overextend ourselves), Tuppler's route will ensure a better understanding of those changes and how to strengthen it during and after pregnancy. The book also contains helpful information about proper nutrition and diet during pregnancy.

Where To Find/Buy:
Bookstores and libraries.

Overall Rating
★★★★
Clear rationale, good explanations of muscle structures, sensible exercise routine

Design, Ease Of Use
★★★★
Illustrations clear and easy to follow (mirror images); text detailed enough to succeed

1–4 Stars

Author:
Julie Tupler, RN
(with Andrea Thompson)
Tupler is a certified personal trainer, fitness instructor, and childbirth educator. She is the creator of Maternal Fitness, a labor-preparation program featuring the Tupler Technique.

Publisher:
Fireside (Simon & Schuster)

Edition:
1996

Price:
$12.00

Pages:
160

ISBN:
0684802953

Media:
Book

Principal Subject:
Pregnancy & Fetal Development

Pregnancy Subject:
Nutrition & Exercise

★★★★

Overall Rating
★★★★
A sensible, knowledgeable, up-to-date guide to nutrition for mothers & mothers-to-be

Design, Ease Of Use
★★★
Easy to use information presented in a friendly style

1–4 Stars

Author:
Mary Abbott Hess, RD, MS, and Anne Elise Hunt

Mary Abbott Hess, "1990–91 President of the American Dietetic Association, is one of the country's leading authorities on diet, health, and nutrition." Anne Elise Hunt "is a home economist, writer, and former food editor at *Cuisine* magazine." They have coauthored another book on feeding young children, as well as a previous edition of this book.

Publisher:
Collier Books
(Macmillan Publishing)

Edition:
1992

Price:
$13.00

Pages:
324

ISBN:
0020654413

Media:
Book

Principal Subject:
Pregnancy & Fetal Development

Pregnancy Subject:
Nutrition & Exercise

Nutrition And Exercise

EATING FOR TWO
The Complete Guide To Nutrition During Pregnancy

 Recommended For:
Pregnancy & Fetal Development

Description:

This book, written by a former professor and registered dietitian and a writer/home economist, seeks to provide an up-to-date, informed guide to nutrition for pregnant women and their babies. It's an updated edition of an earlier book on pregnancy and nutrition, incorporating new recommendations and research findings and translating them into practical advice for mothers-to-be. Chapter 1 introduces us to the womb and how quickly a baby grows, and looks at weight gain during pregnancy: how much is too much, and how much may be too little. Chapter 2 tells how to evaluate yourself in terms of diet and health habits, and chapter 3 introduces "an eating game plan" involving six food groups and the best foods to choose from. Chapter 4–6 discuss proteins, carbohydrates, fats, vitamins and minerals in detail. Chapter 7 focuses on risks and dangers such as food additives, caffeine, cigarettes, alcohol, and drugs. Common and less common health concerns are explained in chapter 8. The last chapter introduces the pros and cons of breast-feeding vs. bottle-feeding, with a chart comparing human milk and infant formula. Some chapters include short quizzes to test your knowledge and to dispel commonly-held myths.

Evaluation:

This book offers valuable advice for mothers and mothers-to-be about nutrition and good dietary habits. Written simply, in a "user-friendly" style, it is easy to read straight through or to flip through to find specific information (e.g. "how much calcium will I need and in which foods can I find it?"). Common dietary myths and mysteries are cleared up or dispelled, and some information here may surprise you (why you may crave clay, mothballs, or laundry starch!). This book goes above and beyond simple dietary information to offer advice on such concerns as morning sickness and edema. It also contains an especially informative and sensitive chapter on the decision whether to breast-feed or bottle-feed your baby—how to evaluate the relative advantages of each, and decide which would be the best option for you and your child. As this book incorporates up-to-date medical findings and requirements for pregnant and lactating women, this should be a "must-have" resource on every mother's shelf.

Where To Find/Buy:
Bookstores and libraries.

Nutrition And Exercise

ESSENTIAL EXERCISES FOR THE CHILDBEARING YEARS
A Guide To Health And Comfort Before And After Your Baby Is Born

★★★

Description:

Noble's 277+ page book, originally published twenty years ago, mirrors her experiences with pregnant and postpartum women along with her lectures and workshops. With her background in physical therapy and women's health issues, Noble has expanded her book to include two new sections one of which explains the principles of exercise and the other reflects the needs of women on restricted activity or bed rest. Her premise is that women should not just focus on childbirth classes alone at the end of their pregnancy. Instead she states that women need to focus on their whole body's needs to meet the challenges brought on by changes during the childbirth years. The 10 chapters of this book focus on exercises for the following areas: the pelvic floor, the abdominal muscles, posture, positions, comfort, relaxation, breathing, and more. Partner exercises, exercises for post-cesarean births, and exercises for women assigned bed rest are also given. Discussions of the physiological functions of particular body muscles during and after birth along with exercises (pictures, narrative) to correct and strengthen them are included.

Evaluation:

First published in 1976, this book has been revised, is now in its fourth edition and has sold over 200,000 copies! That's quite a record for an exercise book and is a testimony that hundreds of thousands of women have found this book helpful. Noble's focus for this exercise guide is not strictly on pregnant women. Rather, she presents information to motivate all women to change their sedentary ways and she helps them to focus on getting their whole body and lifestyle in shape, not just the physical areas that childbirth classes focus on. She argues that while many long-term effects can be felt from the childbirth experience, many ill effects can be avoided simply through prevention if women attend to their bodies prior to, during and after pregnancy. In making this connection, Noble explains a clear rationale for each specific exercise. Also, her book is filled with illustrations, photographs, and summary tables of exercises (prenatal, postpartum, post-cesarean). These are helpful to the reader in and of themselves, but they also fortunately help to soften an often dense writing style. Regardless of such a writing style, this book written by a physical therapist is a very helpful resource for women caring for their own bodies before, during and after pregnancy.

Where To Find/Buy:

Bookstores and libraries, or order direct by calling (508) 432-8040.

Overall Rating
★★★
Places importance on exercising the whole body at all times, not just during pregnancy

Design, Ease Of Use
★★★
Detailed table of contents, useful summary charts, pictures; often dense writing style

1–4 Stars

Author:
Elizabeth Noble

Noble, a graduate in physical therapy and author of 8 books, founded the Women's Health Section of the American Physical Therapy Association. She has "trained over 2,000 instructors in prenatal and postpartum exercise."

Publisher:
New Life Images

Edition:
4th (1995)

Price:
$16.95

Pages:
277

ISBN:
0964118319

Media:
Book

Principal Subject:
Pregnancy & Fetal Development

Pregnancy Subject:
Nutrition & Exercise

★★★

Overall Rating
★★★
Attractive, soothing, provides methods to calm the spirit and soul of a pregnant woman

Design, Ease Of Use
★★★
Well-designed, with clear exercise and stretching illustrations

1–4 Stars

Author:
Janet Balaskas

Balaskas is founder of the International Active Birth Movement and runs the Active Birth Centre in London, where she teaches yoga and preparation for birth and parenthood. She is author of *Active Birth, New Life* and other books on natural childbirth.

Publisher:
Interlink Books
(Interlink Publishing Group)

Edition:
1990

Price:
$12.95

Pages:
95

ISBN:
0940793431

Media:
Book

Principal Subject:
Pregnancy & Fetal Development

Pregnancy Subject:
Nutrition & Exercise

NATURAL PREGNANCY
A Practical Holistic Guide To Wellbeing From Conception To Birth

Description:

The author's intent is "to help you to take responsibility for your own health and harmony in mind, body, and spirit in the months approaching birth." The first chapter contains advice on how to cope with the emotional challenges of pregnancy and how to calm and center yourself using deep breathing and meditation techniques. Following chapters give guidelines for achieving and maintaining a healthful state during pregnancy including the fundamentals of a nutritious diet, step-by-step instructions for basic yoga, and massage sequences to deepen physical awareness and promote body awareness. The final two chapters of the six chapter, 95 page book discuss natural and alternative therapies and "how they can be used safely and effectively to maintain and restore health during pregnancy." These sections cover many of the common ailments that may occur, along with natural remedies. In addition to yoga, meditation, and massage, alternative health care practices covered include osteopathy, reflexology, acupuncture, shiatsu, herbalism, Bach flower remedies, homeopathy, aromatherapy, and hypnotherapy.

Evaluation:

Natural Pregnancy is a beautiful, soothing book. Here one can find yoga, meditative, and deep breathing exercises to restore balance and calm the spirit throughout pregnancy. The book's aim is to approach pregnancy and preparation for childbirth from a holistic point of view. The book's topics are richly illustrated, from yoga positions to massage techniques. The descriptions and suggestions are gentle and appropriate for a wide audience and should not be limited to those already committed to a natural birth; the techniques discussed here—from deep breathing to shiatsu—will give comfort to all pregnant women. In fact, many techniques are suggested for those times when a comfortable position and a good night's sleep seem hard to find. Some of the illustrations and photos provided to illustrate the text's massage techniques are explicit. Those who may be offended by female frontal nudity will want to pass this book by. For most, however, *Natural Pregnancy* celebrates the growth of a life within and the enriched comfort of the mother sheltering that life.

Where To Find/Buy:

Bookstores and libraries.

Loss Of Pregnancy

COPING WITH MISCARRIAGE
A Simple, Reassuring Guide To Emotional And Physical Healing

★★★★

Recommended For:
Pregnancy & Fetal Development

Description:
As the author explains, there are many difficulties attached to coping with and grieving for a miscarriage, complicated "by the invisibility of the death" and the lack of "normal grieving rituals." This book seeks to bridge many of these difficulties and help women heal both emotionally and physically after the trauma of miscarriage. Written primarily with the grieving mother in mind, this book also hopes to sensitize health care professionals to the pain of miscarriage and so they can help their patients deal with the trauma. Using the stories of women who have experienced miscarriage, the author explores such issues as coping with grief, dealing with family, friends, work colleagues and others, physical and psychological healing practices, becoming pregnant again, and specific medical issues causes and treatments available to prevent miscarriage. At the end of the book are appendices with a list of organizations, a table of medical procedures which increase the likelihood of a successful pregnancy, and a glossary of terms.

Evaluation:
Miscarriage is an invisible and often unacknowledged source of grief for many couples. Compounding this difficulty is the fact that not many books are available to help those experiencing this grief deal with it. This book is valuable in this regard. It fully explores both the emotional and the physical healing processes that must take place. Although the author has no first-hand experience with miscarriage, her experience counseling others who have dealt with loss is evident. Of particular interest are the sections on handling older children after a miscarriage—accepting and responding to their own grief which may be profound—and on the healing "rituals" a woman can create in order to mourn a lost baby—seeing and holding her baby, or creating and keeping a memento of the child. The "life stories" chapter offers sensitive accounts of other women who have experienced and coped with losses, and who went on to become pregnant again. Women who have experienced miscarriage will find this book an excellent source of both information and comfort.

Where To Find/Buy:
Bookstores and libraries.

Overall Rating
★★★★
A supportive and informative resource on a seldom-discussed subject

Design, Ease Of Use
★★★★
Very readable; chapters conclude with "questions to ask . . ." & "actions to take"

1–4 Stars

Author:
Mimi Luebbermann
The author is a writer and former pregnancy counselor, with a strong interest in women's issues and family health.

Publisher:
Prima Publishing

Edition:
1996

Price:
$14.00

ISBN:
0761504362

Media:
Book

Principal Subject:
Pregnancy & Fetal Development

Pregnancy Subject:
Loss Of Pregnancy

★★★★

Overall Rating
★★★★
Poignant, practical, warmly comforting, understanding account of the grieving process

Design, Ease Of Use
★★★★
Fully detailed table of contents, summary "points to remember" at end of each chapter

1–4 Stars

Author:
Deborah L. Davis, PhD

Davis is a developmental psychologist who specializes in perinatal bereavement, parent education, and child development. She is also a member of the advisory board for Pen-Parents, the international network for bereaved parents.

Publisher:
Fulcrum Publishing

Edition:
2nd (1996)

Price:
$15.95

Pages:
268

ISBN:
1555913024

Media:
Book

Principal Subject:
Pregnancy & Fetal Development

Pregnancy Subject:
Loss Of Pregnancy

Loss Of Pregnancy

EMPTY CRADLE, BROKEN HEART
Surviving The Death Of Your Baby

 Recommended For:
Pregnancy & Fetal Development

Description:

The author combines her 10+ years of research and clinical work with bereaved parents in her discussion of the grief experienced from different kinds of loss, such as ectopic pregnancies, miscarriages, stillbirths, and infant death; this 268 page book's second edition also includes loss stemming from therapeutic abortions, selective reduction, and death of one or more babies from a multiple birth. The 17 chapters focus not on the separate types of loss but instead on the various facets and phases of the grieving process. Topics included are recovery (grieving, emotional, physical), how to affirm your baby's presence, feelings of failure, anger, guilt, and vulnerability, resolving grief, and "making peace with agonizing decisions." Three chapters focus on various relationships (you and your partner, your family, support networks—friends, healthcare providers, etc.) and how to work through your loss; a new chapter "especially for fathers" is included in this edition. The final five chapters discuss subsequent pregnancies, protective parenting, and more as you "move on." Three appendices include caregiver advice to support those grieving, journal writing tips, and a resource list.

Evaluation:

This comprehensive and poignant account of the grief that parents face when dealing with the loss of their child will make you weep. Although the stories included are more concise than other resources, the honest and heartbreaking accounts of parents coming to terms with their own losses validate each of the author's points. You won't find information here as to "why" you lost your baby. You won't find information on how to avoid losing a future pregnancy. The emphasis here is on emotional support or, as the author states, it is to "let bereaved parents know that they are not alone in their grief." We've reviewed other books that dwell on others' stories, offer questions to ask your caregiver, tests to ask for, and how to get beyond your loss. This book, however, includes stories that we find fresher and more applicable to current times. Many women, due to infertility treatments, are faced with more decisions than ever before, such as pregnancy reduction when multiple babies are not thriving, therapeutic abortions when the mother or baby's health is endangered, and more. We recommend this book in particular for these situations and for anyone in general dealing with the loss of their child.

Where To Find/Buy:

Bookstores and libraries, or order direct by calling (800) 992-2908.

Loss Of Pregnancy

HELP, COMFORT AND HOPE AFTER LOSING YOUR BABY IN PREGNANCY OR THE FIRST YEAR

★★★★

 Recommended For:
Pregnancy & Fetal Development

Description:

The first part of this book, "Working through Grief," is written for parents who lose their baby during pregnancy or shortly after birth. Here, Lothrop shares different loss scenarios (miscarriage, stillbirth, neonatal death, sudden infant death syndrome, adoption, and more) from both a descriptive and a personal perspective. For each type of loss, Lothrop details possible causes and what is endured in experiencing the loss. Throughout these passages, she interweaves quotes from parents who have experienced such losses. The remainder of Part 1 leads the reader through the grieving process. In Part 2, "Caring for the Bereaved," Lothrop shifts her focus to the many groups and individuals who offer support to bereaved parents. This part of the book is reflective of Lothrop's introductory remark that, "Just as a stone thrown into a pond creates ever-widening circles, so sensitivity in hospitals towards parents and their dead or dying children is ever expanding—to the benefit of the parents who are so very dependent on the immediate support they receive." Appendices include a summary of parental rights, questionnaires, meditations, and support information and resources. A bibliography and index are also provided.

Evaluation:

In both the forward and introduction to this book, Lothrop acknowledges that isolation adds a great weight to the burden of sadness that many bereaved parents experience. The reader is continually touched with the numerous quotes of bereaved parents that are then interwoven throughout the book. After providing an overview of most major types of losses, Lothrop then proceeds to offer explanatory information which is thoughtfully and directly conveyed. In this book, parents and supporters are encouraged to honestly acknowledge the loss experience to help further their grieving process to achieve some peace. The tone of the two parts of the book speaks effectively to readers who are seeking "Help, Comfort & Hope"; some medical information is provided, but the book primarily concentrates on how to deal with one's emotions after a baby's death. Readers will also find extensive appendices for further guidance and support. For bereaved parents and for those who are in a position to support them, this book takes great strides towards overcoming that desperate isolation that surrounds a baby's death.

Where To Find/Buy:

Bookstores and libraries.

Overall Rating
★★★★
Thorough, informative, compassionate discussion of the grieving process

Design, Ease Of Use
★★★★
Easily referenced by bereaved parents and their supporters

1–4 Stars

Author:
Hannah Lothrop

Lothrop is the mother of three, including one child that she lost during pregnancy in 1984. She is a psychologist, childbirth educator, grief counselor and lecturer who is a member of the advisory board of SHARE (international support group for bereaved parents.)

Publisher:
Fisher Books

Edition:
1997

Price:
$12.95

Pages:
280

ISBN:
1555611206

Media:
Book

Principal Subject:
Pregnancy & Fetal Development

Pregnancy Subject:
Loss Of Pregnancy

★★★

Overall Rating
★★★
Excellent resource meant to inform and empower the reader; somewhat dated

Design, Ease Of Use
★★★
Well organized; easy to read

1–4 Stars

Author:
Stefan Semchyshyn, MD, and Carol Colman

Dr. Semchyshyn, clinical associate professor of the Seton Hall University School of Graduate Medical Education, a diplomate of the American Board of Maternal-Fetal Medicine, is one of the leading authorities on high-risk pregnancies.

Publisher:
Macmillan General Reference (Simon & Schuster Macmillan)

Edition:
1989

Price:
$9.95

Pages:
242

ISBN:
0020368550

Media:
Book

Principal Subject:
Pregnancy & Fetal Development

Pregnancy Subject:
Loss Of Pregnancy

Loss Of Pregnancy

HOW TO PREVENT MISCARRIAGE AND OTHER CRISES OF PREGNANCY
A Leading High-Risk-Pregnancy Doctor's Prescription For Carrying Your Baby To Term

Description:

In his 242 page book, Dr. Semchyshyn, one of "four hundred doctors in the U.S. certified in maternal-fetal medicine," focuses on the tragedy of miscarriages. The introduction elaborates on his beliefs about medicine and what roles doctors and patients should play. "Partners in Pregnancy," Chapter 4, elaborates by stating that patients and doctors need to learn from each other to make well-informed decisions. Chapter 1 delves into causes of miscarriages and premature births, including infections/illnesses, chromosomal and uterine abnormalities, and more; the next chapter focuses on genetic disorders. Chapter 3 suggests how to choose a doctor and hospital, plan your delivery, deal with insurance, and work-leave. Chapter 5 explains ways to monitor your pregnancy for each trimester—what's normal is coupled with what's not normal. Chapter 8 then explains how your pregnancy can be monitored by your doctor. Other topics included in the book deal with taking care of yourself (home, travel, work), emergency procedures, "new hope for problem pregnancies," support systems to deal with loss and frustrations, and future hopes.

Evaluation:

This book has several facets which make it attractive. First of all, it is written by two persons, one a distinguished obstetrician, the second an award winning journalist. The result of their efforts is a well informed resource written in a clear, easy to digest manner. Secondly, the theme of the book which emerges time and again is on redirecting the focus of obstetrical care from crisis intervention to prevention. As such, its clear purpose is to help couples to become more informed, demanding couples who will settle for nothing less than the best of care during pregnancy. Thirdly, the book contains a wealth of information meant to help women anxious to carry a baby to full-term, whether they have had previous difficulties or not. An especially helpful chapter in this regard is Chapter 9, "New Hope for Problem Pregnancies." The only "negative" about this book is that it was written a decade ago. Much has happened in this field in ten years. To obtain that information, the reader would have to turn to other sources.

Where To Find/Buy:
Bookstores and libraries.

Loss Of Pregnancy

EMPTY ARMS
Emotional Support For Those Who Have Suffered A Miscarriage, Stillbirth . . .

★★★

Description:

This is a spiritually-based look at pregnancy loss and how to cope with the grief of a miscarriage, stillbirth, or tubal pregnancy. The author bases much of her discussion on her own and other women's experiences of losing a child and the emotions and "spiritual battles" they underwent on the path toward healing. This book, in its second edition, has added a new chapter focusing on tubal/ectopic pregnancies based upon reader input; also included is "updated information . . . a new epilogue, and . . . a chapter on . . . letting go of our disappointments and pain." The first half of the book focuses mostly on women's emotional responses (a chapter is devoted to husbands' grieving process), including advice about how to respond to friends and family, and the pain of husbands and older children. The second half of the book offers answers about the types and possible causes of miscarriage, exercise and nutrition after a pregnancy loss, mood swings, tubal pregnancies and stillbirths, beginning another pregnancy, and turning to the Bible for spiritual direction.

Evaluation:

Christian readers looking for a book to guide them through the spiritual anguish of pregnancy loss will find this a supportive resource. The book shows how the author and her husband, both Christians and involved in ministry, turned to the Bible as a source of comfort and guidance through the stages of their healing. The book offers practical information about the medical and technical issues of a pregnancy loss, as well as specific advice (mementos a woman may want to obtain after a stillborn birth—a set of footprints, a photograph taken at the hospital, or the baby's arm bracelet, etc.). Unique to this book and neglected by others is the chapter, albeit brief, on "The Trauma of a Tubal Pregnancy." The anecdotes provided throughout this book of the author's and other women's pregnancy losses are very real and affecting, and there are some helpful insights about pain (". . . The way to let go of our pain is to feel it."). Overall, this book will be most useful for Christian readers looking for inspiration, support and guidance using scripture passages.

Where To Find/Buy:

Bookstores and libraries.

Overall Rating
★★★
Discussion of how to deal with pregnancy loss based upon Bible passages

Design, Ease Of Use
★★
Reference list needs updating (no sources listed after 1983)

1–4 Stars

Author:
Pam Vredevelt
The author has master's degrees in communication and psychology, and is currently a licensed professional counselor at Behavioral Healthcare Northwest in Gresham, OR.

Publisher:
Multnomah Books

Edition:
2nd (1994)

Pages:
171

ISBN:
0880708107

Media:
Book

Principal Subject:
Pregnancy & Fetal Development

Pregnancy Subject:
Loss Of Pregnancy

★★

Overall Rating
★★
Useful for the grieving process; dated medical information

Design, Ease Of Use
★★★
Helpful subtitles, lists of resources, appendix

1–4 Stars

Author:
Jonathan Scher, MD

Dr. Scher, teacher at the Mount Sinai Medical Center and in private practice in New York City, is a "pioneer in the field of miscarriage prevention."

Publisher:
HarperCollins Publishers

Edition:
1990

Price:
$12.50

Pages:
240

ISBN:
0060920564

Media:
Book

Principal Subject:
Pregnancy & Fetal Development

Pregnancy Subject:
Loss Of Pregnancy

Loss Of Pregnancy

PREVENTING MISCARRIAGE
The Good News

Description:

Subtitled "The Good News," this 240 page book presents findings from special clinics, research and new technological developments surrounding the causes of miscarriage and possible treatments. Part One of this three part book details what happens during a miscarriage both physically and emotionally. Several patient anecdotes are offered. Part Two encompasses over half of the book and concentrates on "What has gone wrong? What can be done?" Topics offered include hormonal problems, uterine/cervical abnormalities, mismatches between parents and/or the baby, and more. Part Three deals with the emotional and physical trauma associated with miscarriages and stillbirths. The importance of the grieving process and ways to help those involved with losing a child are addressed; also pointed out are ways others (friends and family) can help, how to help other children cope, and how to arrange for funeral or memorial services. Briefly mentioned are points to consider surrounding the issue of having another pregnancy after a miscarriage. A list of contacts for nationwide support groups is listed at the end of the book.

Evaluation:

This book does an excellent job, through the numerous anecdotes of women who underwent a miscarriage, of illustrating the emotional trauma and devastation that losing a baby can have on disappointed parents-to-be. Consequently, this book can be a helpful tool in offering assistance to those going through the grieving process which miscarriages entail. If the anecdotes in this book can't help one feel the depth of emotions experienced by those who have lost a child, then no book can. It also covers many of the "latest" medical findings although, due to the book's copyright date, some findings need updating and inclusion. A problem with this book, unlike some others on the same topic, is that it lacks any real direction other than providing information. While paying special attention to the grieving process (a strength already noted), it does little to empower the reader to take a proactive role with medical professionals in avoiding a future miscarriage. Other resources will help readers more completely.

Where To Find/Buy:

Bookstores and libraries.

Loss Of Pregnancy

HYGEIA
An Online Journal For Pregnancy And Neonatal Loss

Description:

Hygeia is "an Internet Website committed and devoted to documenting and helping heal the grieving and other aspects of loss related to pregnancy wastage and demise of newborn infants and children, due to any cause." Designed and maintained by an Ob/Gyn and clinical professor in the Yale University School of Medicine, this site features the following: a monthly journal (current medical news, reviews, etc.), the author's complete volume of original "Poems of Grieving and of Hope," a "Visitors Contribution Area" (posted letters and stories), a "Grieving and Sharing Registry" (one for an exchange between users, the other for medical personnel and family members), an area to post memories and mementos like pictures, sonograms, etc. (send in via snail mail, author will post it on the site and then return your items), and a listing of related links, book resources, organizations, and support groups. The articles provided within the journal typically consist of one page of information accompanied by one of the author's poems and background music.

Evaluation:

The author's intent at this website is applaudable. When couples experience the loss of an unborn or stillborn child, often avenues for them to grieve are difficult to find. Medical information needs to be coupled with supportive outlets for expressing grief. We appreciate this site's emphasis on creating a network of families. The problem found here, however, is that the site's design makes it difficult to read the contributed stories due to the lengthy download time necessary to access the entries. Perhaps future design changes will divide the contributions by the type of diagnoses/losses, as does the registry. A visitor to the site must register to gain access to certain areas, which can be intimidating. However, the majority of the website is available to all visitors, regardless of registration. The articles provided in the journal are a bit too concise, more like an impersonal medical text. Use this site to network with others who have experienced similar losses. But, look to other sources for a more thorough and user-friendly discussion of the medical causes and treatments behind pregnancy loss and the loss of a newborn child.

Where To Find/Buy:

On the Internet at the URL: http://hygeia.org/

Overall Rating
★★
Intent is applaudable; good for networking with others but not as a medical resource

Design, Ease Of Use
★★
Navigation is straightforward, but contributions are difficult to access due to site design

1–4 Stars

Author:
Michael R. Berman, MD

Berman has been a practicing obstetrician and gynecologist since 1976. He is an associate clinical professor in the Yale University School of Medicine Department of Obstetrics and Gynecology.

Media:
Internet

Principal Subject:
Pregnancy & Fetal Development

Pregnancy Subject:
Loss Of Pregnancy

★ ★

Overall Rating
★★
Informative yet not easily digested

Design, Ease Of Use
★★
Densely packed information in a terse style

1–4 Stars

Author:
Dr. Kathleen Diamond

Kathleen Diamond has a Ph.D. in biochemistry with a specialty in molecular genetics. Her master's degree is in developmental biology. She has been a Fellow of the National Institutes of Health and the Molecular Biology Institutes. She has experienced miscarriage herself.

Publisher:
Adams Media

Edition:
1991

Price:
$10.95

Pages:
250

ISBN:
155850043X

Media:
Book

Principal Subject:
Pregnancy & Fetal Development

Pregnancy Subject:
Loss Of Pregnancy

Loss Of Pregnancy

MOTHERHOOD AFTER MISCARRIAGE

Description:

This 250 page book is written from the personal and professional perspective of Dr. Kathleen Diamond on the subject of pregnancy miscarriage. The book is divided into three sections as follows: Part 1, Experiencing and coping with a miscarriage; Part 2, Biology of early pregnancy; Part 3, Why did this happen? Explaining and preventing miscarriage. The first section of the book deals with Dr. Diamond's personal experience with miscarriage and her motivation for writing this book. Parts 2 and 3 are filled with detailed information regarding the mechanisms of miscarriage, diagnostics, and the biology involved. A detailed explanation is included on what is currently known about Chromosomal Abnormalities, Abnormal Hormone Levels, Abnormal Uterine Anatomy, other Abnormal Conditions of the Uterus, Infections of Reproductive Tract During Pregnancy, Immune Disorder, Maternal Diseases and Environmental Toxins. This book is targeted to the woman who has experienced miscarriage and would like to inform herself as completely as possible on the topic. A glossary of terms is included as well.

Evaluation:

The author of this book is an expert in genetic research, the mother of two, and has experienced multiple miscarriages. Her personal experiences, anecdotes, and scientific training form a credible foundation for this resource. As expected, a great deal of valuable information is included in this book. A drawback to it, however, is that it is a fairly tough read: people with a background in biology may wade through the explanations on hormones, chromosomes, and abnormalities without difficulty, but others will find it tough going. Also, there is some weakness in the author's ability to communicate issues clearly and succinctly. Although she is obviously unhappy with what she perceives as the current medical professional's reply to a miscarriage ("you cannot do anything, what will happen will happen"), she does not follow through as well as might be wished with sensitive and supportive advise for coping with the aftereffects. Recommendations to "talk it out" simply aren't enough; more focus should be placed on the actual processes of grief and mourning. The main value of this book, then, is that it can serve as a valuable reference on the issues, terminology, and the causes of miscarriage, but it has the mentioned limitations.

Where To Find/Buy:

Bookstores and libraries.

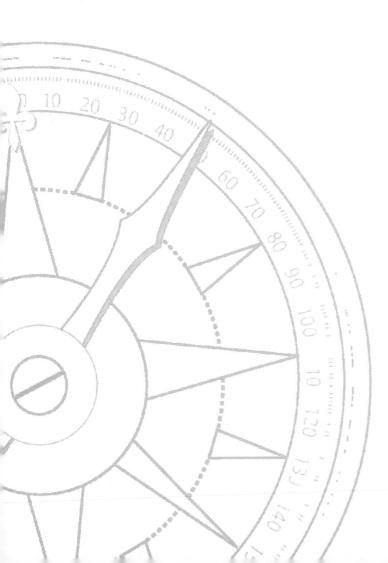

CHILDBIRTH

III

INTRODUCTION

You've made it through nine months of pregnancy, picked out some names, equipped your nursery, and now you're ready for the big event—labor and birth! Your birth will be different than any other birth, but there are many resources available to you as you consider how, where, and with whom you wish to give birth to your baby.

Throughout most of human history, birth was a natural part of life that occurred in the context of the family and the home, usually attended by a woman who had experienced childbirth herself. In the 20th century, however, the setting for most births in the United States shifted to the hospital. Currently though, medical research has confirmed that for a woman with a low-risk pregnancy, giving birth in the setting in which she feels most comfortable may have the best outcome. More recently then, we have seen the resurgence of lower-risk birth settings such as birth centers and home births. High-tech birth is clearly appropriate for some women and some pregnancies, but can cause more problems if technology is used without medical indications. As you consider where to give birth, consider your own philosophy of birth, your comfort level with your body and your support people, and any risk factors or worries you may have about birth.

You should discuss your health provider's "usual" approach to labor—their use of monitors, intravenous fluids, pain medications, episiotomy, etc.—and be sure you have all your questions answered. Tour the facility where you will give birth and meet some of the nurses. You may choose to write a birth plan, but it is best to think of this as a tool for communicating your preferences, rather than a "contract," since unexpected circumstances do arise.

Labor and birth is usually painful, but a woman's ability to cope with the pain reflects her state of anxiety and fear as well. Having support people with you may help you cope with labor without any pain medications. You may wish to consider having a Doula, a trained labor support person, help you with your labor. Taking a warm bath or shower, walking, or rocking can help as well. Don't be afraid to ask that people who will cause you added anxiety not be present during your actual labor. They can wait in the lobby and join you after your baby is born.

When labor pain exceeds a woman's coping ability, or becomes more painful because of complications or the use of medications to induce labor, a woman may choose to use medications to help with the pain. Intravenous narcotics are the most common medication used during labor. They generally ease the pain of the contractions without relieving them totally. They can also help a woman relax between contractions so she can save her strength and focus. Many women find these medications give them a "spacey" feeling, which can be disconcerting. The medicine does get to the baby, which can cause the baby to be sleepy or in very rare cases to be too sleepy to breathe. An antidote is easily available for the baby, so narcotics are considered medically safe.

Epidural analgesia for labor has become more popular. A thin tube is placed in a woman's back near the spinal cord and small doses of pain medicine and local anesthetics flow through the tube and bathe the spinal cord. This leads to excellent pain relief for most women, however it does require that a woman stays in bed connected to a monitor. Side effects can include itching, low blood pressure, and later back pain or leg pain. Several studies have shown that epidural analgesia affects the baby as well. The baby's ability to latch on and suck may not be as well-coordinated, leading to a delay in successful breastfeeding. One study even suggests that the baby's reflexes may be affected as long as 30 days after birth with an epidural. Epidurals can be very helpful, and if you are interested in one be sure to discuss it with your provider. However, keep in mind that they are a medical intervention with associated risks and may not be the best choice in an otherwise normal labor.

Depending on where you give birth, other pain control methods may be available including paracervical block (anesthesia placed near the cervix), intrathecal analgesia (sometimes called "spinal" or "walking epidural"), or other methods. Check with your provider or the birth site to see which therapies are available to you.

First labors, on average, last about eight to twelve hours. People who have told you they have been in labor for three days have generally had a long pre-labor period of contractions that help the uterus get ready for true labor. "Labor" is not just contractions, no matter how painful they may get, but instead labor is contractions leading to cervical change. "Active Labor" is usually not diagnosed until the cervix has thinned out and begins to dilate an average of one centimeter per hour. Most first-time mothers push one to two hours. Subsequent babies tend to come a bit faster—three hours of active labor and 15–30 minutes of pushing on the average. Sometimes, labor will need to be induced or encouraged with medications. Occasionally, if the baby is having trouble or if the mother is exhausted, a vacuum or forceps will be used to help the delivery. In general, you should be able to ask questions and consent to any intervention before it happens, except in an emergency. Discussing possible concerns with your provider in advance will help you work together during your birth.

Some births, now about 20 percent overall in the US, happen by Cesarean section. A Cesarean may be scheduled for breech babies, twins, or other high-risk situations, or may be done urgently in the case of an emergency during labor. Except for true emergencies, women can usually have epidural anesthesia for a Cesarean so they can be awake and see and touch their babies right away. One support person is usually allowed to accompany a woman into the operating room. True emergency Cesareans, such as for fetal distress, may, however, require general anesthesia.

For the first hour after birth, your baby will be alert and learning about you. Ideally, separation of mother and baby should be avoided during this time, even for routine weights and measurements. Within about 30 minutes a baby will begin to search for the mother's breast. Breastfeeding tends to get off to the best start if the first feeding happens during the first hour. Although this uninterrupted hour of bonding helps get moms and babies off to a great start, bonding will happen even if it's delayed.

Natural Childbirth

Several systems have developed over the past few decades to encourage "natural," or non-interventional, childbirth. These include Lamaze,™ Bradley,® and other childbirth-preparation methods. You may find one of these methods fits well for you, or you may want to use a combination of several. Most childbirth-preparation classes now use a Lamaze™ model with some adaptations. Usually, this model focuses on coached breathing and relaxation in labor, and a clear knowledge of what to expect during birth. In addition to labor support and breathing techniques, birth practices such as water birth may appeal to you. All of these ideas can be incorporated into birth in any setting.

VBAC—Vaginal Birth After Cesarean

Obstetricians used to say "once a section, always a section." However, in the past two decades we have learned that most women who have had a prior Cesarean Section can have a subsequent safe vaginal birth. The best candidates for a vaginal birth after a Cesarean (VBAC) have had a previous vaginal birth or had their Cesarean for a reason that is not likely to reoccur, such as a breech baby. About 70 percent of women who have a trial of labor after a prior Cesarean will be able to give birth vaginally. Only women who have had a low-transverse incision (the most common type) on the uterus can safely deliver vaginally, so your provider will need to review the operative note in your past medical history to advise you about this choice. Women who have had more than two Cesareans may be at higher risk for complications from a VBAC.

Usually, these labors proceed normally and uneventfully; if the woman has not had labor before, she will be having her "first labor." The major risk from a VBAC involves rupture of the uterine scar. Without a prior Cesarean, there is about a 0.2 percent risk of uterine rupture; with a prior section, this risk rises to about one percent. If a uterine rupture occurs, it can lead to fetal distress, including neurological damage and even death; it can also require a woman to have a hysterectomy. For this reason, most maternity care providers consider VBAC a relatively high-risk situation. Usually, a woman desiring a VBAC will need closer monitoring and have an intravenous line in case of emergency. However, keep in mind that the first VBACs happened at home, and most of them proceed normally. Most women who have a successful VBAC would do it again, and even many of those who end up with a Cesarean after a trial of labor would have made the same choice.

Some insurance companies have suggested that women should be required to have a VBAC and not be offered a repeat Cesarean. Some obstetricians feel that most women should have repeat Cesareans and only those who absolutely insist should have a VBAC. The best solution probably falls between these two extremes. A woman should discuss her personal risks and preferences for VBAC with her provider and make an informed choice.

We've reviewed numerous resources that can help you as you learn about what happens during childbirth and as you make your childbirth decisions. These resources will help you decide where to have your baby delivered and what form of birthing method best meets your needs. Many of these resources offer up-to-date, in-depth information about the general process of childbirth. Some provide more emphasis on one method of childbirth than another.

After reading these general childbirth resources, you may want more information about specific topics such as delivering a baby with a midwife or doula, having a home birth or water birth, or by using a specific method such as the Lamaze™ method or the Bradley® method. Some general guidebooks will offer you the pros and cons of these childbirth options, but if you're interested in exploring these specific options, we suggest you read some of the childbirth resources we've recommended for having a "natural childbirth."

As in the previous section, we've divided our resource recommendations into several categories to help you focus your search for answers:

We also suggest that prospective parents read the reviews of resources that we recommend in **Section VIII—"Gaining an Overview: All-Inclusive Resources."** These resources address general childbirth issues, but also include descriptions and discussions of pregnancy-related topics as well as offer information on how to take care of your newborn.

Choices in society have prompted a change in the way many women give birth to their babies. Gone are the days of fully anesthetized births, fathers pacing in the waiting room, and a week of recovery in a hospital room after an uncomplicated childbirth. A "passive" childbirth, where everyone in the delivery room made the decisions except the woman giving birth, is no longer the only option. Every woman can now gain the necessary information to control some of the decisions that bring her baby into this world. By arming yourself with knowledge, and by discussing your childbirth options with your health care provider prior to the birth of your baby, you can go through childbirth feeling that you were fully prepared and well-informed.

General Overview

THE BIRTH BOOK
Everything You Need To Know To Have A Safe And Satisfying Birth

 Terrific Resource For:
An overview of the various childbirth choices available to women

 Recommended For:
Childbirth

Description:

"Determining the birth you want and finding out how to get it is what this book is all about," states Sears, a "renowned pediatrician and author," in his Preface. Fourteen chapters make up this 269 page book; they're divided into 3 parts: "preparing for Birth," "Easing Pain in Labor—What You Can Do," and "Experiencing Birth." Part 1 concentrates on a history of birthing practices along with current choices; also given are tips on getting ones body ready for birth and a discussion of tests, technology, etc. that may be involved. Special chapters are devoted to Caesarean sections and VBAC (vaginal birth after Caesarean). Understanding pain and ways to manage it are the focus of Part 2. Part 3 offers information on the best birthing positions, signs of impending labor, and actual labor and delivery. Also provided is information on how to make a birth plan; a sample birth plan is supplied. The final chapter of this part offers 14 birth stories, all different but emphasizing the importance "for a couple to take responsibility for their birth." Anecdotes from the Sears' personal and medical experiences are used throughout.

Evaluation:

The Sears want to empower the reader with "wisdom to get the birth you want, . . . equip you to enter your labor knowing your body, reading its signals, and trusting your responses . . . to a positive birth experience." To that end, they succeed. Throughout this birthing guide, they propose numerous solutions to problems in an effort to offer a "system-fixing, not a system-bashing" book. Mothers-to-be will find the sections on past birthing practices (along with the Sears' personal birth experiences) interesting reading. Well-written sections include the following: the pros and cons of various birthing practices (Bradley, ICEA, ASPO/Lamaze), managing pain (the merits and drawbacks of a medicated birth), choosing a birth team (numerous questions are listed to ask medical professionals and others), composing a birth plan, VBACs, and C-sections. The only weak section deals with "best birth exercises." Little emphasis is given on strengthening abdominal and back muscles. Other resources should be consulted which are devoted solely to this subject. Overall though, there's a gamut of information here that's unbiased and accessible.

Where To Find/Buy:
Bookstores and libraries.

Overall Rating
★★★★
Unbiased clear perspectives on various birthing choices

Design, Ease Of Use
★★★★
Table of contents clearly lists chapter subheadings; text complemented by illustrations

1–4 Stars

Author:
William Sears, MD & Martha Sears, RN

Sears, "one of America's most renowned pediatricians," has been in practice for 20 years and authored 10 books. Currently, he's a clinical assistant professor of pediatrics at USC School of Medicine. His wife is a childbirth educator, registered nurse, & breastfeeding consultant.

Publisher:
Little, Brown and Company

Edition:
1994

Price:
$12.95

Pages:
269

ISBN:
0316779075

Media:
Book

Principal Subject:
Childbirth

Childbirth Subject:
General Overview

★★★

Overall Rating
★★★
Comprehensive, informative and well-written

Design, Ease Of Use
★★★
Clear, well researched and well indexed; heavy textual style at times, no graphics

1–4 Stars

Author:
Diana Korte and Roberta M. Scaer

Korte has won thirty-seven journalism awards. She has been a La Leche League leader and a member of their board of directors. Scaer initiated and co-authored the first survey of women's preferences in maternity care, and serves on the ASPO/ Lamaze board of directors.

Publisher:
Harvard Common Press

Edition:
3rd (1992)

Price:
$14.95

Pages:
360

ISBN:
1558320415

Media:
Book

Principal Subject:
Childbirth

Childbirth Subject:
General Overview

General Overview

A GOOD BIRTH, A SAFE BIRTH
Choosing And Having The Childbirth Experience You Want

Description:

This 360 page book is a resource tool for answering women's questions on childbirth options available in America today. The two authors, who surveyed women to discover exactly what their current beliefs and experiences are, wrote this book aimed at disseminating their findings. The first chapter begins with "What Women Want." This includes: having partners present for labor, delivery, and recovery, being given contact with their babies, receiving effective breastfeeding assistance from their medical professionals, allowing other children to visit, and cooperation and assistance from their childbirth professional in using childbirth techniques. Other topics covered are: sexuality and pregnancy, knowing your options in order to make informed decisions, perspectives on doctors, questions to assist in finding the right doctor, explanations of the interventions doctors favor and why, appreciation of the emotions involved in giving birth, childbirth support groups, and how to get the nurses on your side. A number of appendices offer additional supportive tools for women.

Evaluation:

This book was written by a professional writer and research team, and it shows! Arranged logically and practically, it is filled with personal quotes from women who cooperated with the surveys. In most situations both childbirth perspectives are given, from joyous natural childbirth experiences, to those who were thankful for the drugs and interventions that gave relief and healthy babies. In particular, we respected the amount of attention given the subject of VBACs. Women will find the information given to be useful and supportive. Medical practices are explained and advice on how to overcome obstacles is given along with current research. This book addresses the real issues around a satisfying birth experience—feelings of mastery, of control, of coping well, and of having an active part in the decisions about labor. The information and techniques in this book will assist readers in making the best choices for themselves and their baby.

Where To Find/Buy:
Bookstores and libraries.

III. Childbirth

General Overview

THE CHILDBIRTH KIT
Ideas And Images To Help You Through Labor

★★★

Description:

This resource was created to share techniques and ideas for handling the labor of childbirth with other mothers-to-be. The "kit" includes an 88-page book detailing activities for both the weeks leading up to childbirth and the birth itself, explaining how to use the "waiting days calendar" and the "quick reference cards" used in conjunction with the stages of labor: "early labor," "active labor," "transition," and "pushing." Each card has an image on one side (for example, "rings," "waves," and "bubbles" for the active labor stage) and on the other side a descriptive "visualization," specific techniques (breathing, massage, body positioning), and "triggering" words to help you evoke the image. Each image is closely linked with physical stage of childbirth, so that by evoking the images you can more fully use the techniques on the other side. The authors recommend familiarizing yourself with the techniques and images in the weeks before the birth and using a "birth partner" to help you prepare and to offer support during labor.

Evaluation:

Written by two women who have been through the experience more than once, this resource is a collection of helpful and imaginative techniques and activities to help naturally minimize pain during childbirth and prepare oneself mentally as well as physically. The use of images is especially ingenious, and the techniques themselves are clearly effective. The book takes the view of childbirth as a challenging but absolutely natural human experience, a healthy change from the common view of childbirth as some kind of medical operation or sickness. By using the techniques in this book, perhaps in conjunction with a childbirth class and other resources, a woman may find herself well-prepared for the experience. This resource would be especially helpful for first-time mothers, or for women who anticipate difficulty. Although not all women may respond to all the techniques offered here, this "kit" should certainly inspire women to create a package of their own with personalized images and activities to help them before and during childbirth.

Where To Find/Buy:

Bookstores and libraries.

Overall Rating
★★★
Helpful, detailed techniques for handling pain

Design, Ease Of Use
★★
Interesting "visualization" activities

1–4 Stars

Author:
Marie Fellenstein Hale & Liz Chalmers

The authors, mothers with four children between them, wrote this book to offer women techniques for handling labor from their own experiences of childbirth and feedback from other women who have used these techniques.

Publisher:
Swanstone Press

Edition:
1994

Price:
$22.95

Pages:
88

ISBN:
0964353008

Media:
Book

Principal Subject:
Childbirth

Childbirth Subject:
General Overview

III. Childbirth

★★

Overall Rating
★★
Clear and concise, it uses a logical approach to the argument for homebirths

Design, Ease Of Use
★★
Easy to flip through, but a bit cold in tone

1–4 Stars

Author:
Carl Jones

Carl Jones is a certified childbirth educator and the author of numerous books about baby care and childbirth. He serves as a professional consultant to the American Red Cross.

Publisher:
Carol Publishing Group (Citadel Press)

Edition:
1995

Price:
$12.95

Pages:
267

ISBN:
0806516402

Media:
Book

Principal Subject:
Childbirth

Childbirth Subject:
General Overview

General Overview

CHILDBIRTH CHOICES TODAY
Everything You Need To Know To Plan A Safe And Rewarding Birth

Description:

This 267 page book's goal is to describe the options available in America today for childbirth. Chapter 1 takes a look at the influences that are changing maternity care, from rediscovery of natural health care options to overall dissatisfaction with dehumanizing hospital care. The book's basis is summed up this way: "Your health and your child's depend largely on healthy prenatal habits and good childbirth preparation. Though you will . . . not be able to eliminate all the discomforts of pregnancy and labor, you will increase your chance of enjoying a healthier, happier pregnancy and birth if you observe the(se) . . . steps." The author highlights these steps within each chapter. Chapter topics are as follows: giving birth your way, the experience of labor, planning your birth, obstetric routines and procedures, Cesarean birth, midwifery care, hospital birth choices, birth in a childbearing center, birth at home, and how you can effect a change in terms of future childbirth practices. An extensive resource list is provided as well as a recommended outline of the author's childbirth classes.

Evaluation:

While this book briefly reviews the options available, it is clearly focused on supporting alternative choices to hospitalized care. The outline and bullet-point format makes it easy to flip through this book to the sections that interest the reader. The voice is that of a logical, left-brain thinker, a nice change for some women from the more emotion-centered right-brain books on the market. The author articulates reasons for change in childbirth practices—consumer demands for better, more personal treatment and the women's movement, with its emphasis on women taking control of their own bodies. He also points out the shift in professionals' attitudes toward a more holistic approach to health care, giving equal consideration to the psychological as well as the physical aspects of the birth experience. Still, while pointing out that changes are happening, the writer does not ignore the generally overbearing attitudes of some hospital staff and medical doctors who are still committed to their routines and practices. This book is a useful tool, but should be read in conjunction with other books on the topic.

Where To Find/Buy:
Bookstores and libraries.

General Overview

THE NURTURING TOUCH AT BIRTH
A Labor Support Handbook

★★

Description:

The Nurturing Touch At Birth is an 84 page, 12 chapter book written for labor support caregivers. Chapters include "What's Happening in Labor and Birth," "Let's Talk About Pain," "Communication Skills and Tools," "Touch and Massage," "Innovative Strategies and Techniques," "Implementing Labor Support Strategies At All Birth Sites," and more. The first half of the book is geared more toward the mental, emotional, and relationship aspects of the caregiver's role. The latter half, although not void of those themes, contains more of the physical techniques applied during labor. A chapter on "Healing Arts Modalities" gives suggestions on using aromatherapy, music, water therapy, accupressure, reflexology, and therapeutic touch to help the laboring woman. Other physical strategies for both the mother and caregiver to use during labor are given in Chapters 10 and 11. These include the birth ball, the lunge, pelvic circles and abdominal lift, and more. Some photographs are provided to highlight text. A list of resources is provided at the back of the book. This book does not include an index.

Evaluation:

Perez has made a valiant effort to reach labor support caregivers by attempting to mold their overall approach to helping women in labor. The goal would be to "help shape the maternity care of the future to better suit the needs of women, their babies, and their families." This book works hard at teaching labor support caregivers not only the tangible skills and techniques for helping mothers during childbirth but also the intangible—that is, the caregivers' feelings, attitudes, and mentality. There is much philosophizing in this book, as Perez borrows many philosophical statements from others. She says that "birth education should be based on a biopsychosocial model and the belief that women and their partners have inner strengths and resources which they can employ during labor and birth." This is not your typical book for expectant parents (its target audience is, after all, labor support persons), although expectant parents can glean some information on techniques that can be used during labor. However, readers will need to do much sifting through the philosophical essays to reach advice on practical applications.

Where To Find/Buy:

Bookstores and libraries.

Overall Rating
★★
Author's heartfelt intent is evident, but sometimes the book wanders from its purpose

Design, Ease Of Use
★★
Important practical points often hidden in dense philosophical discussions

1–4 Stars

Author:
Paulina Perez

Paulina Perez is a perinatal nurse consultant and professional labor assistant with 30+ years experience in maternity care. She is the author of *Special Women*, numerous journal articles, and is an internationally known speaker on health care issues.

Publisher:
Cutting Edge Press

Edition:
1997

Price:
$11.95

Pages:
84

ISBN:
0964115980

Media:
Book

Principal Subject:
Childbirth

Childbirth Subject:
General Overview

III. Childbirth

★★★★

Overall Rating
★★★★
Clearly written, relevant information about natural childbirth

Design, Ease Of Use
★★★★
Well-organized and flows well; numerous photos, bulleted tips, and highlighted blocks

1–4 Stars

Author:
Janet Balaskas

Publisher:
The Harvard Common Press

Edition:
1992 (Revised)

Price:
$14.95

Pages:
252

ISBN:
1558320385

Media:
Book

Principal Subject:
Childbirth

Childbirth Subject:
Natural Childbirth

Natural Childbirth

ACTIVE BIRTH
The New Approach To Giving Birth Naturally

 Recommended For:
Childbirth

Description:

Active Birth is a 252 page, 10 chapter book that encompasses some history on childbirth, along with an overview of the stages of pregnancy and childbirth. It instructs expectant parents on how to prepare for giving birth naturally and how women can best use their bodies actively in labor (versus reclined on a bed). Many illustrations and photographs accompany the text. The book begins by defining active birth and comparing it to modern western practice (obstetrically managed birth). Chapter 2 describes the woman's body during pregnancy. Yoga-based exercises, breathing, and massage in preparation for active childbirth are discussed in Chapters 3, 4, and 5, respectively. Labor and birth are discussed in Chapters 6 and 7. Chapter 8 covers water birth. Chapter 9 presents a brief discussion on the woman's body after birth and how to begin breastfeeding. Postpartum exercises are presented in Chapter 10. Included at the back of the book are "Emergency Birth: For the Partner," and a list of recommended readings and resources.

Evaluation:

This is an excellent choice for expectant parents who wish to take an active role in labor and childbirth. A hefty Chapter 3 is devoted to preparing the mother's body for an active birth. The many yoga-based exercises that are taught in this chapter are important to increase the woman's flexibility and strengthen her muscles. In Chapters 6 and 7, a number of different laboring and birthing positions are presented. Also in these two chapters is a good cross-section of personal accounts from many women who share their experiences during labor and birth. However, Chapter 9, "After the Birth," seems to exist just to indulge the reader. Here, an extremely abbreviated discussion is given on what the new mom's body goes through in the moments and days after baby is born, and the subject of breastfeeding is merely touched on (6 pages). This is understandable, since the book's focus is on preparing parents for active birth. The section called "Emergency Birth: For the Partner" will be useful for the support person. A focused resource, this is a great educational tool for a western society dominated by obstetrically managed births.

Where To Find/Buy:

Bookstores and libraries.

Natural Childbirth

THE BIRTH PARTNER
Everything You Need To Know To Help A Woman Through Childbirth

Terrific Resource For:
Birth partners offering support and coaching during childbirth

Recommended For:
Childbirth

Description:

This 241 page book is written specifically for the person assisting a woman during active labor. Organized for easy reference the book is divided into four parts. The first part, "Before The Birth," is an introduction for the birth partner on what to do in the days before the birth. Topics such as meeting with the professionals involved, planning your route to the birthing place, and reviewing a birth plan are covered. Part 2, "Labor and Birth," explains medical terminology one may encounter, and answers questions such as: how long does labor last? How will the mother feel? What does the caregiver do? and How can you help? A "Take-Charge Routine" is given to help partners assist a panicky or scared mother. Part 3 deals with medical intervention and the problems that prompt it. Explanations are given to take the mystery out of the "whys" of doctor intervention. The final section deals with the birth partner's role in the postpartum period. Summaries are provided on what to expect in the first few hours and days for both baby and mother. Suggestions are offered throughout the book on how to be most effective as a birth partner.

Evaluation:

This book is well-organized, professional, and is both supportive and positive for those dealing with potentially distressing situations. The writer includes logical and clear explanations, e.g. why a woman should switch to a high-carbohydrate diet a few days before her expected labor (in a nutshell, fat slows down labor, carbohydrates won't). The interesting amount of detail and the direct relevancy provided in this book makes it a good read for the mother-to-be and her partner before the event. The diagrams, illustrations, and specific pages for each stage of labor, make it a valuable tool for birth partners, for birthing instructors, and for future reference during active labor; the use of darkened edges on pertinent pages will help in locating pages of interest during this busy time. It is a unique resource in that it supports any birth partner, uses minimal rhetoric, and does a great job of making the role of birth partner one that can be fully appreciated as both important and personally rewarding. There is an extensive recommended resources section and a clear index. This book is recommended highly for any birth partner.

Where To Find/Buy:

Bookstores and libraries.

Overall Rating
★★★★
A very useful book for the birth partner, it's intelligent, comprehensive, and supportive

Design, Ease Of Use
★★★★
Illustrations useful; design supports quick reference during active labor

1–4 Stars

Author:
Penny Simkin, PT

Penny Simkin is the mother of four and was present at the birth of two of her grandsons. She has provided labor support for numerous women and has spent more than twenty years teaching and learning from thousands of women and their partners.

Publisher:
Harvard Common Press

Edition:
1989

Price:
$10.95

Pages:
241

ISBN:
1558320105

Media:
Book

Principal Subject:
Childbirth

Childbirth Subject:
Natural Childbirth

III. Childbirth

★★★★

Overall Rating
★★★★
A rare kind of book;
encourages an inner
journey to parenthood

Design, Ease Of Use
★★★★
Breakout topics encourage
contemplation; suggested
projects empower creativity

1–4 Stars

Author:
Pam England, CNM, MA, and
Rob Horowitz, PhD

England, a midwife and registered
nurse, holds a master's degree in
psychology and counseling,
specializing in prenatal birth and
postpartum therapy. Horowitz holds
a PhD in clinical psychology, teaches
Birthing From Within techniques, and
is in private practice.

Publisher:
Partera Press

Edition:
1998

Price:
$19.95

Pages:
309

ISBN:
0965987302

Media:
Book

Principal Subject:
Childbirth

Childbirth Subject:
Natural Childbirth

Natural Childbirth

BIRTHING FROM WITHIN
An Extra-Ordinary Guide To Childbirth Preparation

 Terrific Resource For:
Couples seeking a childbirth experience that encompasses
inward and outer guidance

 Recommended For:
Childbirth

Description:
Birthing From Within is based on pregnancy classes developed
by author Pam England. Her vision: "parents learning through
interactive, creative participation, in a spirit of fun and curiosity."
The book is divided into seven sections: "Beginning Your Journey,"
"The Art of Birthing," "Preparing Your Birth Place," "Being Powerful
in Birth," "Fathers and Birth Companions," "Birthing Through Pain,"
and "Gestating Parenthood." Also included is an afterword, "Birth as
an Adventure," and several appendices: "Special Diets for Special
Situations," "Breech Tilt," "Worksheets for Learning the Pain
Techniques," "Reminder Cards," and "Circumcision." The book
includes many illustrations and original pieces of art, including
"birthing art" produced in "Birthing From Within" classes, and
numerous breakout topic boxes and suggested creative art projects
related to pregnancy. The introduction explains how "Birthing From
Within" classes differ from traditional childbirth classes: the emphasis
on exploring the spiritual, psychological, holistic, and creative
components of pregnancy and childbirth in a non-clinical setting.

Evaluation:
Birthing From Within is not for those parents most comfortable
learning about pregnancy and childbirth in a clinical or uninvolved
setting. This book is for prospective parents and those who are willing
to use all their senses to explore the deeper, primordial connections
that emerge during pregnancy and childbirth. A Zen philosophy flows
through the book and its information, as meditations, birthing art, and
more are interwoven philosophy. The book is an attractive addition to
any pregnancy library, and it presents a philosophy of integrating body
and soul that is gaining greater mainstream acceptance. Some of the
exercises may not appeal to all—one calls for reenactment of the
parental birth, another for using the birth placenta as nourishment
for a tree planted in your child's honor—but there is a wide enough
variety that almost everyone will come away with a greater awe for
the potential for personal and family growth embedded in the act of
procreating. With suggestions as diverse as sharing family birth stories
and traditions, an herbal foot bath ritual for mother, coyote howling,
singing lullabies and journaling, there are riches here for almost everyone.

Where To Find/Buy:
Bookstores and libraries.

Natural Childbirth

GENTLE BIRTH CHOICES
A Guide To Making Informed Decisions About Birthing Centers, Birth Attendants, Water Birth, Home Birth, Hospital Birth

Terrific Resource For:
Alternative childbirth practices and philosophies

Recommended For:
Childbirth

Description:

This 268 page book is written from the perspective of a woman who is not only a registered nurse but has also experienced water birth. The Forward gives an anthropological view of the modern experience of hospitalized childbirth, likening it to initiation into a cult. The author then moves from a historical to a current perspective on childbirth. The focus is on women's goal of taking control away from doctors and their procedures in modern times. Chapter Three works to dispel medical myths currently treated as fact in American society. Chapter Four talks about the effect of social consciousness on wo men and how this has redefined what women want in their birthing experience. Chapter Five goes into detail about midwifery. Chapter Six deals with water births, what they are, where they originated, and general questions about them. Chapter Seven delves into the mind-body connection of how thoughts influence the birth process, and how they can be changed to assist in natural birth and managing pain. This book ends with guides for planning your own childbirth options.

Evaluation:

This book is of particular use to someone who wishes to explore alternatives to mainstream medical care for childbirth. The writing style is clear, intelligent and emotionally moving. The illustrations are well done and provocative. The tone of the book is one of rhetorical support for going against the current "technological medical system." While informative and well-done, it is necessary to caution the reader to be aware that this work has a decided slant that supports the author's perspective on natural birth options. Information is provided on medical history, the development, decline and current rekindling of midwifery, and on current hospital practice, with a definite bias against male doctors and their practices. Interesting and informative as it is, the reader is cautioned to balance this book against other works that detail the advances medicine has made in the interest of healthy pregnancy and childbirth.

Where To Find/Buy:

Bookstores and libraries.

Overall Rating
★★★★
A good overview of alternative childbirth options with a decided "political" tilt

Design, Ease Of Use
★★★★
Well-written and well-illustrated

1–4 Stars

Author:
Barbara Harper, RN

Barbara Harper is the founder of Global Maternal/Child Health Association, a nonprofit organization dedicated to education and research about natural childbirth, including the use of water to ease labor and birth. She is a registered nurse and lectures internationally.

Publisher:
Healing Arts Press

Edition:
1994

Price:
$16.95

Pages:
268

ISBN:
0892814802

Media:
Book

Principal Subject:
Childbirth

Childbirth Subject:
Natural Childbirth

III. Childbirth

Overall Rating
★★★

Surprise ending helps the tape's rather staged practice sessions

Design, Ease Of Use
★★★★

Breathing exercises divided into stages of labor, clearly explained, booklet included

1–4 Stars

Author:
Dr. Art Ulene

This video is presented by The American College of Obstetricians and Gynecologists, and features television medical personality Dr. Art Ulene.

Edition:
1985

Price:
$19.95

ISBN:
156832278X

Media:
Videotape

Principal Subject:
Childbirth

Childbirth Subject:
Natural Childbirth

Natural Childbirth

DR. ART ULENE'S CHILDBIRTH PREPARATION PROGRAM

Description:

The "Childbirth Preparation Program," narrated by Dr. Art Ulene, features breathing exercises for all stages of labor, demonstrates various labor positions, relaxation techniques, massage, and tension techniques. Included at the end of this 52 minute video are actual birth scenes of the couples who earlier in the video demonstrated breathing and relaxation practice sessions. This video, presented by The American College of Obstetricians and Gynecologists, includes an accompanying 24 page booklet that presents the information and techniques shown on the video. Additional topics discussed include selecting a coach/birthing support person, the different stages of labor, communication during labor, use of focal points, and "back labor."

Evaluation:

This at first is an easy video to dismiss. Narrator Ulene talks too fast and his tone is too strident as he leads couples through breathing practice sessions. As he is exhorting couples to relax, the viewer is tempted to urge him to do the same. Also, the couples are too perfect—women perfectly coiffed, studio makeup in place; all participants dressed in white. However, this video holds a surprise, a reward for those practice sessions. The last portion of the 52 minute video is devoted to the actual birth scenes from the couples who earlier demonstrated the breathing practice sessions. Suddenly the reason for the practices comes alive as one moves with each couple into their real-life birth scene, and participates with them in the birth of their child. Not only do we practice labor techniques with them, we are invited to help them welcome a new family member. No stage managing here, only the real-life exhilaration of childbirth. Birth scenes shown include only hospital settings, however they run the gamut from birthing room with an entire family present to delivery room, and from Cesarean to the birth of twins. The video then ends by officially introducing each of the family groups as they give their thoughts on the birthing process.

Where To Find/Buy:

Bookstores, libraries, videotape dealers, or order direct by calling Library Video Company at (800) 843-3620, through FAX at (610) 645-4040, or online at libraryvideo.com.

III. Childbirth

Natural Childbirth

AN EASIER CHILDBIRTH
A Mother's Guide For Birthing Normally

★★★

Description:

Near the beginning of this book, the author states that "becoming a mother is a life transition that our culture greatly underestimates." This workbook is dedicated to preparing a mother-to-be mentally and emotionally for the experience of childbirth and motherhood. Research shows that emotional preparation is essential for an easier labor; central to this book's philosophy is the concept of "pain with a purpose" that is "qualitatively different from other kinds of pain." Chapters 1–4 include preparing your "birth inventory" or overall feelings about the birth, coming to grips with the life transition of becoming a mother, tapping into your own "birth memory," and dealing with feelings from a previous childbirth as well as harmful cultural messages about childbirth. Chapters 5–8 discuss labor preparation techniques including relaxation and visualization exercises for each stage of labor, and how to identify a coping system that will work for you. Chapters 9–10 discuss how to bond with your baby while maintaining relationships with other family members and creating healthy family patterns for the future.

Evaluation:

As more women choose to birth naturally without the aid of drugs and medical intervention, preparing oneself psychologically for the stress of labor becomes an essential part of pregnancy. Even for women who ultimately do use some kind of medical assistance, this book should prove to be an invaluable aid. Its help extends beyond childbirth and labor to include helping you grow accustomed to the idea of yourself as a mother. This seems essential not only for a confident, relaxed birth but also for becoming a confident, relaxed parent. There is not much in our culture that prepares women to become mothers. It is assumed that women will take to it instinctively and blossom unaided into perfect parents. However, many women (especially those who choose to have children later in life) may experience childbirth and motherhood as a difficult transition from previous lifestyles. This book includes not only exercises to gain more understanding of yourself as a prospective mother, but also techniques to cope with and perceive pain as a natural force. This enlightenment will lead to labor and childbirth being seen as a positive experience.

Where To Find/Buy:

Bookstores and libraries.

Overall Rating
★★★
Sensitive and positive approach to childbirth and mothering

Design, Ease Of Use
★★★
Creative techniques presented in a workbook style to be used with your birth partner

1–4 Stars

Author:
Gayle Peterson, PhD

Gayle Peterson, Ph.D., has done research on ways to prevent complications during pregnancy and childbirth, and has also created a prenatal counseling program for women. She is the author of *Birthing Normally* and other books on pregnancy and birth.

Publisher:
Shadow & Light Publications

Edition:
2nd (1993)

Price:
$14.95

Pages:
177

ISBN:
0962523143

Media:
Book

Principal Subject:
Childbirth

Childbirth Subject:
Natural Childbirth

III. Childbirth

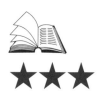

★★★

Overall Rating
★★★
Clear introduction to the role of doulas

Design, Ease Of Use
★★★
Easy to read text; sensitive pictures

1–4 Stars

Author:
Marshall H. Klaus, MD; John H. Kennell, MD; Phyllis H. Klaus, MEd, CSW

The coauthors of this book are known worldwide for their decades of research and devoted effort to make childbirth more humane, more natural and better for babies. Between them they have written *Parent-Infant Bonding*, *The Amazing Newborn*, and others.

Publisher:
Addison-Wesley Publishing

Edition:
1993

Price:
$15.00

Pages:
168

ISBN:
0201632721

Media:
Book

Principal Subject:
Childbirth

Childbirth Subject:
Natural Childbirth

Natural Childbirth

MOTHERING THE MOTHER
How A Doula Can Help You Have A Shorter, Easier, And Healthier Birth

Description:
This 168 page book stresses that today's modern childbirth practices make it more lonely and more psychologically stressful than it need be. The writers of this book have spent the past 15 years studying the effects of restoring women helpers to the labor experience. The results of their study show a marked reduction in the need for medical interventions when a woman uses a doula. This book describes the role of the doula and the physical, emotional, and psychological needs met by employing one. Not a doctor, not a nurse, not a midwife, she is not trained to make any medical decisions. Her role is described as one of support, remaining with the mother through the entire labor and not leaving her alone. She is the mother's link to "normalcy." Details of the authors' studies are included in the text, along with cost-comparison information (eg, the cost of anesthesia vs. a support doula). Examples of doula-supported births are included as are explanations about the difference between husband support and doula support. The book ends with a discussion of support after birth, and how to find and choose a doula.

Evaluation:
This book is beautifully done and communicates a good understanding of the role of supportive women in the childbirth experience. The text is aided by the sensitive photography of Suzanne Arms whose work also appears in several other current pregnancy and childbirth books. Information on studies of doula-assisted and non-assisted births are interspersed throughout with anecdotes. Beyond the text of the book itself, a very interesting section is "Appendix A: The Training of a Doula." This section is straightforward, to the point, and gives one a clear sense of the nature of the doula's role. "Appendix B: Useful Addresses" will also be useful for women wanting more support during labor than perhaps a nervous husband or an overly concerned mother.

Where To Find/Buy:
Bookstores and libraries.

Natural Childbirth

EASING LABOR PAIN
The Complete Guide To A More Comfortable And Rewarding Birth

★★★

Description:

This book is a collection of information about the many methods for managing pain. It begins with a discussion on labor pain offering views both from women who experienced no pain and from women who were in great pain and relieved by modern medical anesthesia. What happens during labor is reviewed, as are explanations for why labor is painful. Chapter 2 reviews myths of painless births, and the role of pain in normal labor. Chapter 3, "Childbirth Education," looks at the development of and benefits arising from the education movement; included are reviews of most of the current ideologies taught today. Chapter 4 proceeds to the heart of the matter—labor—and reviews ten relaxation techniques. Chapter 5 reviews breathing techniques. Chapters 6–12 emphasize a more physical approach to pain relief, including nutrition, acupuncture, acupressure and massage, and more. Chapters 13–16 stress psychological approaches, such as visualization, hypnosis, therapeutic touch, and more. Medical aids are discussed, as is the topic of whether babies feel pain.

Evaluation:

The author, in writing about "The Myth of the Painless Birth," states, ". . . if we could only prepare better, practice more, give birth in the 'right' circumstances, or alter our cultural bias from high tech toward a more 'natural' style of childbirth, then labor wouldn't hurt." This statement points out the exact bias of so many books on the topic today. If we could just prepare perfectly, then everything would be OK. Not so. This book dispels the myth behind those ideologies promoting painless childbirth. And it directs the reader's attention to the techniques that are available for handling the sensations experienced during and after childbirth. Consequently, it is a refreshing, intelligent look at the options available for managing the birth experience and the pain. Written in a clear and straightforward manner, this book could also be recommended for those wishing to learn more about pain management.

Where To Find/Buy:

Bookstores and libraries.

Overall Rating
★★★
An excellent overview of physical and psychological methods of pain management

Design, Ease Of Use
★★
Clear, well-organized, well-referenced and indexed; photographs would be helpful

1–4 Stars

Author:
Adrienne B. Lieberman

Adrienne Lieberman, a mother of two, has been a childbirth educator since 1976. She is the author of *Giving Birth* and the co-author of *The Preemie Parents' Handbook*.

Publisher:
Harvard Common Press

Edition:
2nd (1992)

Price:
$12.95

Pages:
279

ISBN:
1558320431

Media:
Book

Principal Subject:
Childbirth

Childbirth Subject:
Natural Childbirth

III. Childbirth

★★★

Overall Rating
★★★
Strong in explaining merits
and how-tos of the technique;
weak in coaching style

Design, Ease Of Use
★★
Explicit photographs, large
headings; chapters drift;
summary would be helpful

1–4 Stars

Author:
Susan McCutcheon

Publisher:
Penguin Books USA (Plume)

Edition:
2nd (1996)

Price:
$16.95

Pages:
254

ISBN:
0452276594

Media:
Book

Principal Subject:
Childbirth

Childbirth Subject:
Natural Childbirth

Natural Childbirth

NATURAL CHILDBIRTH THE BRADLEY WAY

Description:

"The Bradley Method" is the result of a "movement to return to natural, drug-free techniques in childbirth"; Dr. Bradley endorses this book in the book's preface. Proponents of the technique—also called the Husband-Coached Childbirth—tout a 90%+ success rate; this is compared in the book with a 1% success rate using Lamaze. The 254 page book is divided into four parts: "Getting Ready," "The First Stage of Birth," "The Second Stage of Birth," and "Controversies in Childbirth." The first part offers suggestions for choosing one's doctor and childbirth teacher; also covered are nutrition, birth and labor mechanics, preparatory exercises, and more. Relaxation techniques, "practice plans" for the mother and her coach, getting through labor, and more are given in part 2. Part 3 focuses on pushing. "Master Exercises" are shown for both parts 2 and 3 to prepare for these stages of birth. Part 4 outlines various childbirthing practices (episiotomy, Cesarean surgery, inducing labor, forceps, etc.) and discusses the drawbacks and dangers involved. A brief chapter on breastfeeding is also given (10 pages).

Evaluation:

The purpose of this evaluation is to neither support or refute this method of giving birth. Rather, it reflects the extent to which the authors explain 1) the merits of the method, 2) the rationale for using the technique, 3) the strategies and exercises to manage the pain, and 4) the involvement of the coach in the process. To that extent, this book does a fine job in the first three instances. Also, especially helpful are the abundant, explicit photographs and illustrations. The fourth subject, however, which should be at the center of a text on "Husband-Coached Childbirth," needs more punch. During labor, the coach may be at a loss for words to assist; some explicit vocabulary would have been helpful here. In addition, the chapters' subheadings ramble into one another and you may get lost in the shuffle. Hopefully a future revisions of this book will include a summarizing appendix or chapter that can be accessed during the actual birth (few in the climax of giving birth would be able to find the section they are looking for without some effort). And so, if one wants to try "The Bradley Method," this is the book but it will need to be summarized and annotated before the birth begins.

Where To Find/Buy:

Bookstores and libraries.

Natural Childbirth

THE BRADLEY METHOD® OF NATURAL CHILDBIRTH ★★

Description:

The American Academy of Husband-Coached Childbirth (AAHCC) sponsors this website promoting the "Bradley Method® of Natural Childbirth." Features on their homepage include an outline of the Bradley Method goals, information on how to become an instructor, listings of teacher trainings (dates, places), a recommended pregnancy diet, summaries of course content, and similar material. The underlying philosophy embraces the following ideals: natural childbirth, active participation of the husband as coach, "excellent nutrition," relaxation and "natural breathing," "tuning-in to your own body," breastfeeding, parents' roles in responsibility for the birthplace, procedures, attendants, "consumerism," and more. The on-line pregnancy diet consists of suggested daily requirements, with a "protein counter" listing the amount of protein available in various food sources. The 12 classes taught by Bradley Method® instructors are described in single paragraphs incorporating subjects such as nutrition, the coach's role, labor (first/second stages), birth plans, and potential complications.

Evaluation:

This evaluation neither endorses nor challenges this childbirth method; judgment is based on the cohesiveness and thoroughness of the site. One positive point of this site is its list of protein sources—valuable and convenient for pregnant women to have on hand. Another positive aspect is its outline of the organization's 12-week course in childbirth; most other sites don't volunteer this level of detail. Although the descriptions are brief (generally 3–5 sentences each), they do a good job of highlighting the Bradley Method® philosophy. One can note the importance placed on various aspects of this method, such as the role of the partner, techniques used for relaxation, how to deal with complications, etc. In summary, the site does a credible job in spelling out the philosophy of this method, and the visitor should be able to leave it well-versed in the nature of this method with knowledge about where to go for further information and/or training. This site won't dazzle, but it will inform.

Where To Find/Buy:

On the Internet at the URL: http://www.bradleybirth.com/ or by calling (800) 4-A-BIRTH

Overall Rating
★★
Philosophy vague at times, content is information-oriented

Design, Ease Of Use
★★
Website design straightforward, informational; graphics would enhance the text

1–4 Stars

Media:
Internet

Principal Subject:
Childbirth

Childbirth Subject:
Natural Childbirth

III. Childbirth

III. Childbirth

Overall Rating
★★
Answers basic questions about water birth, but does not go beyond that

Design, Ease Of Use
★★
Easy to read layout, terrific photos which tend to get in the way of reading the text

1–4 Stars

Media:
Internet

Principal Subject:
Childbirth

Childbirth Subject:
Natural Childbirth

Natural Childbirth

GIVING BIRTH UNDERWATER
A Very Gentle Choice

Description:

The Global Maternal/Child Health Association, which incorporated in 1989 to facilitate maternity care reform, sponsors this website to "preserve, protect and enhance the well-being of women and children during pregnancy, birth, infancy and early childhood." At the homepage, a visitor will find an article on why an expectant mother should choose to have a water birth, answers to frequently asked questions, birth stories, books, tub purchase information, and a bibliography. Throughout the website are photographs that depict the images of various water births. Responses to frequently asked questions address specifics of water birth, such as how a baby breathes, when a baby should be taken out of the water, what the water temperature should be, and why water birth is not available in more hospitals. A visitor will find more resources on this topic through the "Books" and "Bibliography" sections. To order any of the books or arrange for purchase or rental of a water birth tub, a visitor can call the telephone number provided.

Evaluation:

The author of the response to one of this website's FAQs states that water birth is more a philosophy of non-intervention than a method of giving birth. It is asserted here that during a medical birth, the doctor takes control of the birthing process, which should instead be left in the control of the mother. Information is given about the organization in general that sponsors the site and how to contact it, but no information is provided about who the people in the organization are. There is a lengthy article on why a woman should choose a water birth, and the website offers many photos taken during various water births around the world. The FAQs are basic, with concise answers. The benefit of this website would be to start an expectant mother on her way to investigating the option of a water birth, but the study should not stop here. The photos provide a view of all that is involved, but once you've seen one or two, you've seen them all. Eventually, they almost seem to get in the way of the information.

Where To Find/Buy:
On the Internet at the URL: http://www.geocities.com/HotSprings/2840

Natural Childbirth

HUSBAND-COACHED CHILDBIRTH
The Bradley Method Of Natural Childbirth

Description:

This 275 page book is written from the first person perspective of a practicing physician in obstetrics. Beginning with his earliest impressions of birth, he expands on the concept of natural childbirth as a humanistic, undrugged approach to parenthood. Dr. Bradley traces the development of his theory and method of childbirth, expands to a description of "Where do fathers fit in?" and then describes his methodology. Chapters 5 & 6 deal directly with his methodology through anecdotes and observations of laboring couples. Chapter 7 covers "The Coach's Training Rules." The rest of the book deals with childbirth-related issues, such as episiotomies, due dates, family relations and postpartum recovery, breastfeeding, natural pregnancy loss, and dealing with pregnancy problems. A chapter is included at the end offering comments and thoughts from fathers who used the Bradley Method. This book is written as a supportive document for couples participating in this particular method of childbirth training and instruction.

Evaluation:

Written in the first person perspective, Dr. Bradley begins with his own orientation to nature and God as the foundation for his work on "natural childbirth." Through 20 chapters he describes how he developed his method, beginning in 1947, with early experiments in undrugged deliveries for unwed mothers. Throughout the book he relates anecdote after anecdote on the benefits of a calming pattern of relaxation, abdominal breathing and loving teamwork between husband and wife as the key to a painless and joyful birthing experience. While interesting from a historical perspective, the book reads like an historical account from a grandfather on what childbirth used to be like and how he helped bring about the perspective in use today. This book will be most interesting to the mothers of women about to give birth naturally, as it will shed some light on changing childbirth perspectives. Those with a deeply religious perspective may enjoy the tone and style of this book as well. Practical and usable information contained in this book, on the other hand, could be summarized in a short pamphlet.

Where To Find/Buy:

Bookstores and libraries.

Overall Rating
★★
Reads more like a novel about childbirth than a how-to guide; anecdotes distracting

Design, Ease Of Use
★★
Wordy, rambling; could be more succinctly written for actual use in the delivery room

1–4 Stars

Author:
Robert A. Bradley, MD

Robert A. Bradley, M.D. has been practicing and promoting "The Bradley Method" of childbirth since 1947. The first edition of Husband-Coached Childbirth appeared in 1965.

Publisher:
Bantam Books

Edition:
4th (1996)

Price:
$11.95

Pages:
275

ISBN:
0553375563

Media:
Book

Principal Subject:
Childbirth

Childbirth Subject:
Natural Childbirth

III. Childbirth

Overall Rating
★★
Information limited to Lamaze organization, philosophy and training

Design, Ease Of Use
★★
Simply designed with clear paths to topics; too much time to download graphics

1–4 Stars

Author:
Lamaze International is dedicated to using Lamaze childbirth methods to promote "natural, healthy, and fulfilling childbirth experiences for women and their families through education, advocacy and reform."

Media:
Internet

Principal Subject:
Childbirth

Childbirth Subject:
Natural Childbirth

Natural Childbirth

LAMAZE INTERNATIONAL

Description:
The motto of Lamaze International, Inc. is to promote "natural, healthy, and fulfilling childbirth experiences for women and their families through education, advocacy and reform." Its website homepage offers information on Lamaze philosophies and background, membership, information on becoming a Lamaze Certified Childbirth Educator, a media center, resource lists, and independent study programs. Lamaze, once known as the American Society for Psychoprophylaxis in Obstetrics (ASPO), promotes the birthing experience of being awake and aware during childbirth, supported by family and friends, with no maternal/infant separation. The resources section lists topics such as a forum on Lamaze, Ten Tips for a Healthy Pregnancy, and Childbirth: Then and Now. The site also offers information about Lamaze conferences. Training opportunities include a new Teen Specialist Training Program for those working with teen mothers, childbirth educator programs, breastfeeding support specialist training, and labor support specialist training. The site includes a cyberstore for Lamaze books, tapes and videos, links to other organizations and training programs, as well as archived articles from the Journal of Perinatal Education.

Evaluation:
This clearly is an informational site, primarily for Lamaze practitioners or those interested in becoming a Lamaze practitioner. The site, hosted by the former American Society for Psychoprophylaxis in Obstetrics, now Lamaze International, Inc., offers only basic information for the expectant or new mother. The site includes information on the history and membership of Lamaze International. It lists workshops and study programs for those seeking training programs. The Resources section does include Ten Tips for a Healthy Pregnancy, which outlines Lamaze philosophies pertaining to midwives, home births, birthing centers, medical intervention and the importance of women gaining control of their bodies. Other resources include discussion forums and links. This site would be particularly helpful for those researching Lamaze philosophies or seeking Lamaze training.

Where To Find/Buy:
On the Internet at the URL: http://www.lamaze-childbirth.com

Natural Childbirth

SPECIAL DELIVERY
A Guide To Creating The Birth You Want For You And Your Baby

Description:

Growing from a manual/tape series that accompanied classes taught by the author, this book focuses primarily on homebirths. The author, founder of the Informed Homebirth/Informed Birth and Parenting organization, combines her research and experiences with Kitzinger, LeBoyer, Peterson, and others in her book's second edition. The 169 pages are divided into 11 chapters; the table of contents detail the contents of each chapter. Chapter 1 gives an overview of the "revolution" taking place concerning childbirth with emphasis on advantages of a homebirth. The next 3 chapters focus on taking care of yourself (diet, exercise), and taking care of your baby during pregnancy. Chapters 5–9 concentrate on labor and delivery—stages of labor, pain management, how partners can work together during labor, complications and what to do, spiritual and psychological aspects (mind-body connections, etc.), and more. The final two chapters focus on the postpartum period for both the newborn and the parents; breastfeeding, and taking care of your baby, yourself, and others are some topics. Most chapters offer various homebirth stories.

Evaluation:

Although the option of having a homebirth is currently gaining more favor these days, there are not many books available to support those parents choosing this method of delivery. Parents for the most part must rely on the services and expertise of a midwife or doula if they choose to have their baby born at home. Useful sections in this book are those outlining complications and emergencies (a handy chart with page notations is provided at the beginning for quick reference), a section dealing with finding and interviewing a midwife, and the chapter on "Tools for Handling Labor" (various exercises for both partners to practice for managing pain). However, the book's general appearance, photographs, and text feel outdated, leaving one doubting the reliability of this method compared to others currently in vogue. Also, although this book does offer convincing arguments for the advantages of a homebirth, all it gives, for the most part, is very basic information regarding labor and delivery. There are more extensive resources than this one on the market which focus on natural childbirth.

Where To Find/Buy:

Bookstores and libraries, or order direct by calling (800) 841-BOOK.

Overall Rating
★★
Argues convincingly for homebirths; basic delivery and labor information presented

Design, Ease Of Use
★★
Textbook style; photographs dated; self-check Qs & charts for recording data

1–4 Stars

Author:
Rahima Baldwin Dancy

Dancy founded Informed Homebirth/Informed Birth and Parenting in 1977 and is an internationally-recognized childbirth educator. She is also a practicing midwife and co-director of The Birth Center (Dearborn, MI). She has also authored two other books.

Publisher:
Celestial Arts Publishing

Edition:
2nd (1996)

Price:
$17.95

Pages:
169

ISBN:
0890879346

Media:
Book

Principal Subject:
Childbirth

Childbirth Subject:
Natural Childbirth

★★

Overall Rating
★★
A unique retrospective, informative and detailed, especially for midwives

Design, Ease Of Use
★★
Well illustrated, well written, but far too "busy"

1–4 Stars

Author:
Ina May Gaskin

Ina May Gaskin is a midwife, mother of five, and a member of a group of midwives who provide prenatal care and attend births for a community currently consisting of 300 people. This community is called The Farm and was founded in 1971 near Summertown, Tennessee.

Publisher:
Book Publishing Company

Edition:
3rd (1990)

Price:
$16.95

Pages:
479

ISBN:
0913990639

Media:
Book

Principal Subject:
Childbirth

Childbirth Subject:
Natural Childbirth

Natural Childbirth

SPIRITUAL MIDWIFERY

Description:

Three books appear to be combined in one, giving the reader a unique perspective on the people and the midwives who inhabit a community called The Farm in Tennessee. The first book is a collection of stories from the midwives, birth mothers, and fathers, who first gathered together in 1971 as hippies in California. The experiences that led these women to become midwives, the trials and lessons they learned, and their unique spiritual views are revealed in this collection of stories. The second part incorporates the beliefs and principles of the people in this self-sufficient community and is a guide for the pregnant woman on prenatal care, preparing for the birth and the newborn, postnatal care, and more. The last section of this book is a primer for midwives. It takes the reader through things like: anatomy, the baby and its life support system, prenatal care, determining the baby's position in the pelvis, physiology and management of normal labor at home, tending to the baby at birth, follow-up care of the mother and baby, injuries and repairs, and a host of problems and complications a midwife may encounter.

Evaluation:

A unique book, this work takes one back to the 1970s with a force that must be read to be believed. In the first part, birth stories are shared in the language of that time. Intimate photographs of midwives and families are included that complete the flashback process. The subsequent section, offering the viewpoints of "The Farm" community members, how they care for each other, and their spiritual responsibilities, naturally sets up the final section of the book, the midwife primer. These stories and suggestions all support the decision to have a midwife attend the birth. This book also instructs a midwife on what her responsibilities and attitudes need to be for creating a "spiritual birth" experience. The final section is reassuring in its medical detail and attention to such things as prenatal testing, sterile environments, and what to do about complications (including getting medical advice and when to take women to hospitals). This book offers a very different look at childbirth; the text, unfortunately, is many times a distraction.

Where To Find/Buy:

Bookstores and libraries, or order direct by calling (800) 695-2241.

Natural Childbirth

WATER BIRTH INFORMATION

Description:

The Waterbirth website is "dedicated to the belief that every mother has the right to have the birth experience she wants, and to educate parents and birth care professionals about the extraordinary value of water labor and waterbirth to everyone concerned." At the site, visitors are given 15 options, several of which contain information about the site's designer, its production company, and other areas not directly related to waterbirth. The remainder of the site offers the following: mothers' personal waterbirth stories (long and short versions), general information about waterbirth, the benefits of waterbirth, how to prepare for waterbirth (your mind, the tub, the water, the birthing room, birth positions, dealing with debris, etc.), and a photo gallery containing more information about waterbirths via point and click pictures. A list of resources is offered, along with the "Water Baby" video, available through email or snail mail. Links also are provided to other child-related sites.

Evaluation:

The review and ratings of this site neither endorse nor challenge this method of childbirth; judgment is based on the cohesiveness of the website. Although this site contains elements not offered at other birthing methods' sites, more input will be needed to help in weighing the advantages of a waterbirth. Unusual topics at this site include how to prepare for a waterbirth, along with personal accounts of mothers using this method. Most other sites, in fact, could benefit from this personal input. The colorful graphics are a plus. The main criticism of this site is the lack of information on who sponsors it. All that the visitor receives is information on the site's designer, her beliefs, and promotional info on her other videos. Since a waterbirth spa ad is up-front and center on the site's homepage, is the site sponsored by a manufacturer? There are other resources that are more objectively informative than this one.

Where To Find/Buy:

On the Internet at the URL: http://www.well.com/user/karil/

Overall Rating
★★
Personal accounts of waterbirth deliveries, scant information on goals and rationale

Design, Ease Of Use
★★
Despite site's promotional nature, it's easily navigated

1–4 Stars

Publisher:
Point of View Productions

Media:
Internet

Principal Subject:
Childbirth

Childbirth Subject:
Natural Childbirth

III. Childbirth

III. Childbirth

Overall Rating

★

An anti-medical treatise on the use of midwives and at-home births

Design, Ease Of Use

★★

Site is straightforward; points difficult to discern without careful reading

1–4 Stars

Media:
Internet

Principal Subject:
Childbirth

Childbirth Subject:
Natural Childbirth

Natural Childbirth

THE FARM MIDWIVES
Summertown, Tennessee, USA

Description:

The Farm, started by Stephen and Ina May Gaskin and their followers in 1971, is "the largest working commune in America." The group was founded on the principles of "pronatalism, midwifery, and synergistic marriage, spiritual enlightenment. . . ." Ina May Gaskin is considered to be the "mother of authentic midwifery." The Farm's website offers several editorials, results of their home birth study, an interview with Ina May, the history of The Farm from the 1970s to the present, and a request for donations. Featured editorials include the following topics: "Boots At The Door" (a plea for legalizing midwifery); "Insurance Industry . . ." (a plea for health care for all); and "The Safety of Home Birth: The Farm" (a comparison of birth statistics between the Farm and those of a local hospital). The interview with Ina May focuses on her comparisons of maternity care systems in other countries to the U.S.'s, along with basic health care comparisons. The study is presented in full, with results highlighting that "under certain circumstances, home births . . . can be . . . as (safe) as . . . hospital deliveries."

Evaluation:

The U.S.'s determination to solve its medical crises, coupled with the current push for women to take a more proactive role in childbirth and pregnancy, make midwifery a "hot" topic. Advocates will enjoy reading the site's editorials (when you look past the typos); they have a decidedly anti-medical tone. Although the study concludes that home births with an attending midwife were as safe as those attended by physicians in a hospital setting, no evidence is offered that they are necessarily better. The most valuable features of the study are comparisons made between home births and hospital births in terms of the number of births that were "assisted" (C-section, forceps, vacuum extractor), the rate of C-sections, and the number of babies injured at birth (women with prior C-sections along with others, however, were omitted from this study). Women searching for convincing evidence to seek a midwife may get some support here, but they must look elsewhere for a more thorough treatment of the subject.

Where To Find/Buy:

On the Internet at the URL: http://www.thefarm.org/charities/mid.html

THE VBAC COMPANION
The Expectant Mother's Guide To Vaginal Birth After Cesarean

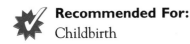

Recommended For:
Childbirth

Description:

Chapter 1 describes the advantages of a VBAC—Vaginal Birth After Cesarean—and includes information about Cesareans and VBACs in other countries. Chapter 2 describes women's common fears and suggests ways to cope with those fears. Chapter 3 helps a woman plan for a VBAC based on her individual Cesarean history, and Chapter 4 discusses common medical insurance options. Chapters 5 and 6 give tips on finding a "VBAC-friendly" health care provider and birthing center, and Chapter 7 provides information for a woman's birth partners. Details of a VBAC delivery are contained in Chapter 8, and Chapter 9 focuses on encouraging a woman to enjoy her birthing experience. Appendices include charts of VBACs, Cesareans, and infant mortality rates from a number of countries, and a resource directory listing organizations and contact information. A bibliography is provided for those who seek more information. Women's stories, illustrations, and lists of techniques complement the text.

Evaluation:

This is a book to be considered by any woman interested in a vaginal birth after a Cesarean birth history. The author's aim is clear—to provide the information a woman needs to make an appropriate decision based on her own medical history. Information is presented in a supportive and empowering manner that encourages women and their partners to reach the best birthing decision for them. "Take only what you want from this book, and ignore the rest," the author urges in her introduction. Despite its rather utilitarian name, *The VBAC Companion* covers important territory many other books on the subject do not. One example is the frank and supportive discussion aimed at sexual abuse survivors and how they can ensure that their birth experience proceeds smoothly and joyfully in light of their history. This is a book full of common sense and caring. The author hastens to say she is not a physician, but she obviously is someone sensitive to the needs of pregnant women. The presentation of material, the women's stories, and line illustrations that are included offer a book that will be a valuable companion for many pregnant women and their families.

Where To Find/Buy:
Bookstores and libraries.

★★★★

Overall Rating
★★★★
Provides clear, sensitive, complete information without stridency

Design, Ease Of Use
★★★★
Attractive, easy to read, soothing illustrations

1–4 Stars

Author:
Diana Korte

Diana Korte is the author of *Every Woman's Body* and co-author of *A Good Birth, A Safe Birth*. The winner of more than 40 awards for medical journalism, she writes on parenting for the *Los Angeles Times* Syndicate. She also hosts a public-radio interview program.

Publisher:
The Harvard Common Press

Edition:
1997

Price:
$12.95

Pages:
240

ISBN:
1558321292

Media:
Book

Principal Subject:
Childbirth

Childbirth Subject:
VBAC

III. Childbirth

★★★

Overall Rating
★★★
Positive, practical help for women hoping to birth naturally after a cesarean

Design, Ease Of Use
★★★
Effective blend of personal anecdote, advocacy, and specific techniques

1–4 Stars

Author:
Karis Crawford, PhD, and Johanne C. Walters, BSN, RN

Karis Crawford, Ph.D., is an independent writer and women's health advocate. Johanne C. Walters, B.S.N., R.N., is an obstetric nurse and childbirth educator. Both authors have experienced childbirth through C-sections and VBACs.

Publisher:
Blackwell Science

Edition:
1996

Price:
$14.95

Pages:
255

ISBN:
086542490X

Media:
Book

Principal Subject:
Childbirth

Childbirth Subject:
VBAC

Vaginal Birth After Cesarean

NATURAL CHILDBIRTH AFTER CESAREAN
A Practical Guide

Description:
Two women with professional and personal experiences in childbirth (both had normal childbirths after cesareans) wrote this 255 page book in the belief that women can experience a natural birth even if they have had one or more cesareans. This book offers advice, suggestions, and support for women who wish to try a vaginal birth after a cesarean. Accounts of the authors' eight births and numerous other women's experiences are shared in chapter 1 and throughout the book. Chapter 2 discusses the medical side of cesareans, including the rise in surgical interventions during birth, the risks attendant on cesarean surgery, and the myths and fears that may steer women towards C-sections. The third chapter is composed of 20 questions to determine your chances for delivering vaginally. Types of caregivers are discussed in the next two chapters, and chapters 6–8 take us through the journey from pregnancy to labor and through delivery. Chapter 9 discusses the repeat cesarean. The last chapter discusses how to sort out your feelings after birth and includes a "labor checklist" to note symptoms and solutions for the stages of labor and birth.

Evaluation:
It is incredible to note, as the foreword points out, that "From the 1960s to the 1970s the United States cesarean rate zoomed from 4% to over 25% with no improvement in mother or baby outcomes that could be directly linked to the higher rates." Reasons include the increasing unwillingness of medical practitioners to accept lengthy, difficult labors, and that most women who once had a cesarean were almost certain to have another. Although it looks as if changes in the health care industry are beginning to reverse this trend, this book should certainly fill a necessary role in educating and advocating for women who wish to birth naturally. The authors smoothly weave personal narrative, medical information, visualization and relaxation techniques, and emotional support in this book. But most effective is how they model what real women can do for themselves both in the delivery room and outside of it. For women hoping to deliver vaginally after a cesarean, this book may be of real help.

Where To Find/Buy:
Bookstores and libraries, or order direct by calling (800) 215-1000 or 617-876-7000.

Vaginal Birth After Cesarean

BIRTH AFTER CESAREAN
The Medical Facts

★★★

Description:

The author's extensive research on VBAC (vaginal birth after cesarean) includes "the world's largest study of normal birth after cesarean section." He is convinced that "for the majority of women normal birth after cesarean section is both safe and likely to succeed." This book was written to give an accurate, honest account of what is today "the most common major operation performed in the United States." In a Q & A format, this book responds to questions a woman may have about VBAC. The first three chapters discuss the medical facts about C-sections and a brief history of the operation up until modern day. Chapters 4–5 focus on the risks and benefits of VBAC. Chapter 6 discusses the reports of medical organizations and other groups to help you "make the decision." Pregnancy and labor after a C-section comes next, followed by a look at special situations (breech, twins, etc.). The last three chapters focus on birth alternatives, the doctor's role, and the future of birth in a modern world. A list of resource groups, organizations, and medical statements and reports on VBAC from the U.S. and around the world are given in the appendices.

Evaluation:

This is a persuasive case for VBAC in a straightforward question and answer format. Women considering VBAC will find the sheer number of facts, statistics, and report findings quoted here in its favor both convincing and heartening. Although this book focuses on the medical side of VBAC and offers little in the way of psychological/emotional support or advocacy for women, the fact that it contains so many positive facts and was written by a respected doctor should be profoundly reassuring. This author is neither on the side of "intractable doctors" that seek to dissuade women from VBAC nor on the side of "irate childbirth activists." Flamm's reference point is taken from the middle, allowing the facts to speak for themselves. And along with the "facts," the book presents a sensitivity to childbirth, and especially VBAC, being as much an emotional event as it is a physical challenge. As such, it can be a knowledgeable and helpful companion for women who are discerning whether their next birth can and should be a successful VBAC.

Where To Find/Buy:

Bookstores and libraries.

Overall Rating
★★★
A factual and accurate rendering of the success of VBAC

Design, Ease Of Use
★★
Digestible question and answer format

1–4 Stars

Author:
Bruce L. Flamm, MD

The author is director of research at the Kaiser Permanente Medical Center in Riverside, CA, and associate clinical professor of obstetrics and gynecology at the University of California, Irvine. He has published extensively on cesarean-related topics.

Publisher:
Fireside (Simon & Schuster)

Edition:
1990

Price:
$11.00

Pages:
197

ISBN:
0671792180

Media:
Book

Principal Subject:
Childbirth

Childbirth Subject:
VBAC

III. Childbirth

Overall Rating
★
Heavy on birthing horror stories and personal opinion

Design, Ease Of Use
★★
Straightforward layout and design

1–4 Stars

Author:
Andrea Frank Henkart

Henkart holds an MA in psychology from Sonoma State University. She is a holistic health educator, a certified childbirth educator, and cofounder of the Marin County chapter of the International Cesarean Awareness Network.

Publisher:
Bergin & Garvey
(Greenwood Publishing Group)

Edition:
1995

Price:
$14.95

Pages:
178

ISBN:
0897892941

Media:
Book

Principal Subject:
Childbirth

Childbirth Subject:
VBAC

Vaginal Birth After Cesarean

TRUST YOUR BODY! TRUST YOUR BABY!
Childbirth Wisdom And Cesarean Prevention

Description:

This book consists of 12 essays written by eight authors about childbirth and issues surrounding Cesarean sections. Contributors include author/editor Henkart, who wrote eight of the essays; Robbie E. Davis-Floyd, a cultural anthropologist; Gina Maria Alibrandi, a registered nurse specializing in maternal-child nursing; Donna Germano, a psychotherapist specializing in post-traumatic stress syndrome and women's issues, and a founder of Hospice in America; Jeannine Parvati Baker, author, midwife, astrologer, herbalist, and speaker; John Gray, author of *Men Are From Mars, Women Are From Venus*; author Robin Lim; and Marilyn Fayre Milos, a registered nurse and founder of the National Organization of Circumcision Information Resource Centers. Appendices include: Questions to Ask Your Care Provider, Ideas for Your Birth Plan, Affirmations for Childbirth Preparation; Things You Can Do to Avoid Unnecessary Cesareans, and Sources of Further Information. Also included are a bibliography and suggested reading list, as well as two forewords, by Nancy Wainer Cohen and Michel Odent, MD.

Evaluation:

Henkart opens this book with the stories of her own two traumatic birthing experiences and seems determined throughout to emphasize the negative aspects of all births that do not meet the rigid expectations of what she calls "purebirth . . . a birth that is completely free of medical intervention . . . I was introduced to childbirth by a silent knife," she writes. "It crept up on me when I least expected it." Not all the essays are as uniformly frightening. One focuses on the need for better childbirth education, another cries out against the perceived inhumanity of circumcision. The bright spot of the book is John Gray's Chapter 11, "The Husband's Role in Pregnancy." His writing is clear and insightful. He suggests birth partners be prepared for the communication style differences between men and women so that their childbirth experience can be as positive as possible. It is unfortunate that prospective parents would have to read through so much fear-evoking surrounding material to get to Gray's contribution. "My innermost goal has been to affect healing of birth in a loving and gentle way," writes Henkart in Chapter 16. Yet her message throughout is one of fear, pain, and intolerance.

Where To Find/Buy:

Bookstores and libraries.

Vaginal Birth After Cesarean

THE EXPECTANT PARENT'S GUIDE TO PREVENTING A CESAREAN SECTION

Description:

The Expectant Parent's Guide to Preventing a Cesarean Section is presented in seven chapters that include "The Rising Cesarean Rate," "Indications for a Cesarean Section," "How Unnecessary Cesareans Are Made," "Ten Steps to Take during Pregnancy to Prevent a Cesarean," "Cesarean Prevention during Labor," "Vaginal Birth after a Previous Cesarean," and "If a Cesarean is Necessary." The book offers resource lists, a list of additional suggested reading material, and an index, as well as a foreword by Donald Creevy, MD. Most sections include lists of tips and points pertaining to each individual subject.

Evaluation:

This is not a book for prospective parents seeking unbiased information about Cesarean sections. This author has a strong point of view: physicians in the U.S. perform too many Cesarean sections, and most healthy women can deliver vaginally. Unfortunately, Jones too often dips into the wells of fear and distrust to make his points. Even the book's chapter titles and subheadings invoke fear instead of educated enlightenment. Consider just a handful of subtitles found early in the book: "Wildfire," "Surgical Birth Trauma," "Physical Trauma to the Mother" (with, he gleefully informs us, increased risk of death, pain, and illness), and "Emotional Trauma to Both Parents." Perhaps most insidious of all is the author's apparent determination to make a woman distrust her physician's and caregiver's competency and advice, suggesting they may try to trick her into an unneeded medical procedure. While vaginal birth is by far the preferred method of childbirth and VBACs are something to work toward, one is hard pressed to see what is accomplished by instilling fear within a pregnant woman rather than positive support and substantial knowledge.

Where To Find/Buy:

Bookstores and libraries.

Overall Rating

★

Sensationalistic, fear-inducing, one-sided

Design, Ease Of Use

★

Even chapter titles and subheading sections seem to encourage mistrust

1–4 Stars

Author:

Carl Jones

Jones, a certified childbirth educator, is author of 10 books about childbirth and parenting, including *Mind Over Matter* which "introduced guided imagery to the childbearing public." He serves as consultant to many organizations, including the American Red Cross.

Publisher:

Bergin & Garvey
(Greenwood Publishing Group)

Edition:

1991

Price:

$12.95

Pages:

159

ISBN:

0897892232

Media:

Book

Principal Subject:

Childbirth

Childbirth Subject:

VBAC

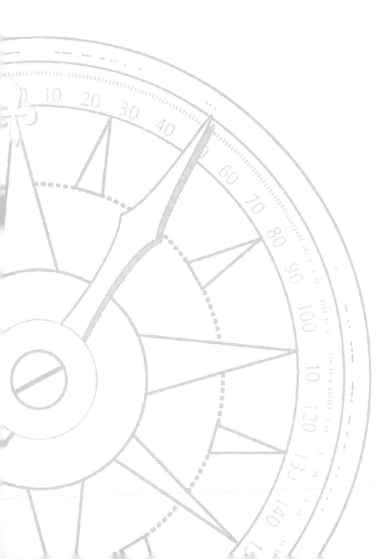

POSTPARTUM
MATERNAL CARE

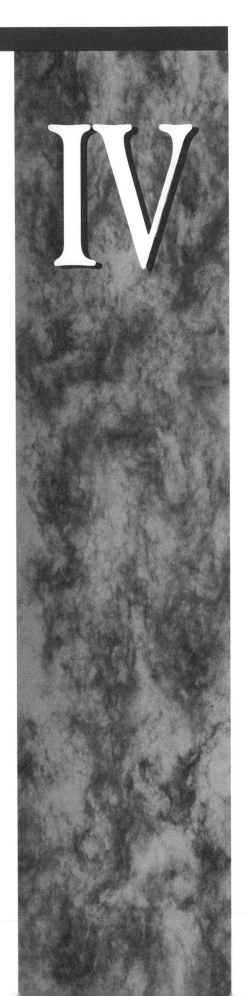

IV

INTRODUCTION

In most human cultures throughout history, new mothers have been honored and cared for by their extended families. In traditional Korean culture, for example, new mothers stayed in bed for a month after giving birth. Unfortunately, in our modern culture with limited involvement by extended families, most mothers face the tasks of taking care of both themselves and their newborns without much support or assistance. Even when helpful family or friends provide assistance or advice for newborn care, we have lost our cultural traditions of supporting and caring for the mother, not just the baby.

After a vaginal birth, most mothers need about four to six weeks for their bodies to recover from the pregnancy. The uterus needs to contract back to its pre-pregnancy size, the placental site needs to heal, the blood volume should return to normal, and the joints loosened by a special hormone during pregnancy must get solid again. This physical recovery takes longer especially if the mother is anemic after the birth, if any complications such as high blood pressure or diabetes have occurred during pregnancy, or if the perineum has had significant injury from a tear or episiotomy during childbirth. Some mothers, whose doctors recommended bed rest before childbirth, will find they need extra time to recover their stamina. And those mothers who have undergone a Cesarean birth, which is considered major abdominal surgery, will require a minimum of six weeks before the mother should lift anything. Most mothers who have had a Cesarean or an episiotomy will also be advised to wait until their postpartum check-up to resume strenuous exercise or sexual activity. However, "medical disability" from work usually lasts only six to eight weeks, clearly an inadequate length of time for a woman's full emotional and physical recovery after giving birth.

Until the last ten or fifteen years, women commonly stayed in the hospital for up to a week after childbirth. They were fed and cared for by nurses, and allowed a few days to recover from birth. While these extended hospitalizations (with the baby usually in the hospital nursery) did not help breastfeeding initiation, they did allow the mother a bit more supported time before she was on her own with her baby. However, nowadays, with the average hospital stay being less than 48 hours for a vaginal birth and 72 hours for a Cesarean birth, a woman needs to plan for a support system at home after her discharge from the hospital. A new mother should carefully consider whom she wants with her at this time. Ideally, her at-home support people will share her commitment to breastfeeding and understand her need to care for her baby herself. The support person's main duties should be to feed the mother, keep her supplied with plenty of water, rock the baby when the mother needs a break for a nap or a bath, and to "run interference" for any external stresses that may present themselves. This ideal person may be the baby's father, but more often is another woman who has lived through this transitional time herself—a grandmother, a mother, an aunt, a friend, or a Doula.

The first few weeks after giving birth present many physical and emotional changes. A huge hormonal shift, a sore bottom, and exhaustion from giving birth, are accompanied with the necessary tasks of learning how to care for a newborn, learning how to breastfeed, and getting acquainted with a whole new human being and understanding their needs. Understandably this can lead to feelings of being overwhelmed! The "baby-blues," a period of tearfulness and depressed mood, affects about 85 percent of new mothers during the first few weeks after birth. For some mothers, however, these "blues" can become more severe or extended, eventually leading to postpartum depression or postpartum obsessive compulsive disorder. Symptoms of these more severe disorders may include an inability to sleep (even when the opportunity presents itself!), a drastic change in eating patterns, pervasive thoughts of suicide or of harming the baby, or an overwhelming and incapacitating fear that someone or something else will hurt the baby. If any of these symptoms occur, a new mother should not hesitate to get help by calling her healthcare provider or contacting a local crisis service.

For most mothers, however, those early weeks at home with their newborn babies are joy-filled "baby-honeymoons." Put aside all those plans you had for everything you were going to accomplish during your "vacation," and just enjoy your new baby. Don't turn down any offers of food or housecleaning, do turn down most offers for babysitting, sleep when the baby sleeps, and try to find someone willing to pamper you for a while!

Following this section are our recommendations for those resources that explain what happens during the postpartum period after childbirth and its possible effect on you physically, emotionally, and socially. These resources will alert you to what's normal, what's not, possible danger signs to be aware of, how to find daily support to help you during this period, and how to find professional help if needed. Be sure to read our full-page reviews of these resources to find the ones that can best serve your needs.

Additionally, fathers who are in need of guidance and support to help them during this period may wish to read our recommendations in **Section V—"Specifically for Fathers."** Although most of these resources focus on the father's transition, some of these resources also offer suggestions to fathers on how to understand and help their partner during this sometimes stressful period.

★★★★

Overall Rating
★★★★
Most comprehensive guide to dealing with and understanding postpartum "blues"

Design, Ease Of Use
★★★★
Summaries given before each chapter, numerous case examples, checklists, and more

1–4 Stars

Author
Ann Dunnewold, PhD and Diane G. Sanford, PhD

Dunnewold, a psychologist, specializes in women's mental health issues, including prenatal and postpartum adjustment, pregnancy loss, infertility, and PMS. Sanford, a psychologist, educator, and mother, is nationally recognized for the treatment of postpartum disorders.

Publisher:
New Harbinger Publications

Edition:
1994

Price:
$13.95

Pages:
275

ISBN:
1879237806

Media:
Book

Principal Subject:
Postpartum Maternal Care

POSTPARTUM SURVIVAL GUIDE

 Recommended For:
Postpartum Maternal Care

Description:

As the authors of this 275 page self-help book state, "This book was written to let you know that having a baby is a tough adjustment: feeling lost or down or nervous is completely understandable." Citing research that says 50–80% of all new mothers experience the "blues" with 10–20% experiencing long-lasting negative feelings, this book delves into postpartum depression, how to take care of yourself, and ways to cope. A continuum of reactions to new parenthood is the topic of chapter 2 including checklists, descriptions, and case examples for: normal postpartum depression, postpartum mania, postpartum panic, obsessive-compulsive reaction, and post-traumatic stress. Chapter 3 focuses on biological, psychological, and relationship risk factors that can cause postpartum difficulties; questionnaires are provided. The next 3 chapters focus on how new parents can take care of themselves, including a chapter for "single mothers, older mothers, adoptive mothers, and families with infertility issues." Other chapters discuss professional help, prenatal planning tips to reduce postpartum feelings, and more.

Evaluation:

New mothers sometimes have difficulty with feelings of self-blame, disillusionment with motherhood, and isolation. Knowing you aren't alone and hoping that you'll eventually get beyond this period may help, but it isn't enough. Fortunately, this book takes you much further than the chapter provided in most childbirth books on the subject of postpartum "blues." You'll find tools and strategies within each chapter to help you manage your feelings and move forward. For example, if you're feeling overwhelmed or powerless, the authors suggest that you "single out one area in which you do have control, and in which you are accomplishing something . . . write this down on a notecard and post it . . . pat yourself on the back . . . take things one day at a time . . ." Another suggestion when you feel your identity is lost is to think of yourself as a pie chart with various segments such as mother, wife, teacher, etc.; while one segment at the moment is the largest, the rest are still there. If someone you know is suffering alone or needing emotional support after having a baby, do them a favor. Offer them an empathetic ear and this book.

Where To Find/Buy:

Bookstores and libraries.

THIS ISN'T WHAT I EXPECTED
Recognizing And Recovering From Depression And Anxiety After Childbirth

★★★★

 Recommended For:
Postpartum Maternal Care

Description:

Authors Kleiman and Raskin draw on their own experiences as medical professionals and mothers to discuss postpartum depression and related anxiety disorders triggered by pregnancy. As many as 30 percent of women experience some degree of post-pregnancy anxiety, the authors say, and their suffering too often is misunderstood. The book describes the syndrome of postpartum depression and includes checklists of both depression and panic disorders to allow readers to early on gauge their own level of concern. One chapter is written specifically for a woman's partner; another is devoted to helping mobilize support from a spouse, family and friends. The book also addresses unresolved issues with a woman's parents that may be affecting her sense of personal esteem as she struggles with postpartum depression. The authors also describe stages of recovery and common concerns that may emerge as a woman recovers. Included are a number of checklists and assessments, including the authors' own Raskin-Kleiman Postpartum Depression and Anxiety Assessment.

Evaluation:

Readers will find solid information, reassurance and common sense here. The book's plain packaging may cause some bookstore browsers to pass it by, but that would be a mistake. Despite the unimaginative cover, the book presents 288 pages of straightforward information any woman suffering from a postpartum anxiety disorder can use immediately. Readers will learn the latest scientific theories about possible causes of postpartum anxieties and depression and when to seek emergency help. They'll discover how to get through the day when every hour seems impossible. "Get out of bed, even if you feel like you can't," is first on an empathetic list that also urges setting aside time for crying, if needed, and nurturing oneself. Quirky chapter titles, easy reading of on-target information and patients' stories pull readers along. Who among us could pass up Chapter 5, "I'm Tired, Fat, Ugly, and Still Wearing My Nightgown at Noon," which turns out to offer a new mother fighting depression dozens of ways to nurture herself even when she hasn't the energy to comb her hair. Self-help is the book's focus, and healthy self-empowerment is its aim making this one of the best for helping someone dealing with postpartum depression.

Where To Find/Buy:
Bookstores and libraries.

Overall Rating
★★★★
Full of practical straightforward advice based on the authors' self-help program

Design, Ease Of Use
★★★★
Particularly approachable with bulleted lists, self-assessment questions, and more

1–4 Stars

Author
Karen R. Kleiman, MSW and Valerie D. Raskin, MD

Kleiman, a licensed clinical social worker, is founder of the Postpartum Stress Center (Philadelphia). Raskin, a psychiatrist, was director of the Pregnancy and Postpartum Treatment program (Department of Psychiatry) at the University of IL College of Medicine.

Publisher:
Bantam Books (Bantam Doubleday Dell Publishing)

Edition:
1994

Price:
$12.95

Pages:
297

ISBN:
0553370758

Media:
Book

Principal Subject:
Postpartum Maternal Care

★★★★

Overall Rating
★★★★
A beautiful, useful and compassionate book for surviving your first year as a mother

Design, Ease Of Use
★★★★
Clear color illustrations; highlighted inserts useful for self-help tips

1–4 Stars

Author
Sheila Kitzinger

Sheila Kitzinger is the author of twenty-two books, including the bestselling *The Complete Book of Pregnancy and Childbirth*. She has an international reputation as a social anthropologist, researcher, and women's advocate on pregnancy.

Publisher:
Charles Scribner's Sons

Edition:
1994

Price:
$13.00

Pages:
302

ISBN:
0684825201

Media:
Book

Principal Subject:
Postpartum Maternal Care

THE YEAR AFTER CHILDBIRTH
Surviving And Enjoying The First Year Of Motherhood

 Recommended For:
Postpartum Maternal Care

Description:

The Year After Childbirth is 302 pages long and divided into fourteen chapters. The book begins with an introductory overview of the challenges and changes a woman can expect to face in the coming year. Then each chapter takes a different aspect of a woman's experience and expands on it. The topics included are: how your body changes with childbirth, learning to enjoy your body again, movement and exercises, understanding the strains and possible damage to the pelvic floor, bladder and vagina and what to do about it, breastfeeding, nutrition, depression in mothers, recognizing the personality of your child, the development of father's feelings, changes to your identity and relationships, and information on resuming your sex life. The final chapter is titled "Coming up for Air" and focuses on what a new mother can do to care for herself amid the stresses of caring for another. This book includes a glossary of terms, reference notes, a list of "helpful organizations," and an index. This book is intended to be a practical tool for the potentially stressful first year of parenthood.

Evaluation:

This book is a must read for any first-time mother. Up-to-date and concise, it is also insightful and compassionate. Beginning with information from what is normal bleeding and what is not, to the physical maladies that linger after labor, this book offers complete support with clear advice of what a woman can do to help herself. Detailed information on such things as: the pelvic-floor muscles; how to avoid surgeon-recommended "repairs;" problems inherent with episiotomies; and other information concerning why one may not want particular medical treatments. Other issues of motherhood, including depression and its causes, are also given thorough and up-to-date treatment. This work also contains a beautiful chapter on fatherhood. In short, the book addresses many more challenges than are reviewed here; and each is easily referenced, well-illustrated and practical. A lovely book to look at as well as to read, this one will sit on the nightstand and be well-thumbed.

Where To Find/Buy:

Bookstores and libraries.

OVERCOMING POSTPARTUM DEPRESSION & ANXIETY

Description:

The author uses her background as a nurse and psychotherapist, as well as her own firsthand experience, to provide information regarding postpartum mood disorders, an often misunderstood and seldom-discussed consequence of having children. ". . . There was little discussion about the adjustment period following the birth and no mention of how devastating postpartum blues can be, let alone the possibility of more severe depression," she writes. These 129 pages include eight chapters, an appendix/resource list, a bibliography and an index. Peppered throughout the book are firsthand accounts of women who have experienced different types of mood disorders. Discussions include the background and history of the study of postpartum mood disorders, the lack of awareness and information available to new mothers, risk factors, typical symptoms and classification methods. Specific chapters are included which briefly discuss the different types of anxiety and depression along with a list of symptoms typically experienced in each disorder. The effects on the new baby and other family members, particularly spouses, also is addressed.

Evaluation:

This book is a useful primer for those who may be experiencing a postpartum disorder and are seeking information about what is happening to them. Throughout, the author offers a good balance of medical explanation, experiential knowledge, and practical advice. Medical descriptions are clear and understandable to a lay person, thorough without being overwhelming. Descriptions are short and to the point, a bonus to someone who is suffering and seeks readily accessible information. The author addresses the importance of getting professional, medical help and does not downplay the potential seriousness of the problems. In addition, common sense self-help methods are included and serve as useful reminders to a woman who may need simple advice. A comprehensive index serves as a quick reference tool for finding specific information provided within the book. What makes this book stand out is that it covers a lot of useful information in a short time. Information is clear and succinct, making it a good starting point for anyone who is searching for a foundation of knowledge regarding postpartum mood disorders.

Where To Find/Buy:

Bookstores, libraries, or order direct by calling (800) 352-2873.

★★★

Overall Rating
★★★
Excellent primer balances medical information, experience, and commonsense advice

Design, Ease Of Use
★★★
Short, concise chapters; bullets, boxed highlights, narratives; comprehensive index

1–4 Stars

Author
Linda Sebastian

Sebastian is a psychiatric nurse with 25 years of experience. An Advanced Registered Nurse Practitioner, she provides outpatient therapy, medication management, and education for professionals about postpartum depression and anxiety.

Publisher:
Addicus Books

Edition:
1998

Price:
$12.95

Pages:
129

ISBN:
1886039348

Media:
Book

Principal Subject:
Postpartum Maternal Care

IV. Postpartum
Maternal Care

★★★

Overall Rating
★★★
Informative, intense, a bit vague at times due to the subjective nature of the illness

Design, Ease Of Use
★★★
Numerous narratives from mothers; chapters are well-organized, topics well-indexed

1–4 Stars

Author
Sharon L. Roan

Roan is a journalist and a mother. She has received many awards for her research, and she is the personal health columnist for the *Los Angeles Times*.

Publisher:
Adams Media

Edition:
1997

Price:
$9.95

Pages:
246

ISBN:
1558507655

Media:
Book

Principal Subject:
Postpartum Maternal Care

POSTPARTUM DEPRESSION
Every Woman's Guide To Diagnosis, Treatment, & Prevention

Description:

Roan has not herself experienced postpartum depression, but she has been both personally and professionally affected by it. As a newspaper reporter, she came to know a woman who killed her infant while suffering postpartum psychosis. Within her personal social circle, half suffered postpartum depression to the point that it "shattered" lives. Roan believes that many women (and others in their life) are caught unaware and unprepared to deal with postpartum depression. Within this resource's 246 pages, Roan offers ". . . Information and solutions these women need, through the advice of the top experts in the field and the personal experiences of dozens of women who have recovered from this postpartum illness." In the first half of the book, the reader is educated about depression in general, and postpartum in particular. Throughout the book, there is an emphasis on private/nonprofessional measures to help the PPD sufferer; professional interventions are also highlighted. The book acknowledges some ramifications for the entire family of a PPD sufferer. An 8 page "Resource" guide, bibliography, and more are given.

Evaluation:

This book conveys the harsh realities of PPD; it would most likely be too overwhelming for any reader who is already a victim. But for others (a pregnant women, a friend, a spouse, an in-law, etc.) who want to gain an understanding of the topic, this book will offer insight. While Roan does state that a minority of women suffer from PPD, she describes so many severe situations that the reader may feel threatened. Roan's findings may be accurate, but it may unnecessarily alarm prospective mothers believing that this condition will virtually happen to them after their baby is born. More unsettling is Roan's assertion that this is not a condition fully understood, easily treatable, or completely acknowledged within the medical community. Roan does provide a useful resource guide to help the reader obtain help for an individual situation. Readers will find comfort in the author's thrust to the reader to understand as much as possible about PPD, accept the reality, look for treatment if need be, and offer support for those suffering from PPD.

Where To Find/Buy:

Bookstores, libraries, or order direct by calling (800) 872-5627, or (617) 767-8100 in Massachusetts.

AFTER THE BABY'S BIRTH . . . A WOMAN'S WAY TO WELLNESS
A Complete Guide For Postpartum Women

★★

Description:

This book is intended as a guide for postpartum women, written from the author's perspective and experience as a mother of five children. Chapters describe the physical and psychological phases a woman may experience during the postpartum period, from birth through year four. There are four main parts to this 308 page resource. Within Parts One and Two are sections which cover breastfeeding and breast care, postpartum pelvic health, and toning exercises for the postpartum mother. Other sections address such issues as health care, exercises, infections, and the return to sexual activity. An exercise section to help a woman tone and stretch her body includes explanations and drawings for illustrative purposes. Part Three—the health section—includes chapters on healing touch, Eastern philosophies of women's health, and the Ayurvedic lifestyle. The last part of the book includes information and shared stories regarding various "issues of the heart," including bonding, postpartum blues, single mothers and children who have died.

Evaluation:

The author, a mother of several children, uses her experiences from the traditions of her home in Hawaii along with a lifestyle that leans more toward the organic. Although there is much useful information regarding breastfeeding and general health, it is important for the reader to keep in mind that the author writes mainly from her own perspective, without taking into account much individuality between women. The tone in several parts of the book seems to dictate to a woman what to feel. The discussions regarding postpartum pelvic health and toning exercises are especially useful. Additionally, the breastfeeding and breast care section covers every aspect of the topic including the physiology behind lactation. The book is comprehensive and informative. The chapter on the Ayurvedic lifestyle is interesting, but seems best suited for another book. This book offers some practical advice along with moral support and encouragement to a postpartum woman. It would be especially useful to women who practice or desire a more natural lifestyle.

Where To Find/Buy:

Bookstores and libraries.

Overall Rating
★★
Promotes a natural lifestyle, with comprehensive information on breastfeeding

Design, Ease Of Use
★★★
Good layout, easy to read; many illustrations

1–4 Stars

Author
Robin Lim
Lim, the mother of five, has written for "Mothering" magazine and many local publications in her home state of Hawaii.

Publisher:
Celestial Arts

Edition:
1991

Price:
$14.95

Pages:
308

ISBN:
0890875901

Media:
Book

Principal Subject:
Postpartum Maternal Care

IV. Postpartum Maternal Care

★★

Overall Rating
★★
Much background on various topics, balanced with useful, practical information

Design, Ease Of Use
★★★
Wordy at times, but excellent resource lists are provided at the end of each chapter

1–4 Stars

Author
Sally Placksin

Placksin has written, produced, and narrated many national radio programs, including the documentary "Mothering the New Mother" for National Public Radio's Horizons series. She has received various grants and awards and is the mother of two children.

Publisher:
Newmarket Press

Edition:
1994

Price:
$15.95

Pages:
328

ISBN:
1557041784

Media:
Book

Principal Subject:
Postpartum Maternal Care

MOTHERING THE NEW MOTHER
Your Postpartum Resource Companion

Description:

This book is about the care and comfort necessary for new mothers. The author asserts that American society expects the transition to new motherhood to be accomplished effortlessly and without support when, in reality, many new mothers feel overwhelmed by the life changing experience of giving birth. Many wide-ranging issues are covered in the book's nine chapters: realistic expectations of a new mother's feelings after childbirth, postpartum rituals in different cultures, support and assistance during the postpartum weeks, breastfeeding, postpartum depression, returning to work, staying at home, and helping siblings deal with a newborn. Resources are listed at the end of each chapter, rather than at the end of the book. First-person experiences and testimony illustrate the author's points. The author, who compiled her information in part by collecting questionnaires from new mothers, discusses in depth the concept of a doula, or a mother's helper. Advice on "creating a postpartum plan" is offered in the final chapter in which the author assists the reader in creating a support network using worksheets and checklists.

Evaluation:

There is much attention given to background, personal testimonials, and history of the various subjects the author addresses. However, the "practical, useful" information is wisely separated from the main body of the text by the use of sidebars, so that the reader can choose what level of information to focus on. Chapters also are divided into short, relevant subsections. The detail the author provides is quite comprehensive, although not concise, and fairly easy to understand. Some may find that there are too many statistics and too much history given without enough practical, working knowledge provided. This book's most valuable asset for new mothers and fathers is the resource list at the end of each chapter. Each entry includes contact information along with detailed descriptions of what the resource includes. These resources, however, will be more beneficial to those who desire and have the time to coordinate background information with practical how-tos. This resource is better suited for those who support postpartum mothers; those wanting more immediate help may need to rely on other more succinct resources.

Where To Find/Buy:

Bookstores and libraries.

COMPOSING MYSELF
A Journey Through Postpartum Depression

★★

Description:

Shaw says, "It seems paradoxical to say that my writing has been, in some way, close to a scream. Not that it is one, but that it's been trying to make sense of what it was that took me beyond words." Shaw begins her personal narrative story by describing her relationship and life with her husband around the time their first daughter was born. Life during this time was harmonious. Then, within 10 days of giving birth to her second daughter, life became miserable and confusing. The remainder of this book ponders Shaw's personal feelings and experiences relating to her severe postpartum depression. She was hospitalized, given ECT (electroconvulsive therapy), medications, and assigned psychiatrists. Professionals encouraged Shaw to try to forget the experience, yet she wanted to reach an understanding and requested referral to a psychologist. Eventually, she used her inheritance to fund private counseling. Both her writing and her counseling have brought her some peace, or as she states, "Nevertheless it has been by way of words—my words—that I have gradually taken hold of my life."

Evaluation:

Presenting a unique view of the topic of postpartum depression (PPD), this is the story of Shaw's personal journey. Readers drawn to this book because of an interest in learning about PPD will fully realize the author's message that help is not readily available, and that there is no easy cure. Because Shaw details both of her pregnancies, it may seem clear to PPD information seekers that she experienced extreme depression by apparent chance. Shaw conveys on nearly every page that, at least in her case, the most effective treatment was introspection/psychotherapy. Although Shaw's depression was triggered by the birth of her second child, this story focuses less on pregnancy, instead emphasizing honestly knowing oneself through all of one's life experiences. This story is embellished with imagery and sensory detail which help to translate the tremendous sadness, emptiness, and aloneness that Shaw had to work through. For those who would prefer to read a personal narrative of PPD rather than a more medically-based description and treatment of PPD, this book will offer insight and a possible course of action. Others may feel more comfort in a resource that offers narrative stories and more easily accessed information.

Where To Find/Buy:

Bookstores and libraries.

Overall Rating
★★
Personal journal of one woman's struggle with PPD and possible treatments

Design, Ease Of Use
★★
Reads as a novel, a relatively chronological introspective; no cross-referencing or index

1–4 Stars

Author
Fiona Shaw
Shaw suffered one year of postpartum depression which forced her and her infant into hospital care. She lives in northern England and is now working on her first novel.

Publisher:
Steerforth Press

Edition:
1998

Price:
$24.00

Pages:
210

ISBN:
1883642973

Media:
Book

Principal Subject:
Postpartum Maternal Care

★★

Overall Rating
★★
Useful for those considering hormone therapy

Design, Ease Of Use
★★
Clearly presented, numerous personal stories provided; tone somewhat formal and aloof

1–4 Stars

Author
Katharina Dalton with Wendy M. Holton

Dalton is an international authority on premenstrual syndrome and postnatal depression (PND). She is also a pioneer of hormone therapy.

Publisher:
Oxford University Press

Edition:
3rd (1996)

Price:
$15.95

Pages:
206

ISBN:
0192861859

Media:
Book

Principal Subject:
Postpartum Maternal Care

DEPRESSION AFTER CHILDBIRTH
How to Recognize, Treat, And Prevent Postnatal Depression

Description:

In the introduction, PND is defined as "the first occurrence of psychiatric symptoms severe enough to require medical help occurring after childbirth and before the return of menstruation." Dalton stresses early identification of symptoms, including anticipation of and preparation for PND before a baby is born. Based on her area of expertise, Dalton emphasizes treatment of PND through the use of hormone therapy. The book begins by explaining the role of hormones in the body. Then, several chapters detail symptoms of PND: "The Blues," "Black Depression," "Endless Exhaustion," "Irrational Irritability," "Not Tonight, Darling," "Psychosis," and "Infanticide and Homicide." While Dalton distinguishes between the "blues," "depression," and "premenstrual syndrome," she relates each one as a hormonal condition. Interspersed amid the medical teachings, the reader will find quotes from individual sufferers. The book concludes with an explanation of the hormonal treatments that are available, along with placing responsibility on professionals and nonprofessionals to identify when a woman needs treatment for PND.

Evaluation:

While acknowledging that there can be psychological factors, Dalton expresses faith in hormone therapy to successfully treat PND. The opening discussions of hormones and their role in the body is educational for the reader; the graphs and charts included here are effective, as are illustrations in a later chapter correlating PND and PMS. The author's historical overview and discussion on mental illness and PND helps the reader to understand the experts' scheme for the understanding and treatment of PND. While this book offers good insight into the topic of PND and how it can be treated with hormone therapy, there is only limited mention of other treatment possibilities. Also, even though personal quotes are inserted throughout the text, there is a rather formal and professional tone to this book which may deter some readers. Considering that this book was originally published in England, many of the "Useful Addresses" and "Further Reading" listings are also to be found outside of the USA. Primarily useful for those considering hormone therapy, others interested in a discussion of other possible treatments will need further back-up resources.

Where To Find/Buy:

Bookstores, libraries, or order direct by contacting Oxford University Press, Inc., 200 Madison Avenue, New York, NY 10016.

SHOULDN'T I BE HAPPY?

Description:

Misri has written this 340 page book as a resource for mothers and their network of supporters. Following the birth of her first son, Misri was supported in her postpartum period by Indian tradition. At that time, her mother and a family assistant came from India for six months to nurture mother and baby. In contrast, Misri points out that in the industrialized West, we should consider giving "distinct recognition and support to women in the postpartum period." To that end, this book considers many possible problems of the postpartum period (psychological, medical, and obstetrical) as well as some specific events (miscarriage, fetal abnormalities, congenital defects, death, depression and mood disorders, breastfeeding and psychiatric illness, and marital upset). Misri fears that, and offers her rationale why, many suffer in silence. While the general focus of the book is based on psychiatric counseling, alternatives such as medications and electroconvulsive treatment are also considered in "Part II—Getting Professional Help." Along with her insights, patients' stories are included throughout the book.

Evaluation:

As with many books available on "emotional problems of pregnant and postpartum women," this book was written to help the reader acknowledge, accept, and cope with postpartum depression (PPD). As described in the book's title, Misri gives some good rationale to illustrate the cultural and individual motives for denying postpartum problems rather than dealing with them. Her book describes how closely the mother's self-perception and consequent emotional state are connected to her perceived success or failure as a mother. She does a fine job at outlining the varying emotional problems of pregnant and postpartum women. However, the patient stories she includes do not particularly convey the intensity of those emotions or personal struggles; they tend to serve as mere illustrations of psychological influences and the effects they can impart. Misri also makes certain judgements about mothers that appear biased and not well-founded, especially in regards to breastfeeding. No resource list is included to connect the reader with a professional who might help. This book was clearly written from a psychiatric point-of-view and adheres to that reference point throughout the book.

Where To Find/Buy:

Bookstores and libraries.

Overall Rating

★

Information does not come across as particularly solid, influential, or stimulating

Design, Ease Of Use

★★

Logical organization with Q and A segments, personal stories; rather clinical tone

1–4 Stars

Author

Shaila Misri, MD

Misri (mother of two) is a clinical professor of psychiatry and obstetrics/gynecology at the University of British Columbia (Vancouver, Canada). She also serves as the Director of the Reproductive Psychiatry Program at St. Paul's Hospital.

Publisher:
The Free Press
(Simon & Schuster)

Edition:
1995

Price:
$23.00

Pages:
340

ISBN:
002921405X

Media:
Book

Principal Subject:
Postpartum Maternal Care

IV. Postpartum Maternal Care

Overall Rating

★

Focuses on mothers who kill their children, melodramatic, with little practical info

Design, Ease Of Use

★

Chapters barely touch on each subject, focusing instead on sensationalized case histories

1–4 Stars

Author

Arlene M. Huysman, PhD

Huysman is a practicing clinical psychologist specializing in mood disorders with more than two decades of professional experience. She is listed in *Who's Who in Medicine and Health Care* and is well-known in the field of medical investigative reporting.

Publisher:
Seven Stories Press

Edition:
1998

Price:
$23.95

Pages:
191

ISBN:
1888363703

Media:
Book

Principal Subject:
Postpartum Maternal Care

A MOTHER'S TEARS
Understanding The Mood Swings That Follow Childbirth

Description:

This book almost exclusively addresses postpartum mood disorders that manifest themselves in psychotic episodes. The author, a practicing psychologist with a background in mood disorders, began studying this issue when a number of cases gained national media attention. The stated purpose of the book is as a primer on the subject of postpartum depression. Throughout are detailed stories of women who have suffered from various forms of this illness. A detailed explanation of the process a hormonal system goes through during pregnancy is included, and the signs and symptoms of postpartum depression are listed for the reader. The author discusses characteristic traits of women who kill their children, and profiles instances in which a woman's partner, who also may suffer from mood disorders, assists the postpartum depressive woman in committing acts of psychotic behavior. Lastly, a resource list is provided to women who seek assistance. This list includes professional organizations, books, and videos. A description of each resource is included, along with addresses and phone numbers.

Evaluation:

The author states, "This book is written to educate and comfort women concerning the normal hormonal changes which take place after the birth of a baby." Unfortunately, it fails to educate and comfort on all fronts. The author's focus is on the small number of women suffering from postpartum depression who exhibit psychotic behavior. The author states that one in 1,000 new mothers develop a postpartum depressive psychosis. The focus of this work is on the extreme of those cases. In addition, too many cited examples have nothing to do with postpartum depression at all. One cites a grandmother who killed her grandchild. While any woman with depression who has thoughts of harming herself or another should get help immediately, this book seems to assert that, if a woman has postpartum depression, she will kill her child. There is little practical, rational advice; the majority of the work consists of recitations of case studies with too often incomprehensible medical explanations. The last chapter on getting help does offer some practical advice. Alas, this chapter was not written by the author.

Where To Find/Buy:

Bookstores and libraries.

SPECIFICALLY
FOR FATHERS

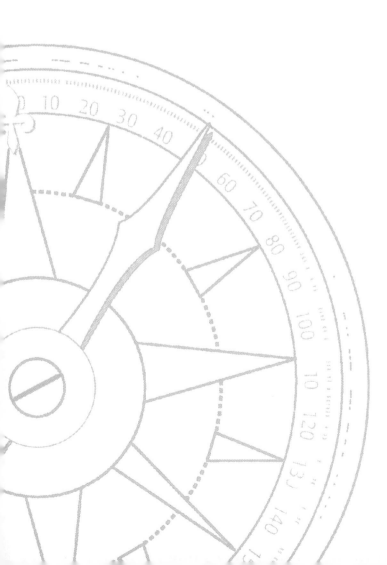

INTRODUCTION

No, it isn't just women who have babies. Fathers clearly can share in the experience. More and more research suggests that fathers play an essential role, both biologically and developmentally, in the growth of their children from the minute they are conceived and later on throughout their children's lives.

Fathers-to-be should join their partners in quitting smoking, and avoiding alcohol and any other toxic exposures before their partners get pregnant. Fathers should continue to avoid cigarettes both during the mother's pregnancy and after the baby is born, since it's been shown that passive exposure to smoke can harm both the growing fetus and the new baby. In fact, recent studies have linked second-hand smoke inhalation by a baby with sudden infant death—SIDS. Fathers will want to be healthy and offer support to their partners in making healthy choices as well. Sometimes during pregnancy, some fathers in fact show such "sympathy pains" for their partner that they can even develop physical symptoms of pregnancy that mimic the mothers' symptoms!

Although a mother plays an integral part in conceiving and giving birth to a baby, a father plays an important role in the development of his baby as well. A baby can actually hear her daddy's voice through the mother's abdomen during pregnancy, and she will then turn to his voice preferentially after she is born. Within a few days after being born, a baby will come to know and recognize her daddy's face as well. Eventually, by the time a baby is only a few months old, daddy is usually associated with "fun," and a baby will respond with clear unbridled screams of delight whenever she becomes aware of her daddy's presence nearby.

Unfortunately, our culture tends to equate feeding with love, and fathers of breastfed babies are often concerned that they will be excluded from this part of the relationship. It is true that fathers are not biologically equipped to feed babies the way nature intended. But dads can do many, many other things just as essential for their baby's development that help cement their growing bond and attachment. For example, research and current evidence have shown that babies who are fed, but not touched, will die—so snuggling is obviously at least as important as food! Dad can be the primary diaper-changer and bather, he can have some great snuggle time with his newborn baby, and later on when the baby gets older, he can be the one who gets covered with baby oatmeal! (Many families do introduce bottles at some point, so dad can do that too if he feels he really needs to.)

And a new dad can show his partner and baby how much he loves them by making sure the mother is well fed, has plenty of water to drink, and is able to find opportunities to sleep so her body can make enough milk for breastfeeding their new baby.

Some recent research suggests that the interactions of both parents with their baby contribute important but varying facets to their child's development. Mothers in general tend to nurture their babies and children, emphasizing the need to be connected to others and safe. Fathers, on the other hand, in general tend to offer encouragement while emphasizing independence. Children, then, who experience both of these styles usually grow up feeling loved and secure, but are also able to take risks and grow.

The resources we recommend in this section do an exceptional job of assisting you during your transition to fatherhood. These resources offer both quick and detailed tips and advice to make your discovery a pleasant journey, while not ensuring that it will be a smooth learning experience! Not only do these resources describe what you should pack in YOUR bag for the hospital, but they also offer ideas on how to keep your relationship strong and connect in new ways with your partner while you learn how to care for your new baby. Several resources offer pointers and checklists on how to financially prepare before and after your baby is born, how to cope with combining work and family life, how to deal with possible major lifestyle changes (from two-income to one-income, buying a home, etc.), how to understand the emotional changes you might face, and more. As always, read the full reviews to find the resources that best serve your needs and individual circumstances.

Additionally, fathers who are in need of additional information or support to help understand their partners' postpartum period may wish to read our recommendations in **Section IV—"Postpartum Maternal Care."**

★★★★

Overall Rating
★★★★
Perfect mix of humor and practical, realistic information and advice

Design, Ease Of Use
★★★★
Well thought-out topics and sections, with lots of handy worksheets and lists

1–4 Stars

Author:
Everett De Morier

De Morier conducts a series of adult education workshops. He lives in Vestal, New York, with his wife Debbie, and their two sons, Nicholas and Alexander. He also is the author of *Crib Notes for the First Year of Marriage: A Survival Guide for Newlyweds.*

Publisher:
Fairview Press

Edition:
1998

Price:
$14.95

Pages:
178

ISBN:
1577490738

Media:
Book

Principal Subject:
Specifically For Fathers

CRIB NOTES FOR THE FIRST YEAR OF FATHERHOOD
A Survival Guide For New Fathers

 Recommended For:
Specifically For Fathers

Description:
De Morier aims to offer a comprehensive guide for new fathers on a variety of topics in his 10 chapter, 178 page book. Included is an index, and each chapter concludes by offering a resource list and De Morier's "crib notes" of advice. The author says in his introduction, "I hope you will find it to be a light, informative view of what happens when you become a father. The goal is to give you ideas about what to expect and what to prepare for, and to direct you to resources that will make the change easier to bear and more enjoyable." In meeting those goals, the author has included chapters on topics such as: helping out the new mom, getting organized, safety in the home, and expectations on the part of the new parents and others. Separate chapters focus on financial concerns, such as debt, budgeting, saving and investing, as well as buying a home. As an interactive bonus, there are worksheets throughout, especially in the financial sections. Many firsthand experiences are recounted by the author about his wife and two young sons. Humor is used as a medium to keep the reader entertained while providing information.

Evaluation:
Finally, a how-to book that is fun to read! From beginning to end, the author, a master humorist as evidenced by this book, has managed to provide the perfect mix of entertaining reading and plenty of practical advice. For example, he states in his introduction that he and his wife obviously "had too much disposable time and money on our hands, and too many hours of REM sleep each night. Because suddenly, we were trying to have children." The "About the Author" section is written from his 3-year old son's perspective—"Our father is a writer and lecturer, although the idea of someone actually paying him to talk is completely beyond [us]." As entertaining as the book is, it also provides a comprehensive overview of what men may expect and plan for when becoming a new parent. The information provided is more realistic than idealistic, although some information (feeding baby solid foods at 3 months) is not recommended. The chapters are divided into well-planned topic areas, then further divided. Topics include everything from babyproofing the home and pampering the new mom to financial planning. A great primer for any man (or woman) expecting a first child, it provides details without drowning the reader in technicalities.

Where To Find/Buy:
Bookstores, libraries, or order direct by calling (800) 544-8207.

THE EXPECTANT FATHER
Facts, Tips, And Advice For Dads-To-Be

 Recommended For:
Specifically For Fathers

Description:

This 215 page book uses a guidebook design to lead first-time fathers through the first year of becoming a parent. It focuses on the benefits to fathers of being active and involved before and after the birth of their child. In the introduction, the four key topics used for each chapter are explained. Each chapter then provides month-by-month coverage of these topics: what she's going through, what's going on with the baby, what the new dad is going through, and tips for the father on how to stay involved. Also provided are discussions on topics dealing with the unexpected—ectopic pregnancy, miscarriages, and birth defects. Many chapters also include advice to fathers-to-be on ways to show their partner that they care, including exercises that can be done together, communication skills to be cultivated, and more. A variety of activities to prepare the father for upcoming changes in lifestyle include such topics as: financial planning, family and medical leave planning, birth announcements, birth classes, birth plans, nursery plan, emergency plans, and care giver plans.

Evaluation:

This book, written by two collaborating professional writers, fills a noticeable gap in the baby-book market with this guidebook for fathers. The information is presented in a straightforward, practical manner that should appeal to men. Many concerns that come up for both parents, but are often a higher priority for men (like taxes and insurance), are handled in factual and helpful inserts. Most pregnancy books deal with the birth experience from the mother's perspective leaving the father looking over her shoulder wondering what he should be doing. This book takes the approach of informing expectant fathers on exactly what issues must be decided (circumcision, preterm labor/preterm birth, etc.), how and what to do if he finds himself delivering his child, and so on. A father's view of normal hospital delivery procedures and what decisions he should expect to make is covered in detail. Dads will find helpful tips of what to do after the baby comes home, including tips on how to soothe a crying infant. This book is well-done, comprehensive, and a "must buy" for new dads.

Where To Find/Buy:

Bookstores and libraries. Videotape (45 minutes) is also available for $19.98 by calling Total Marketing Services, Inc. at (800) 262-3822.

★★★★

Overall Rating
★★★★
A very useful, factual and informative book for first-time fathers

Design, Ease Of Use
★★★★
Clear, easy to read, well illustrated

1–4 Stars

Author:
Armin A. Brott and Jennifer Ash

Armin A. Brott has written on fatherhood for the *New York Times Magazine, Newsweek, American Baby* magazine, *Parenting* magazine, and the *Washington Post.* Jennifer Ash is the author of *Private Palm Beach* and a contributing editor to *Town and Country.*

Publisher:
Abbeville Press

Edition:
1995

Price:
$10.95

Pages:
215

ISBN:
1558596909

Media:
Book

Principal Subject:
Specifically For Fathers

★★★★

Overall Rating
★★★★
Will instill confidence in fathers to help them define their roles within the family

Design, Ease Of Use
★★★★
Succinct; detailed table of contents, subheadings within chapters; whimsical drawings

1–4 Stars

Author:
S. Adams Sullivan

Sullivan, a writer, illustrator, and artist, works at home allowing him to spend long hours with his children, sharing projects and pleasures, many of which found their way into this book. He is also the author of *The Quality Time Almanac.*

Publisher:
Main Street Books (Doubleday/Bantam Doubleday Dell)

Edition:
2nd (1992)

Price:
$17.95

Pages:
391

ISBN:
0385426259

Media:
Book

Principal Subject:
Specifically For Fathers

THE FATHER'S ALMANAC

 Recommended For:
Specifically For Fathers

Description:
Published originally in 1980 to invoke an argument for "involved fatherhood," this revision notes changes in the role fathers play nowadays. This 391 page book is separated into 12 chapters, about 30 pages each. Chapter topics focus on: pregnancy and childbirth, baby care, fathers' jobs, family issues (working, stay-at-home, divorce, siblings, etc.), "providing" (childcare, safety, insurance, fix-it, etc.), daily events (baths, bedtime, reading, etc.), outings and special events, teaching and discipline, learning and playing with kids (games, activities,), working with kids ("handyman's helper," cooking, etc.), and "keeping a record" (photographing, videotaping, etc.). The table of contents lists major subtopics within chapters and bold headings are used for further divisions. The author has included his own black line illustrations throughout along with photographs of fathers with their children to introduce each chapter. A 16 page index completes the book along with a reference section to further reading.

Evaluation:
What a perfect addition to the family library! Sullivan offers fathers the chance to see themselves as more than "babysitters," more than a "breadwinner," more than a stand-in for mom. By presenting common hurdles and problems that fathers face and offering bite-size tidbits of advice to help fathers deal with those problems, the author has accomplished what he set out to do: instill confidence in fathers so they will be and stay involved. From instructions for how to make a teepee to how to deal with absences due to business trips, this guide offers succinct and well-constructed tips for making fatherhood an enjoyable experience. The author's illustrations are charming, but not sickeningly cute. The only area that is treated lightly concerns that of child development. Fathers will need other resources to supplement this topic. Focused on the questions, needs, and abilities of fathers, mothers, however, will also benefit from its content. This resource deserves a real place of honor within the family home.

Where To Find/Buy:
Bookstores and libraries.

NEW FATHER BOOK

 Recommended For:
Specifically For Fathers

Description:

The authors, collectively the fathers of five children, have put together a book that covers childhood from pregnancy through a child's early years. The first portion tackles the issue of what it takes to be a good dad. Other topics in this 96-page book include pregnancy, birth, the first two weeks, the first year, and the toddler and preschool years. The appendix is written especially for moms. It addresses five myths between mothers and fathers, such as "Household duties should be shared 50-50," and offers six tips for a mother to use when dealing with a new father, such as "Don't 'rescue' your husband." Every chapter offers many sidebars and lists, such as "10 Ways to Make Time for Your Children," "What's a Man To Do?" (when mom's in labor), and "Eagle's Eye View of Your Baby's First Year." The authors use firsthand experiences to illustrate their subjects. The last chapter addresses issues faced by fathers who adopt, are divorced, widowed, or single parents, as well as those who are stepfathers. A comprehensive index is included at the end of the book.

Evaluation:

This book's success rests heavily on the authors' experience as fathers. While light on technical information, the book's greatest assets are the real-life tips, tricks and strategies the authors have learned and incorporated throughout. The text is not overloaded with medical information; there's just enough to inform. The book's other great strength is that on almost every page there is a sidebar discussion, chart, or list to highlight or supplement the topic being addressed. Chapter 1 asks—and answers—the question, "What makes a good dad?" It makes a good argument for a model of fatherhood that includes a supportive partnership with the mom and deep involvement in the child's life. Advice offered includes real-life information, for example, "Ideas and techniques that sounded great in (childbirth) class may be worthless during the real event. The key is to be flexible and improvise." Horn and Rosenberg stress the importance of prioritizing responsibilities. This book, while geared a little toward the "white-collar" professional, is a good resource for helpful information on pregnancy, childbirth, and childcare.

Where To Find/Buy:

Bookstores and libraries.

★★★★

Overall Rating
★★★★
Excellent real-life advice from experienced fathers, light on technical information

Design, Ease Of Use
★★★★
Great to thumb through for information on-the-spot; many useful sidebar articles

1–4 Stars

Author:
Wade F. Horn, PhD, and Jeffrey Rosenberg, MSW

Horn is a clinical child psychologist who has held a number of private and public positions focusing on children's issues. He is the father of two teenage girls. Rosenberg is a father of three, including two-year old twins.

Publisher:
Better Homes and Gardens Books (Meredith Books)

Edition:
1998

Price:
$9.95

Pages:
96

ISBN:
069620617X

Media:
Book

Principal Subject:
Specifically For Fathers

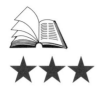

★★★

Overall Rating
★★★
"Sound bites" of advice offering 36 tips on concerns new dads may have

Design, Ease Of Use
★★★★
All topics—"Keys"—listed in table of contents; short, concise text for busy dads

1–4 Stars

Author:
William Sears, MD

Sears, "one of America's most renowned pediatricians," has been in practice for 20 years and authored 10 books. Currently, he's a clinical assistant professor of pediatrics at USC School of Medicine.

Publisher:
Barron's Educational Series

Edition:
1991

Price:
$6.95

Pages:
152

ISBN:
0812045416

Media:
Book

Principal Subject:
Specifically For Fathers

KEYS TO BECOMING A FATHER

Description:

The stated theme of this book is that, as more fathers are becoming involved in child care, the father's relationship with his child is different than a mother's (but equally important). Sears' guide addresses the concerns that fathers face as they take on new roles with their children. Sears shares "uniquely male nurturing tips" that he himself has learned through fathering eight children. There are 36 "Keys" in this 152 page book, all of which are listed in the table of contents; these topics usually are covered in 2–3 pages. Topics include the following: fathering during pregnancy, fathering with a newborn, how to handle a fussy baby, relationships with your wife, how to juggle career and parenthood, helping your son or daughter develop healthy masculinity or femininity, being a single father, playing with your baby (3 months intervals to one year), disciplining your baby/child (increments from birth), and fathering older children (1–3 years old, 3–6 years old, 6–11 years old, teenager). A question and answer section is supplied at the end of the book listing 10 questions posed from fathers and Sears's responses.

Evaluation:

This book is not simply for fathers. Mothers, by reading this book, can get a better idea how (and why) fathers respond differently to their children. Sears speaks quite candidly about mistakes he has made, revelations he has gleaned, and the great joys and satisfactions he has received from his experiences as a father. No doubt any father will appreciate Sears's candor and feel supported without being babied—no psycho-babble here. The book's short, concise "Keys," although not written in great depth, offer just enough for busy fathers who might be reluctant to sit down and read a book on parenting. Although some of Sears's suggestions, such as working at home, easing back on work demands, etc., may not work with many fathers' careers, he does offer many thoughts on how to juggle fatherhood and careers; these tips are useful for working mothers too. His section on being a single father, however, seems weak; also, tips on how to be a "house husband/father" are missing. Hopefully these areas will be strengthened in future editions.

Where To Find/Buy:

Bookstores and libraries.

PREGNANT FATHERS
Entering Parenthood Together

★★★

Description:

This 188 page book is the result of an ongoing effort by psychologist Jack Heinowitz to add perspective to the experience of fatherhood. Initially the topic of his graduate dissertation, this is the second edition of *Pregnant Fathers* and represents the author's 20 year involvement in the subject. Beginning with an introduction to the idea of a father "being pregnant," it progresses in an orderly way. Topics include chapters on feelings and needs of expectant fathers, getting involved in the pregnancy, relationship changes, sex and the pregnant couple, relationship communication skills, the birth itself, and adjusting to the new member of the family. Exercises are included to assist an expectant father with coming to grips with his emotions and needs. Information on how to improve his ability to relate these internal experiences to the others in his life is regularly spaced throughout the book. The book closes with self-help tips, a list of regional support organizations, and additional references and suggested reading.

Evaluation:

This book will be a useful resource for a first-time father as he navigates through his own internal experience of impending fatherhood. It is well-written, intelligent, and sensitive. It clearly illustrates how fatherhood is viewed in America, how this perspective has begun to shift in the last 20 years, and what changes are recommended in order to improve on it today. Contemporary expectant fathers, it says, need to be sensitive, involved and nurturing. And, in order for this model to work, the book proposes that fathers must do some "internal work" during pregnancy for this transformation in their identities to occur smoothly. The book's style is well-balanced and thoughtful; it's easy to read and well-illustrated. Consequently, it is a recommended companion to other books for the first-time father who wants to understand and master his own emotional issues created by pregnancy.

Where To Find/Buy:

Bookstores and libraries.

Overall Rating
★★★
Sensitive, thought-provoking; unique perspective on the father's role during pregnancy

Design, Ease Of Use
★★★★
Well written, well laid out, interesting

1–4 Stars

Author:
Jack Heinowitz, PhD
Heinowitz began working on the concept of pregnant fathers as the topic of his graduate thesis in psychology. For the past 20 years he has maintained his interest and involvement in the topic through Parents As Partners in San Diego and through his writing on the topic.

Publisher:
Parents As Partners Press

Edition:
2nd (1995)

Price:
$14.95

Pages:
188

ISBN:
0964102404

Media:
Book

Principal Subject:
Specifically For Fathers

★★★

Overall Rating
★★★
Good succinct advice and info for men wrestling with emotional aspects of fatherhood

Design, Ease Of Use
★★
Consistent chapter format, but icons are annoying; photographs would be a nice addition

1–4 Stars

Author:
Marcus Jacob Goldman, MD

Goldman trained in general psychiatry at Harvard Medical School where he also completed the Gaughan Fellowship in forensic psychiatry. He has taught psychiatry and behavioral health at Harvard and currently practices geriatric psychiatry.

Publisher:
Prima Publishing

Edition:
1997

Price:
$15.00

Pages:
228

ISBN:
0761504524

Media:
Book

Principal Subject:
Specifically For Fathers

THE JOY OF FATHERHOOD
The First Twelve Months

Description:

Written "by a man for men," this 228 page book aims to provide new fathers with information on the possible emotions, thoughts, and behaviors that they may experience. With the exception of the first chapter which deals with labor, delivery, and the postpartum period, the book includes twelve other chapters divided month-by-month for a baby's life from birth to 12 months of age. The author uses a consistent format for each of these chapters with subheadings highlighting: what's new with baby, "focus," what's new with mom, what's new with dad, "being there for your baby," and growing together (a one paragraph summary of the chapter's important points). Icons are used in the margins to mark each of these sections. The focus sections contain how-to instructions, questions and answers, clinical information, and advice on topics that concern new fathers, such as colic, getting in shape, anger management, how to maintain relationships with friends, and more. Each chapter includes a Q & A segment and various tips are offered in the margins. An appendix gives information about common childhood ailments.

Evaluation:

The consistent format works well here making it a breeze for busy days to find information. New fathers will also appreciate the focus sections as they wrestle with practical concerns such as safety issues, saving money for baby, and other topics. The author also does a great job of summing up a baby's development in one paragraph packages that can be easily digested. Cartoon strips are interspersed throughout allowing humor to be interjected within the scope of the chapter's topic. Especially appealing about this resource is its effort to present the varying emotions new mothers and new fathers may experience along with ways to make those emotions a bonding experience rather than a divisive one. However, there are two problems with this book: the icons the author uses (amateur, distracting, and cluttered) and the lack of how-to pictures or photographs to make some of the childcare tasks a bit easier. Overall, however, fathers confused about their new roles will appreciate this author's welcome tips and concise answers to their questions.

Where To Find/Buy:

Bookstores, libraries, or order direct by calling (916) 632-4400 or contacting Prima Publishing at P. O. Box 1260, Rocklin, CA 95677.

PARENTS'™ BOOK FOR NEW FATHERS

★★★

Description:

This book is an installment in the Parents'™ Magazine Baby and Child Care Series. The author covers the process of becoming a father from the decision to have a child, through birth and the first year. He also includes information for special situations, including adoptive and single fathers. At the end of the book are two appendices, one on infant development and the other a resource list that covers a range of pregnancy and baby-care topics. Four chapters in this 14-chapter book discuss basic pregnancy issues, from how to make a baby to the more technical issues of medical problems that can occur during pregnancy. In addition to technical medical information, the author covers what emotions a father-to-be can expect to feel, how to handle worries about the baby, and what possible changes may occur in a new father's relationship with his wife. Other chapters include information regarding the birthing process, the first few weeks of a newborn's life, establishing new family routines, the difficulties of being a parent, bonding and playing with a baby, and providing adequate childcare.

Evaluation:

While this book is a wealth of information on almost every topic imaginable, the format leaves a little to be desired. The layout is that of a paperback novel, with few visual breaks. It is best suited for a reader who wants extremely comprehensive, detailed information, and has the time and stamina to read the book cover to cover, or at least chapter by chapter. It is not a book to thumb through while looking for specific information. The author uses testimony from other fathers to illustrate the topics. Chapter 3 begins similar to a course on Health 101: How to Make a Baby, and ends with the various stages of fetal development. Obviously, this book is meant for an expectant father who begins knowing nothing and wants to know everything. In that, the author does well in covering the range of information from the technical to the emotional. Unexpectedly, Chapter 11 is a delightful chapter on bonding and playing with baby, and Chapter 10 takes a realistic look at the frustrations and stresses of becoming a parent. This book is a dry read, but offers well the "nuts and bolts" of pregnancy and baby care.

Where To Find/Buy:

Bookstores and libraries.

Overall Rating
★★★
Much useful information, from the technical to the emotional

Design, Ease Of Use
★
Chapters are long, with not much to break them up

1–4 Stars

Author:
David Laskin

David Laskin is the father of three daughters, which include twin baby girls. He has written about infant development and many other topics in books and magazines.

Publisher:
Ballantine Books
(Random House)

Edition:
1988

Price:
$4.95

Pages:
407

ISBN:
0345337077

Media:
Book

Principal Subject:
Specifically For Fathers

V. Specifically For Fathers

★★

Overall Rating
★★
Light reading of topics well worth consideration, might put off some reluctant new dads

Design, Ease Of Use
★★
A quick and easy read with one page inspirational quotes; advertising in back distracts

1–4 Stars

Author:
Jeanne Murphy

Murphy says that the suggestions made in this book are opinions which are true to the best of her knowledge. A parent herself, Murphy has also written a three book series entitled "Baby Tips for New Moms."

Publisher:
Fisher Books

Edition:
1998

Price:
$6.95

Pages:
135

ISBN:
1555611699

Media:
Book

Principal Subject:
Specifically For Fathers

BABY TIPS FOR NEW DADS
Baby's First Year

Description:

This book is written for first time fathers who have yet to understand the possible effects that parenting can have on the marriage relationship. Before the book begins, Murphy gives notice that, "The suggestions made in this book are opinions and are not meant to supersede a doctor's recommendations." Nevertheless, the book does not particularly address medical issues. Instead, each page is a message or quote provided to offer teachings about new life situations (challenges) that arrive with the baby. Chapter topics include "Hormones and How to Handle Them," "The Monumentally Sensitive Issue of Weight," "What to Do and Say," "What Absolutely Not to Do and Say," and "Other General Survival Tips." In these passages, the demands of parenthood are described from the mother's point-of-view. The reader is told, for example, that "Being a good dad and husband isn't the result of a gene. It's the result of commitment." This book also contains the following: an index, a contest, a very brief first year interest/activity summary, a guide to resource organizations, catalog information, and coupons.

Evaluation:

At first glance, this book seems to display the attitude that the mother will typically give it her all to meet her baby's needs, while the father may have a tendency to be a bit more selfish. Taken too literally this book could be discouraging to the reader, but Murphy's writing style is very lighthearted and easily considered by the reader. On the whole, the book conveys many of the new transitions and demands put upon the mother who is having her first child. Sometimes the scenario is a bit exaggerated (for example the chapter on "Hormones and How to Handle Them"), but the reader is entertained and gets the message. The reader is encouraged to resist putting his own needs first ("Remember: In the back of your wife's mind, she is probably thinking, 'One baby is enough,' so don't act like a baby") and asked to give 100% ("It's better to give your wife a reason to say 'thank you' than it is for you to find a way to say 'I'm sorry'"). This book provides good medicine for late-blooming fathers.

Where To Find/Buy:
Bookstores and libraries.

FATHERS & BABIES
How Babies Grow And What They Need From You, From Birth To 18 Months

Description:

This 1993 step-by-step manual aims to "teach both practical skills and child development theory." It includes five major sections with a preceding introduction. Chapter One includes information and advice on newborns: feeding, how to handle and soothe an infant, bathing, changing diapers, and more are covered. Chapter Two discusses child care for infants 1 to 6 months. Sleeping and eating idiosyncrasies, discipline, dressing, bathing, some developmental milestones, and other topics are contained in this section. Chapters Three, Four, and Five cover similar topics of infant care but in a progressive age-specific format from 6 to 9 months, 9 to 12 months, and 12 to 18 months of age, respectively. Additional information and advice is provided on the following topics: beginning walking, shyness, first words, safety and childproofing, how to keep your patience, toilet training, activities to do with your child, infant toys, birthday parties, recipes, and more. There is no index.

Evaluation:

This is a well-intentioned guide targeting an audience (fathers) who might appreciate concise information. However, much more depth could have been added to this resource without sacrificing brevity. Lightly touching on just the very basics, this book gives fathers a sampling of what its like to be a primary care provider. The problem is that, in so doing, it sometimes delivers the message to the reader in dumb-downed fashion—"If your baby likes to poke, watch out for your eyes." Other examples include how to determine when a child is able to sit so that the father no longer needs to prop them up or how to change a baby at someone else's house. The author does provide some helpful advice and information, such as offering baby a toy to play with while changing their diaper, ways to babyproof the home, and fun activities and games. The book is written in a humorous vein, with extensive use of black and white line illustrations. Worth the read? Other resources serve fathers' needs better. Use them instead.

Where To Find/Buy:

Bookstores and libraries.

Overall Rating
★★
Too concise and hodgepodge—fathers are capable of assimilating more in-depth info

Design, Ease Of Use
★
Index would have contributed immensely; no detailed help from table of contents

1–4 Stars

Author:
Jean Marzollo

Jean Marzollo graduated from the University of Connecticut and the Harvard Graduate School of Education. She previously has written parenting articles for such magazines as Scholastic's *Let's Find Out*, *Parents Magazine*, *Family Circle*, and *Working Mother*.

Publisher:
HarperPerennial (HarperCollins)

Edition:
1993

Price:
$12.50

Pages:
235

ISBN:
0060969083

Media:
Book

Principal Subject:
Specifically For Fathers

V. Specifically For Fathers

★★

Overall Rating
★★
Reads like a textbook, with no experiential advice

Design, Ease Of Use
★
Chapters are a little disorganized, but generally well laid out; visual aids absent

1–4 Stars

Author:
Gene B. Williams
No information given

Publisher:
Avon Books

Edition:
1997

Price:
$12.00

Pages:
318

ISBN:
038078906X

Media:
Book

Principal Subject:
Specifically For Fathers

THE NEW FATHER'S PANIC BOOK
Everything A Dad Needs To Know To Welcome His Bundle Of Joy

Description:

This 318 page, 16-chapter book is intended to provide basic information on the various issues facing expectant fathers. The first 10 chapters focus on the pregnancy, from basic anatomy to labor and birth. The three trimesters of pregnancy are discussed, as well as the physical and emotional changes the mother can expect to experience, and the stages of development of the fetus. Explanations of what to expect during doctors' visits and while in the hospital are also included. In these chapters, the author describes what problems may arise during the various stages of pregnancy, labor, and birth. Other chapters include issues such as the mother's recovery, what to expect from the first few hours of a baby's life, what happens during follow-up doctors' visits, and other issues of particular concern to new fathers. The last chapter is written for the mother, describing to her what a new father goes through emotionally. An appendix on massage goes into detail about how to give the expectant or new mother a healthy, comfortable, and relaxing massage; no illustrations are given. A comprehensive glossary completes the book.

Evaluation:

The author's viewpoint in this book is that a father's role in pregnancy is important, but ultimately third in importance to the child and the mother. He stresses that focus should be on the child and mother throughout pregnancy and the first few months following birth, but that a large part of the mother's well-being depends on having a supportive, understanding father present. Therefore, much of this book is a description of what the mother is going through during the pregnancy, labor, and birth processes. More than half of the book addresses pregnancy. The last few chapters turn to other issues, such as physical recovery, dealing with the newborn, and visits with doctors. The information provided, however, is most basic. There are few creative tips or bits of advice offered. This book feels, and operates, more like a textbook, void of empathetic support, and without belief that the author has actually experienced his topic. It is the last chapter, which advises expectant moms about what expectant fathers may go through, that finally offers a unique perspective. That, as well as the appendix on massage, makes the book worthwhile. Other resources, however, do a better job at describing a father's experience and emotions.

Where To Find/Buy:

Bookstores, libraries, or order direct by calling (800) 762-0779.

SHE'S HAVING A BABY–AND I'M HAVING A BREAKDOWN

What Every Man Needs to Know—And Do—When The Woman He Loves Is Pregnant

Description:

In this 177 page book, Barron sends 237 messages to the reader. Each message is conveyed in a sentence (bold type) and then there is a paragraph or more of detail. These messages are for expectant fathers who, as Barron declares, will go through many personal and experiential changes as they become new fathers. Even during pregnancy, the father-to-be may have intense feelings and reactions that come as a surprise. Although written for fathers, Barron says that his book will help both men and women understand how a father-to-be is likely to experience pregnancy, delivery, and early fatherhood. Interspersed amid these messages, the reader will find many lists: "10 Great Moments of Pregnancy and Early Fatherhood," "10 Responses to the News That She's Pregnant Your Wife Doesn't Want to Hear," "10 Things a Father-To-Be Fears Most About Pregnancy," "12 Last Hurrahs For You and Your Wife," and more.

Evaluation:

The book begins in a very upbeat and heartfelt manner by listing "10 Great Moments of Pregnancy and Early Fatherhood." This positive outlook prevails even though Barron continually shares the opinion that fathers may not get much acknowledgment because "the world is still catching up to the involved father-to-be." Although the 237 numbered messages contained in the book address many topics in a helpful manner, the overall message of the book seems to be one of encouragement, not information. Reading this book is a bit like listening to a close friend who's already experienced what the reader is about to embark upon; this may be a tone, however, that might put some men off. The lists that are periodically found are funny; the lists will be especially funny once the reader has experienced parenthood. The lists usually refer to those things that parents don't mind "suffering" for the gift received—their child. While the comical aspects of this book are prevalent, it is Barron's positive outlook that naturally combines the humor and the reality of the pregnancy and parenthood experiences. Good transition support here for new dads which will be best appreciated when combined with other more informational resources.

Where To Find/Buy:

Bookstores and libraries.

Overall Rating
★★
Wonderful cover-to-cover reading for support, not thorough with medical details, etc.

Design, Ease Of Use
★
Not easily referenced by contents, no index; bold text helps highlight author's points

1–4 Stars

Author:
James Douglas Barron
Barron lives in New York City and Connecticut with his wife and their two children. He grew up in the Midwest.

Publisher:
Quill (William Morrow)

Edition:
1998

Price:
$10.00

Pages:
177

ISBN:
0688158250

Media:
Book

Principal Subject:
Specifically For Fathers

Overall Rating

★

Pep talk for expectant fathers with little useful advice

Design, Ease Of Use

★

Random design and content; there is no list of subjects provided, no index

1–4 Stars

Author:
Greg Jones

This book was compiled, designed, and produced by Marquand Books, Inc. and edited by Greg Jones. No information is provided about the editor.

Publisher:
Running Press Book Publishers

Edition:
1997

Price:
$9.95

Pages:
60

ISBN:
0762401923

Media:
Book

Principal Subject:
Specifically For Fathers

THE EXPECTANT FATHER'S HANDBOOK
A Simple Guide To Your New Life

Description:

This guide for new fathers is presented in 27 chapters; one for an introduction and one for each letter of the alphabet. Each chapter is intended to address various topics to assist a new father in adjusting to life with baby. The introduction asks the question, "What Kind of Father do you want to be?" It encourages fathers-to-be to make the pregnancy "couple-focused" instead of mother-focused, and offers tips to include the father in the pregnancy and childbirth experience. The remaining chapters, A–Z, discuss issues from anxiety about baby clothes to a sudden yearning to visit the zoo. Included are discussions on the emotional aspects of fatherhood, advice on how to become and remain involved, and encouragement to show an expectant father the attention and congratulations typically bestowed on the mother. In this 60-page book, chapters are typically one or two pages long, with the remaining pages devoted to photographs and quotes offered as either a tip or as a father's perspective on a particular issue.

Evaluation:

It seems there is a reason this book lists an editor, but does not list an actual author. The majority of the content is a hodgepodge of one or two lines of unorganized advice, thrown together in 26 chapters. None of the chapters, with the exception of chapters "B" and "J" have a specific subject. The chapters themselves essentially share the same thesis: an expectant father should be prepared, recognize that there will be many varied emotions to experience, ask questions, and communicate with his partner. All good messages. In fact, this book is more of a pep talk on becoming a father than a resource for actual practical information. All "chapters" are only a few paragraphs long and emphasize their topic by enlarging all words in bold that begin with the letter for that particular chapter. For example, the "B" chapter exclusively deals with what to "Buy" for "Baby" and is somewhat useful. The "J" chapter discusses the "Jealousy" an expectant father may feel toward his unborn child and suggests he "Joke" with his male friends who have children. However, there is very little practical, on-the-ground advice offered in this guidebook.

Where To Find/Buy:

Bookstores and libraries.

HOW TO PAMPER YOUR PREGNANT WIFE

Description:

Written to advise the reader on ways to pamper their wife, this book begins by listing some of the signs of pregnancy relating these indications to how the husband might feel about it. In the remainder of this "trimester-by-trimester crash course in pregnant relations," the author focuses on how husbands can honestly acknowledge their concerns while supporting their wife's pregnancy. Some concerns of the mother-to-be are conveyed: waistline, hormones, lifestyle, and others. The first trimester of pregnancy is described as a transitional period for both parents; dealing with miscarriage is mentioned as a possibility. Within the second chapter (focusing on the second trimester), the text is supported by a bibliography where medical conditions and procedures are introduced. Generally, Schultz shares personal insight related to in-laws, sex, folklore, superstitions, etc. The last chapter of the book covers the third trimester and topics related to delivery. Again, the reader is told what to expect in the way of sex, superstitions, and fulfilling his role as supportive husband (offer massage and understanding!)

Evaluation:

The reader should appreciate the author's acknowledgment of a new father-to-be's feelings. As this book conveys, it is also worthwhile for the reader to consider the mother-to-be's concerns too. Although Schultz cites that material for this book came from a variety of sources ("interviews with pregnant wives, doctors, lawyers, therapists, mothers-in-law, mothers, . . ."), the book's tone is as if an older person is giving advice to a younger person, which may put some readers off or feel as if they are being talked down to. Reading the entire book will offer some idea of what to expect, but some of the specific experiences detailed are either irrelevant or are overly dramatized. Readers are told to be comforting or commanding depending on the situation being described. However, the advice to direct the mother, rather than to encourage her, might not be welcome or appreciated by the mother. Similarly, the author makes certain assumptions (such as the wife doing the cooking), which gives the book a rather dated and subordinating feel, as also evidenced by the book's title. Other sources address both the prospective mother's and father's concerns. We recommend those over this one for support and information.

Where To Find/Buy:

Bookstores, libraries, order direct by calling (800) 338-2232 or (612) 930-1100 (in Minnesota), or Fax a request to (612) 930-1940. It can also be ordered through Meadowbrook Press at 5451 Smetana Drive, Minnetonka, MN 55343.

Overall Rating
★
Tone of this book is outdated, not extremely entertaining or informative

Design, Ease Of Use
★
No index for referencing, nothing outstanding about the book's organization

---

1–4 Stars

Author:
Ron Schultz and Sam Schultz

Ron Schultz and his father, Sam, have collaborated on more than a dozen children's television projects. Both Ron and Sam have published numerous books on various topics.

Publisher:
Meadowbrook Press
(Simon & Schuster)

Edition:
1996

Price:
$7.00

Pages:
103

ISBN:
0881661690

Media:
Book

Principal Subject:
Specifically For Fathers

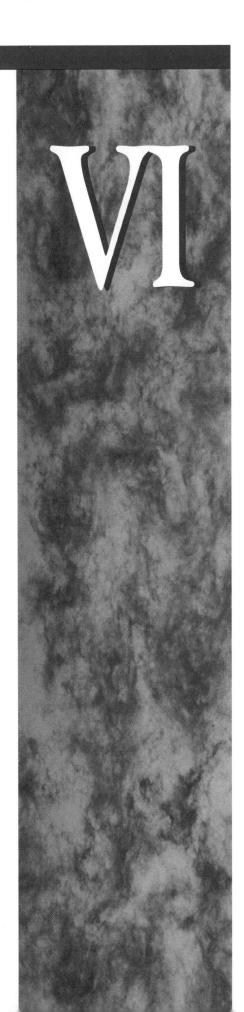

YOUR NEWBORN

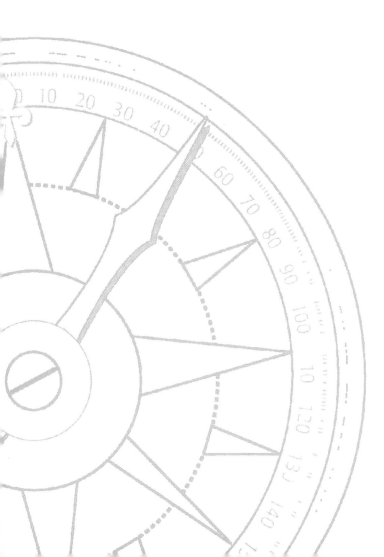

INTRODUCTION

The first time you hold your baby in your arms and your eyes meet, you will see your future and be amazed. Newborns are just incredible little creatures. We once thought newborns were passive creatures who ate, slept, peed, pooped, and waited to grow up so they could then do something. We now know that babies are learning before they are born, and that this process accelerates at the time of birth. For example, newborns know their mothers by smell as soon as they are born. They recognize their father's voice and will turn to it preferentially after birth. And within a few days, they can recognize the faces and voices of the special people in their lives. Babies come hard-wired with all the reflexes they need to survive. They can and do exert control on their environment through their sleep states, their cries and fusses, and by gazing deeply into their parents' eyes.

Despite all these amazing skills, babies remain entirely dependent creatures. It is our responsibility as parents to figure out all those signals, to respond to them appropriately, and to keep the baby safe and healthy. New parents will begin to develop a parenting style that fits for their family and their baby. No single book about babies or child care will likely "fit" for you in every situation, so choose a few that you are generally comfortable with, and pick and choose advice that works for you.

One thing you will definitely need to consider while you are pregnant is whom you will choose to be your baby's health care provider. If you are seeing a family physician for your pregnancy, or have a family physician that provides your primary care, he or she will likely be delighted to care for your baby as well. If you have a midwife or obstetrician, you will need to choose a pediatrician, family physician, or nurse practitioner to care for your new baby. Ask for recommendations from people who already have children and check with your insurance company to see who will be covered. It is a good idea to make an appointment to get acquainted with the baby's provider some time during the last trimester of pregnancy. Ideally, choose someone who practices at the hospital where you will deliver so that you won't have to arrange for another provider for your baby's initial hospital care.

Parents of new boys have an additional decision to consider—whether or not to have their baby circumcised. There is no medical indication for circumcision. One large military study suggested a 0.2 percent risk of complications from circumcision, primarily bleeding and local infection, and a 0.2 percent risk of complications related to being uncircumcised, primarily penile or urinary tract infections. Boys in Europe and throughout the world are generally only circumcised for religious reasons. We have no evidence to suggest that uncircumcised boys have any psychological troubles related to peer or family comparisons, nor do we have any evidence that there is long-term psychological harm from the procedure. Consider carefully that you are making a decision about cosmetic surgery for someone who can't directly consent, and be sure to educate yourself fully about the procedure and its risks and possible benefits.

Baby Care

So now that you have total responsibility for this new little person, what do you do?

Mostly, you love the baby, you keep the baby safe, you feed the baby, and you keep the baby reasonably clean.

You may choose books from any of several experts, but remember, you are the expert about YOUR baby. Your major job is to get to know your baby's signals and learn to trust your instincts as parents. Educate yourself about the normal developmental stages of babyhood so you can recognize and encourage your baby as you pass through them together. Celebrate and enjoy each stage, because they do pass quickly.

Many new parents have questions and concerns about the health of their baby and how they will know their new baby is sick. Newborns snort, sneeze, hiccup, make funny faces, and sleep a lot. If your baby is doing these things more than he or she usually does, you may want to watch for other signs of illness. Fever (over 100 degrees rectal) is never normal in a baby less than two months old, and requires consultation with your health care provider. Most babies should see their health care provider within a few days of discharge from the hospital, and again at about two weeks. New babies should regain their birth weight by two weeks of age. Your provider will recommend a schedule of health exams and immunizations, usually about four to six visits during the first year.

Breastfeeding

More and more research confirms what we've always known—breastfeeding is best for babies and mothers. Human milk is the best food for human babies. It contains all the proper nutrients in the proper amounts, as well as many components that help the baby's gastrointestinal system and immune system develop. Because we have large heads for our body size, human infants are born the most immature of all the mammals; we are, in effect, designed to "finish gestation" through breastfeeding. Research studies suggest that babies who are breastfed have lower rates of gastrointestinal and respiratory infections, lower rates of some childhood cancers and diabetes, and higher IQs and school performance compared to formula fed babies. And, mothers who breastfeed have a lower risk of uterine, breast, and ovarian cancer. Many other health effects of breastfeeding are just beginning to be documented. In addition, the breastfeeding relationship enhances the bond between mother and child.

Although most women know "breast is best," we live in a society with many barriers to successful breastfeeding. Most women in human history have grown up watching their mothers, sisters, and cousins breastfeed. In our current culture though, most women do not grow up learning how to breastfeed by watching others do it. Breastfeeding is "natural," but it's also clearly a learned skill. Babies have the reflexes to breastfeed, but they have to practice to get good at it as well. Educate yourself about breastfeeding during your pregnancy, find support people who share your commitment to breastfeeding, and try to find a support group of breastfeeding women.

Ideally, the first breastfeeding will happen just after the birth of your baby. Nature has given us a few days to learn the skills. Fortunately, babies are born with extra fluid on board, so all they need is the nutrition-packed, but low volume, colostrum for the first few days. Most mothers notice their milk supply then increasing about day three. And most mothers find their nipples a bit tender in the first few weeks when the baby is first latching on. However, once the milk is in and flowing, it should not hurt to breastfeed. Sore nipples during a feeding indicate something is wrong with the baby's latch or position. New babies usually need to eat eight to twelve times per day. They will have increasing urine and stool output over the first few days. By the fifth day, babies should have at least three large, yellow bowel movements and at least six to eight wet diapers daily.

Over the first few weeks, you and your baby will get better and better at breastfeeding. Most mothers find the first two to three weeks of breastfeeding challenging. Babies often have a first growth spurt at about three weeks and another at six to eight weeks. During growth spurts the baby will want to eat almost continuously. This is a particularly vulnerable time for mothers to think they don't have enough milk. However, the supply and demand system of nursing works itself out efficiently—the more the baby eats, the more milk the mother makes. It's very important to avoid supplemental bottles, however, since that may indeed lead to inadequate milk supply. The mother's body will respond to the baby's hunger and catch up to baby's need within a few days.

Mothers who will return to work often wonder if it's worth it to breastfeed. Clearly, any breastfeeding is better than none (and more breastfeeding is better than less). Some mothers will choose to wean before returning to work, others will combine breast- and formula-feeding after returning to work, and others will be able to work near their babies and/or express milk so they can continue full breastfeeding. In all of these cases, the best way to get started is to breastfeed exclusively at first. Even if you find you are unable to continue, you will help your baby get off to the best possible start.

If breastfeeding presents challenges or concerns, mothers can get help from mother support groups such as La Leche League or from lactation consultants. Ask the lactation consultant about his or her training and experience, just as you would any health care provider. The most recognized credential for lactation consultants is International Board of Lactation Consultant Examiners certification.

Choosing A Caregiver

The majority of mothers of preschoolers in the United States have reentered the work force. Consequently, more and more babies and children require care while their mothers are at work. Those of us who advocate for children continue to work for appropriate maternity and paternity leave, and for adequate, safe child care for those who need it. Making a good choice for your baby or child will help you feel more comfortable and confident with combining your work and parenting. Some families are able to juggle their full- or part-time jobs so that Dad can care for the baby when Mom is at work. More and more Dads are serving as the main at-home parent. Families also find ways to telecommute or work at home. For most employed mothers, however, some type of child care will also be necessary.

When choosing a caregiver, look for safety first. Next, concentrate on finding a situation that will support your parenting style and the type of care you want for your baby. Try to find a location near your workplace so you can visit during the day. Many mothers like to spend their lunch hour or breaks with their babies, which can make combining employment and breastfeeding much easier.

In-home "nanny" care can be very expensive, but is a good option especially for a young infant. Some families choose au pairs or use a nanny service; these agencies screen the applicants but also charge a fee. If you hire a nanny directly, be sure to check out his or her background thoroughly and check all references. Ask about their experience and philosophy of child rearing. Families who have found a nanny that fits their style and stays with them for a long time

VI. Your Newborn

usually love this type of arrangement. For others, it can be a frustrating process of turnover and rehiring. Be sure to investigate tax issues and also immigration issues if you will be hiring a foreign national.

Child care centers range from dismal to excellent. Children in larger, well-established centers usually receive more stimulation and educational focus than in other settings. When investigating a center, ask about staff training and turnover, and about health practices such as hand washing and administration of medications. Check out the license of the center and be sure they have not had any significant complaints filed with the regulatory agency. Visit the center and observe how the caregivers and children interact. What is the discipline style? Do infants get prompt attention or are they left in cribs to cry? Centers have many advantages—the center is always open even if one of the caregivers gets sick, they usually have at least some trained or certificated early childhood teachers on staff, and they tend to provide care for a wide range of ages.

Day care provided in a caregiver's home may have the widest variation in quality, and requires close scrutiny. Many day care homes provide loving, attentive care in a smaller setting with fewer children than a day care center. Most states license home day care providers who care for more than one child from another family, so investigating licensing and complaints will be important here, too. Look for a safe, loving environment with age-appropriate activities for the children in the home.

Whoever cares for your baby will need to know your preferences and desires for care. Developing a close relationship with this person who is sharing your baby's life can help you feel more comfortable with your choices and the daily transitions. Be sure to give your caregiver specific instructions about sleeping, eating, response to crying, etc. Be especially sure that your caregiver knows about the recommendation that babies sleep on their backs to lower the risk of SIDS.

Crying And Sleeping

New babies have only one sure way to communicate when they need something—cry. Crying is a survival skill for babies; the ones that don't cry at all often are the ones who die of starvation without anyone knowing they were hungry! You will quickly become knowledgeable about your own baby's cries. You will learn what means "hungry," what means "lonely," what means "ouch," and what just means "I've had enough of this!" Almost all new babies have a fussy time of day, often in the early evening, which probably reflects their immature neurologic system hitting the day's limit of new experiences. This fussy period usually diminishes by the time a baby is three months old.

"Colic," or incessant crying by a baby who appears to be in pain, can be very frustrating and overwhelming to parents. Trying to determine why the baby is crying may not be very productive after the first few unsuccessful attempts. Tried-and-true methods, some of which might actually work for your baby and some of which won't, include rides in the car, warm baths with mom or dad, vacuuming (white noise) with the baby in a carrier, or just handing the baby off to a sympathetic grandparent for a while. If you have a colicky baby, try to remember, "This too shall pass," and keep up your strength and stamina by supporting each other.

One of the most common questions asked by parents of young babies concerns sleeping "through the night." Sleeping patterns again reflect survival skills. New babies are just not designed to sleep long stretches of time, nor to sleep all alone. Babies don't know whether they have been born in the African bush or in suburban America. All they know is that they need to be warm and safe and have access to food. For most babies, that means sleeping with mom. New babies need to eat frequently, so "snack and snooze" may be the best pattern for growth. You might be interested to know that even "sleeping through the night" is defined in most research studies as sleeping a five-hour stretch between midnight and five a.m. Also, babies who sleep more deeply and independently may be at higher risk for SIDS.

Parents do need to balance baby's physiology with their own need for restorative sleep. Some parents will find they get the most sleep if they share sleep with their babies; others need to have some time alone in bed to get enough sleep. This is one area where you need to figure out what works for your family and not worry about doing it the way "everyone else" does. (Everyone else sleeps with their babies at least part of the time even if they don't tell you about it, by the way.) And if people ask, just smile and say, "My baby sleeps just fine, thank you."

Equipment And Supplies

It seems these days that babies come with an amazing amount of "stuff." Babies actually don't need any "stuff." They simply need mom's breasts, dad's arms, and lots of love from both parents. However, some of the "stuff" does actually make parenting easier. Soft baby carriers ease the strain on parents' arms and backs, and allow life to continue easily with baby in tow. Later, a backpack can be tremendously helpful for a family on the go. Breastfed babies are quite portable—just a diaper or two in a bag, and you're off! If you're bottle-feeding you will want to investigate larger diaper bags and portable bottle warmers. Bottle-feeding families will need about a dozen bottles, unless they want to wash bottles more than once a day.

As for clothing, some cotton T-shirts (the ones that cover the diaper and have a snap crotch are best), a few sleepers, and a nice outfit or two will be plenty for a newborn. Babies grow very fast, so don't spend a lot of money on newborn-sized clothes. Hand-me-downs and clothes borrowed from your friends' babies can round out baby's wardrobe.

In considering diapers, there's the big debate of cloth versus disposable. However, with the new Velcro diaper covers and also the availability of diaper services, cloth may be almost as convenient as disposable, and it is clearly easier on the environment. Many families choose to use cloth diapers at home and disposables on the road. There can be so much laundry associated with a new baby, that an extra load of diapers isn't usually overwhelming.

All families who travel by car will need an approved car seat. If you buy or borrow a used seat, make sure it meets all current safety regulations. Also, keep in mind that any car seats that were involved in an automobile accident should never be reused due to possible internal damage and loss of integrity. Car seats for newborns should face the rear. The middle of the back seat is the safest place for baby to ride. Never put a baby in the front seat in a car with air bags.

Most families will want a bassinet or crib for baby to nap in, although the floor can work well, too. If you buy or borrow a crib, make sure it meets current standards. Slats should be close together and there should be no "points" or snags on which clothing can get caught. The mattress should fit firmly against the sides of the crib. For those who will have the baby with them in bed, a side-rail (designed for children's beds, but very useful for shared beds) or a special extension attached to the side of the bed can help families share sleep with more comfort.

All of the other "stuff" is purely optional—swings, strollers, even the nursery. You may even want to wait to redecorate a whole room until your child is old enough to make some of the choices, unless you like to redecorate frequently! (Those cute pastel bears and bunnies just don't seem to appeal to school-aged kids.) Keep toys simple and bright.

If someone gives you something or lends you something, great. If it makes you happy to see baby stuff in your home, by all means get it. Otherwise, wait until after your baby is born and see what "stuff" will make your life with baby easier and more enjoyable.

In the pages that follow, we have included resources that focus on your life with your newborn and decisions you will face. We have divided these resources into the following six categories to help focus your search for answers:

Take the time to carefully select the best resources for you. Share them with your partner, the parent of your child. You want to make the right decisions for yourself and your family, and these resources can help you feel confident about the choices you make.

General Overview

★★★★

Overall Rating
★★★★
Outstandingly comprehensive and illustrative, a must-have for any new parents

Design, Ease Of Use
★★★★
Companion booklet lists all "chapter" subtopics; real-life demos; concise and interesting

1–4 Stars

Publisher:
Vida Health Communications

Edition:
1987

Price:
$39.98

Media:
Videotape

Principal Subject:
Your Newborn

Newborn Subject:
General Overview

BABY BASICS (VIDEOTAPE)
The Complete Video Guide For New And Expectant Parents

 Terrific Resource For:
The how-tos of infant care and development (through a videotape)

 Recommended For:
Your Newborn

Description:

Focusing on the care and development of newborns and infants, this 110 minute videotape is divided into eight "chapters" with an accompanying booklet listing all subtopics. Combining professional advice and sample footage of four new families, this videotape takes parents through their newborn's life from birth onward. Chapters One and Two discuss "the newborn at birth" along with postpartum care of the mother. Chapter Three describes the newborn and new parents' first days at home with details about emotional adaptations, changes in the newborn, reflexes, development, signs of overstimulation, sleep states, and swaddling. "Daily Care" is the topic in Chapter Four with information about bathing, diapering, dressing, circumcision and umbilical care, and more. Chapter Five includes breastfeeding how-tos (positions, problems, expression, storage) and bottlefeeding information. Chapter Six focuses on "Health and Safety" with information on check-ups, immunizations, illnesses, and more. Chapter Seven discusses babies' cries and sleep patterns, while Chapter Eight describes babies' growth and development.

Evaluation:

The price tag is not exactly cheap, but this is the closest new parents will get to having a visual owners' manual to baby care. In fact, it will be like having a pediatrician/mother/close friend on hand offering the best advice and information every step of the way as new parents struggle "on the job." The footage is excellent with real life demonstrations in every case. The companion booklet is very well-thought out suggesting that parents start their VCR counter on "O," view the tape, and then record the counter number next to each subtopic listed in the booklet. This will make for quick easy access for busy new parents who haven't the time to scan through the tape's two hours looking for the information they need. The advice is up-to-date (despite its listed copyright date), and compiled from health care professionals, child development specialists, educators, and parents. The segment on breastfeeding in particular was outstanding offering advice and support for a subject that most often is learned visually but not often presented in that form. This video is a must whether as a gift for new parents, the focus of a parent education class, or to help train a child care provider.

Where To Find/Buy:

Bookstores, libraries, videotape dealers, or order direct by calling (800) 524-1013.

General Overview

CARING FOR YOUR BABY AND YOUNG CHILD
Birth To Age 5

 Recommended For:
Your Newborn

Description:

This 670 page reference book contains advice from the American Academy of Pediatrics and is broken into two parts. The first part contains advice on basic care from infancy through age five, along with guidelines and milestones for physical, emotional, social, and cognitive growth. Early chapters address such issues as: preparing for a new baby, birth and the moments after (in a hospital), basic infant care, and the basics of feeding a baby. In Chapters 5–12, advice is grouped by age and stage, i.e. newborn, the first month, one month through three months, four months to seven months, eight months to twelve months, the second year, the third year, the fourth, and the fifth year. Each of these groupings address growth and development, basic care, family, health watch, safety check, immunizations, and more. A chapter each is devoted to how to keep your child safe and how deal with part-time childcare issues. The second part of the book, with "guide words" at the top of the page, is a thorough medical reference guide for child-related topics (behavior, eyes, skin, etc.). A great many illustrations, information boxes, and tables are given.

Evaluation:

The American Academy of Pediatrics sponsored this book with contributions from 70+ "pediatric specialists and a six-member AAP editorial review board," making it a baseline standard for child care and pediatric medical information in America today. Beautifully illustrated and nicely designed for readability, this book has all the touches that publishers use to make a book easy to look at and digest. Where other books take a question and answer approach to providing information, this book lines up its topics and hands out advice in a straightforward and authoritative manner. In this way, it covers the same information as similar books on this topic, but seems to do it in a much more readable and inviting way. If one is making a choice on a first year baby book, this may well be **the** book.

Where To Find/Buy:

Bookstores and libraries.

★★★★

Overall Rating
★★★★
Comprehensive guide to children's physical, emotional, social and cognitive growth

Design, Ease Of Use
★★★★
Clear, concise, well-illustrated, and direct; excellent index

1–4 Stars

Author:
Steven P. Shelov, MD, FAAP

The Feeling Fine Programs and the American Academy of Pediatrics, an organization of 45,000 pediatricians dedicated to the health, safety, and well-being of infants, children, adolescents, and young adults, developed this book as the first of a three part series.

Publisher:
Bantam Books

Edition:
2nd (1993)

Price:
$17.95

Pages:
670

ISBN:
0553371843

Media:
Book

Principal Subject:
Your Newborn

Newborn Subject:
General Overview

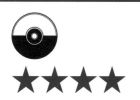

Overall Rating
★★★★
An informative look at how important quality care is on a child's brain development

Design, Ease Of Use
★★★★
Well-laid out CD-ROM; visually appealing and slick presentation; easy navigation

1–4 Stars

Publisher:
The Reiner Foundation
(Families & Work Institute/IBM)

Edition:
1997

Media:
CD-ROM

Principal Subject:
Your Newborn

Newborn Subject:
General Overview

General Overview

I AM YOUR CHILD (CD-ROM)
The First Three Years Last Forever

 Recommended For:
Your Newborn

Description:

This national public awareness campaign (funded by The Reiner Foundation, IBM, Families and Work Institute, and others) aims to make early childhood development a top priority based upon new research regarding brain development. Four options are available on their CD-ROM. "Brain Facts" highlight how undeveloped a child's brain is at birth. As the brain develops, the child's experiences and attachments within the first 3 years directly impact his emotional development, learning abilities, and how he functions later. Parents' "most pressing questions" and responses from "experts" are listed under "Parent Questions." "Ages & Stages" detail child development from prenatal to age three with "top experts" (Brazelton, Bowman, Koop, Perry) offering their child development advice and insight via downloadable QuickTime movie clips. Also given are ten "Key Guidelines" that summarize the experts' advice. A list of summarized resources and references is also available. An index is also provided.

Evaluation:

Opportunities exist every day to contribute to the healthy development of a baby or child's brain through experiences, affection, and other ways, and this CD-ROM reinforces this message. With recent attention focused on the plight of our nation's children and the lack of quality childcare, this campaign is timely. This CD-ROM offers "ten guidelines that can help parents and other caregivers raise healthy, happy children and confident, competent learners." The guidelines aren't novel ("talk, read, and sing to your child," "use discipline as an opportunity to teach," etc.). But, coupling them with the latest in brain research gives parents rationale for giving and demanding quality care for their child especially during those important first three years. This CD-ROM takes its position seriously; there are no "chats," humor, or a lighthanded look at parenting. It's free (with a $5.00 shipping and handling fee) and quantities are limited. Those seriously interested in children's welfare will be enlightened.

Where To Find/Buy:

Contact the I Am Your Child Campaign by calling (202) 338-4385, by FAX at (202) 338-2334, or through the mail at 1010 Wisconsin Ave., NW, Suite 800, Washington, D.C. 20007. There is a $5.00 shipping and handling fee.

General Overview

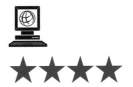

I AM YOUR CHILD (INTERNET)

 Recommended For:
Your Newborn

Description:

Founded by Rob Reiner, Michele Singer Reiner and others, this national "public awareness and engagement campaign to make early childhood development a top priority for our nation" offers eight options at the website homepage. "Key Issues" and "Brain Facts" highlight how undeveloped a child's brain is at birth. As the brain develops, the child's experiences and attachments within the first three years directly impact his emotional development, learning abilities, and how he functions later. Parents' "most pressing questions" and responses from "experts" are listed under "Parent Questions." "Ages & Stages" detail child development from prenatal to age three, and "top experts" (Brazelton, Bowman, Koop, Perry) offer their child development advice and insight via downloadable QuickTime movie clips. A list of summarized resources also is available. For those interested in working on behalf of children, two options offer information on this site's campaign, along with ways for communities to promote the cause.

Evaluation:

With recent attention focused on the plight of our nation's children and the lack of quality childcare, this campaign is timely. If you're a working parent with a child in daycare, you won't be guilt-tripped here. This site offers "ten guidelines that can help parents and other caregivers raise healthy, happy children and confident, competent learners." The guidelines aren't novel ("talk, read and sing to your child," "use discipline as an opportunity to teach," etc.). But, coupling them with the latest in brain research gives parents rationale for giving and demanding quality care for their child, especially during those first three years. Opportunities exist every day to contribute to the healthy development of a child's brain through experiences, affection and other ways, and this site reinforces this message. You won't find chats here, you won't find humor or a light-handed look at parenting. This site takes its position seriously. Those seriously interested in the welfare of children should visit and become informed, too.

Where To Find/Buy:

On the Internet at the URL: http://www.iamyourchild.org/

Overall Rating
★★★★
An informative look at how important quality care is on a child's brain development

Design, Ease Of Use
★★★★
Well-laid out site; downloadable QuickTime movie clips require lots of hard disk space

---

1–4 Stars

Publisher:
Yahoo!.com

Media:
Internet

Principal Subject:
Your Newborn

Newborn Subject:
General Overview

★★★★

Overall Rating
★★★★

An informative look at how important quality care is on a child's brain development

Design, Ease Of Use
★★★★

Good balance between scientific/research jargon and how-tos; engrossing footage

1–4 Stars

Publisher:
The Reiner Foundation (New Screen Concepts)

Edition:
1997

Price:
FREE

Media:
Videotape

Principal Subject:
Your Newborn

Newborn Subject:
General Overview

VI. Your Newborn

General Overview

I AM YOUR CHILD (VIDEOTAPE)
The First Years Last Forever

 Recommended For:
Your Newborn

Description:
Developed through the financial support of Johnson & Johnson and presented by The Reiner Foundation, this video focuses on how the experiences of a child's first three years can affect their brain development. Child professionals (Brazelton, Koop, Bowman, Siegel, Perry) discuss how parents can have a profound effect on a baby's ability to think, move, feel, communicate, and more based upon their interactions with their baby and child. Coupling footage of parental interactions with new research in brain development, this approximately 30 minute video is divided into seven segments: Bonding and Attachment, Communication, Health and Nutrition, Discipline, Self-Esteem, Child Care, and Self-Awareness. These child development specialists recommend parents: respond to a baby (touch, sing, read, tune in to their cries and nonverbal language), get good prenatal care and child health care, offer predictable boundaries and limits, value the child, find quality childcare, and more. The video highlights the parental-child connection as the most important because "with the right start, you can stay in touch for the rest of their lives."

Evaluation:
With recent attention focused on the plight of our nation's children and the lack of quality childcare, this video arising from the "I Am Your Child" campaign is timely. This video and its accompanying website offer guidelines for parents and caregivers to raise healthy, happy children and confident, competent learners. The guidelines aren't novel ("talk, read, and sing to your child," "use discipline as an opportunity to teach," etc.). But, coupling them with the latest in brain research gives parents rationale for giving and demanding quality care for their child especially during those first three years. Although there are no "chats," humor, or a lighthanded look at parenting, this video would be excellent for parent education classes for prospective parents. It's free (with a $5.00 shipping and handling fee) and quantities are limited. Opportunities exist daily to contribute to the healthy development of a child's brain through experiences, affection, and other ways, and this video reinforces this message.

Where To Find/Buy:
Contact the I Am Your Child Campaign by calling (202) 338-4385, by FAX at (202) 338-2334, or through the mail at 1010 Wisconsin Ave., NW, Suite 800, Washington, D.C. 20007. There is a $5.00 shipping and handling fee.

General Overview

THE JOY OF TWINS AND OTHER MULTIPLE BIRTHS
Having, Raising, And Loving Babies Who Arrive In Groups

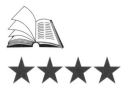

Terrific Resource For:
Raising and taking care of twins or multiples

Recommended For:
Your Newborn

Description:

The author states that this 324 page resource grew out of her belief that "twinship is a gift: to parents who can learn they are far more capable that they ever dreamed . . ." There are 12 chapters in this parenting guide. Chapter 1 explains how multiple births occur, while Chapter 2 discusses how parents can understand and take care of themselves and their babies after birth. Chapters 3 and 4 offer the "how-tos and whys" of feeding, and developing attitudes and routines through the first year. The next four chapters include information on mothercare, family adjustments, going back to work, and language ability. Developing a sense of identity is the focus of Chapter 9. A quick-reference list is offered in chapter 10. Chapter 11 deals with premature births and chapter 12 offers tips on how to deal with more than two babies. A reader questionnaire, a list of resources, a bibliography, and an index complete the book. Sidebar tips are given in bold, along with numerous black and white photographs throughout.

Evaluation:

This book strives to offer a realistic and positive outlook to parents of multiples. This guide, taking a look at the most "recent research," shows parents options they may not have considered in raising their children. Myths about having multiples are dispelled throughout this resource helping parents cope with the advice and comments of others. The book is meant to be used as a "browse through" to fetch useful ideas when parents don't really have time to sit down and read. The index is extensive allowing for easy access to specific topics. There is an incredible 8 page bibliography, and the "Resources" section lists: useful organizations for parents of multiples; information sources for childbirth, infant and new mother care; parent and marriage support groups; baby equipment; and additional periodicals and publications. While this guide does not spend too much energy on any one topic, it touches on the important primary issues, mainly parenting twins. As a quick reference, this book offers a good deal of information and support.

Where To Find/Buy:

Bookstores and libraries.

Overall Rating
★★★★
This resource offers fundamental information with a positive approach

Design, Ease Of Use
★★★★
Sidebar tips, numerous black and white photos; extensive resource and bibliography section

1–4 Stars

Author:
Pamela Patrick Novotny

Pamela Patrick Novotny is a journalist whose work has appeared in many magazines and newspapers. She currently teaches writing at the University of Colorado. She is the parent of five children, two of which are twins.

Publisher:
Crown Trade Paperbacks (Crown Books)

Edition:
2nd (1994)

Price:
$16.00

Pages:
324

ISBN:
0517880717

Media:
Book

Principal Subject:
Your Newborn

Newborn Subject:
General Overview

VI. Your Newborn

★★★★

Overall Rating
★★★★
This complete guide includes advice from child development experts & professionals

Design, Ease Of Use
★★★★
Side tabs for each age group; extensive index; reader friendly

1–4 Stars

Author:
Laura Walther Nathanson, MD, FAAP

Nathanson, M.D., is board Certified in Pediatrics and Peri-Neonatology. She earned her B.A. from Harvard and her M.D. from Tufts Medical School. She has handled over 100,000 office visits, more than twice as many phone calls, and says she still hears something new.

Publisher:
HarperPerennial (HarperCollins)

Edition:
1994

Price:
$20.00

Pages:
502

ISBN:
0062731769

Media:
Book

Principal Subject:
Your Newborn

Newborn Subject:
General Overview

General Overview

THE PORTABLE PEDIATRICIAN FOR PARENTS

 Recommended For:
Your Newborn

Description:
Reflecting recommendations from professional organizations (American Academy of Pediatrics, American Academy of Pediatric Dentistry, etc.) and child development researchers (Burton L. White, Erik Erickson, Jean Piaget, etc.), this 502 page resource offers a month-to-month guide to children's physical and behavioral development from birth to 5 years of age. Part I encompasses most of the book and discusses "The Well Child." The 11 chapters within this part focus on a given age range; topics that are discussed within each chapter include: a narrative description of the age group, separation issues, setting limits, health and illness, day to day issues (developmental milestones, sleep, growth, teeth, feeding and nutrition, activities, etc.), "windows of opportunity," and more. Part II focuses on "frightening behaviors" (fever, inconsolable crying, etc.), first aid, and bodily ailments. Part III offers six essays from a pediatric's point of view. Part IV offers pediatric "Handouts" designed to alleviate disagreements between parents, relatives, and caregivers. Part V is a glossary of medical terms. A 17 page index is also provided.

Evaluation:
By using her background as a pediatrician coupled with studies by well-known child development researchers, Dr. Laura Walther Nathanson allows parents to see growth and changes from the child's point of view. She then strongly encourages parents to view their child's pediatrician as a team player who should be interested in informing, but not advising, parents. With her experience of over "100,000 office visits and more than twice as many phone calls," she is able to give detailed, age appropriate information regarding medical and developmental questions. And, if the reader is still in doubt, she encourages them to seek professional advice. This resource, then, is a most unusual book—parents won't find many better resources available that offer a variety of professionals' advice and suggestions in one neat affordable package.

Where To Find/Buy:
Bookstores and libraries.

General Overview

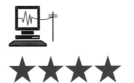

MOMS ONLINE (AOL)
A Home For Moms In Cyberspace

★★★★

Terrific Resource For:
Advice and support for new moms through online dialogs with other moms

Recommended For:
Your Newborn

Description:

Found on AOL using the Keyword: Mom's Online. Several options are available at Moms Online's homepage, "A home for Moms in cyberspace." "Chat" and "Message Boards" offer forums for moms to discuss parenting issues. The "Daily Alexander" is a running chronicle about raising a four-year old boy and a baby girl, and being a working mom (Dad contributes an article on Wednesdays). The "Daily Sphinx" is a daily game of three questions related to maternal trivia. "Hot Tips" consists of contributions from moms on various subjects ranging from choosing a pediatrician to limiting TV-time. "Weekly Magazine" features a new mom in "Mom of the Week," along with her perspectives in raising children, strengths, and weaknesses, etc. It also offers essays written by various moms, "The Guidance Council," crafts, and articles on various other topics. Other links include a weekly poll, an advice link called "Ask the Pros," and "The Baby Namer." Two other major links are "The Daily Dish," an index of recipes and kitchen tips submitted by moms, and "Time Out, The Virtual Spa for Moms," which includes "comfort corners," humor, and creative projects. A "Teen Center" is available for parents with teens as well as "Homeschooling Center."

Evaluation:

This website's strength lies in its unusual format—its use of journals, articles, and submissions from moms. Trust is placed in moms as experts, a refreshing stance for moms who often feel defeated, overly advised, or powerless. Moms are invited to chat with one another, discuss issues, offer "hot tips," submit articles, nominate moms for "Mom of the Week," ask questions, and offer feedback to the site, making this an inviting place to air frustrations and voice celebrations. Moms can even find a link pertinent for their needs, when it is time to take a brief mental break from life as a parent. A database of recipes and kitchen tips submitted by moms is available for any occasion, even those quick, low-fat, recipes with few ingredients that all hurried moms love to have on hand. Reading the ongoing saga of life with a four-year old and a baby, and how one family works through its problems makes this website come alive. What one will not find here are hard facts or objective information; parents will need to find that information elsewhere. However, Moms Online is a friendly, fun, and supportive home for moms needing a lift in their day.

Where To Find/Buy:

Found on AOL using the Keyword: "Mom's Online"; also found on the Internet at the URL: http//www.momsonline.com/

Overall Rating
★★★★
An active community of moms, packed with useful and fun information

Design, Ease Of Use
★★★
Novel use of journaling and essays by moms; easy-to-follow layout

1–4 Stars

Media:
Online Service

Principal Subject:
Your Newborn

Newborn Subject:
General Overview

VI. Your Newborn

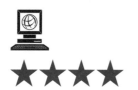

★★★★

Overall Rating
★★★★
An active community of moms, packed with useful and fun information

Design, Ease Of Use
★★★
Novel use of journaling and essays by moms; easy-to-follow layout

1–4 Stars

Media:
Internet

Principal Subject:
Your Newborn

Newborn Subject:
General Overview

General Overview

MOMS ONLINE (INTERNET)
A Home For Moms In Cyberspace

 Terrific Resource For:
Advice and support for new moms through Internet dialogs with other moms

 Recommended For:
Your Newborn

Description:

Fourteen options are available at Moms Online's homepage, "A home for Moms in cyberspace." "Chat" and "Message Boards" offer forums for moms to discuss parenting issues. The "Daily Alexander" is a running chronicle about raising a four-year old boy and a baby girl, and being a working mom (Dad contributes an article on Wednesdays). The "Daily Sphinx" is a daily game of three questions related to maternal trivia. "Hot Tips" consists of contributions from moms on various subjects ranging from choosing a pediatrician to limiting TV-time. "Weekly Magazine" features a new mom in "Mom of the Week," along with her perspectives in raising children, strengths, and weaknesses, etc. It also offers essays written by various moms, "The Guidance Council," crafts, and articles on various other topics. Other links include a weekly poll, an advice link called "Ask the Pros," and "The Baby Namer." Two other major links are "The Daily Dish," an index of recipes and kitchen tips submitted by moms, and "Time Out, The Virtual Spa for Moms," which includes "comfort corners," humor, and creative projects.

Evaluation:

This website's strength lies in its unusual format—its use of journals, articles, and submissions from moms. Trust is placed in moms as experts, a refreshing stance for moms who often feel defeated, overly advised, or powerless. Moms are invited to chat with one another, discuss issues, offer "hot tips," submit articles, nominate moms for "Mom of the Week," ask questions, and offer feedback to the site, making this an inviting place to air frustrations and voice celebrations. Moms can even find a link pertinent for their needs, when it is time to take a brief mental break from life as a parent. A database of recipes and kitchen tips submitted by moms is available for any occasion, even those quick, low-fat, recipes with few ingredients that all hurried moms love to have on hand. Reading the ongoing saga of life with a four-year old and a baby, and how one family works through its problems makes this website come alive. What one will not find here are hard facts or objective information; parents will need to find that information elsewhere. However, Moms Online is a friendly, fun, and supportive home for moms in cyberspace.

Where To Find/Buy:

On the Internet at the URL: http://www.momsonline.com/

General Overview

THE BABY BOOK
Everything You Need To Know About Your Baby—From Birth To Age Two

★★★

Description:
Pediatric specialists and parents of 8, Sears and his wife present their parenting philosophy as it relates to the practice of raising children in this 689 page, 28 chapter book. Detailing their parenting style—"attachment parenting"—in chapter 1, Sears uses this as a foundation for the remainder of the book. You will find 5 parts to this book focusing on topics for parents of newborns through age 2. These 5 parts deal with "Baby-Care Basics" (giving birth through the early weeks); "Infant Feeding and Nutrition" (breastfeeding, bottlefeeding, solid foods, toddler feeding); "Contemporary Parenting" ("babywearing," nighttime parenting, parenting the "fussy or colicky baby," working outside your home); "Infant Development and Behavior" (0–6 months, 6–12 months, the second year, toddler behaviors, toilet training); and "Keeping Your Baby Safe and Healthy" (baby-proofing, checkups, immunizations, medicines, self-help home care, lifesaving procedures, and first aid). Personal anecdotes from their own children as well as patients are used by the authors for illustration purposes throughout the text.

Evaluation:
A conscientious new parent has zillions of nagging questions, e.g. "should I let my baby cry or should I pick her up? Should I let the baby sleep with me or should he sleep alone? Should I breastfeed my baby or bottlefeed?" Different experts answer these questions in different ways since there are several schools of thought and differing philosophies about raising a child. The Searses describe "attachment parenting" here as one in which parents use five "tools" to "get connected to [their] baby" which include, connecting early with one's baby, reading and responding to her/his cues, breastfeeding, "wearing" the baby, and sharing sleep with one's baby. This book, then, is for those who believe that a baby who forms a strong attachment to their caretakers (trusting them to fulfill all his or her emotional, social and physical needs) will feel secure and self-confident. Whether one buys into Sears' parenting style or not, their medical advice and behavioral descriptions are universally useful, in particular their section on how to handle a baby with colic. Some of their medical information (immunizations in particular), however, needs to be updated.

Where To Find/Buy:
Bookstores and libraries.

Overall Rating
★★★
The "bible" for those who enjoy a philosophy of non-authoritarian parenting

Design, Ease Of Use
★★★★
Anecdotes interspersed throughout; table of contents lists subtopics; extensive index

1–4 Stars

Author:
William Sears, MD & Martha Sears, RN

Sears, "one of America's most renowned pediatricians," has been in practice for 20 years and authored 10 books. Currently, he's a clinical assistant professor of pediatrics at USC School of Medicine. His wife is a childbirth educator, registered nurse, & breastfeeding consultant.

Publisher:
Little, Brown and Company

Edition:
1993

Price:
$21.95

Pages:
689

ISBN:
0316779059

Media:
Book

Principal Subject:
Your Newborn

Newborn Subject:
General Overview

VI. Your Newborn

★★★

Overall Rating
★★★
Great all-inclusive guide; immunizations discussion needs updating

Design, Ease Of Use
★★★★
500+ color photographs, drawings, graphs, & charts; color coding makes for easy access

1–4 Stars

Author:
Miriam Stoppard, MD
Miriam Stoppard, M.D., is the author of many bestselling books on pregnancy and childcare.

Publisher:
Dorling Kindersley
(Carroll & Brown Limited)

Edition:
1995

Price:
$29.95

Pages:
352

ISBN:
1564588505

Media:
Book

Principal Subject:
Your Newborn

Newborn Subject:
General Overview

General Overview

COMPLETE BABY AND CHILD CARE

Description:
This 352 page reference contains six major chapters. Chapter 1 contains behavior and health information about newborn babies. The second chapter deals with a child's everyday care including their environment, feeding, dressing, bathing, crying/comforting, and sleeping. Children's development (physical, speech and language, and mental), teeth, vision, hearing, and social behavior are a few of the topics in Chapter 3. The fourth chapter focuses on family life and discusses such topics as organization, separation and divorce, and multiple births. Children with special needs are addressed in Chapter 5, and the final chapter contains information about medicine and health care. Each topic is separated into four age groups (young baby, older baby, toddler, and preschool child), with color-coded bands given to access key information for each gender and age group. Illustrations and photographs guide parents through suggested routines. The book includes a first aid section, contact info for organizations, and an index.

Evaluation:
The word for this visually appealing book is simply, "WOW!" Case studies, tips, extensive illustrations, and graphs are just the tip of the iceberg in describing this very well-presented guide. The book has made every effort to touch all aspects of child care, and has done an excellent job, although some updating needs to be done in terms of immunizations. The information is intelligent, with in-depth advice on topics as diverse as bathing a baby, to coping with disorders such as epilepsy and dyslexia. Special panels on the side of the page highlight and explain the differences in caring for and the differences in development between boys and girls in many areas. Case studies provide new insights, while medical facts help answer common parental questions. New parents will find Dr. Stoppard's commonsense approach informing, reassuring, and inspiring. This guide's index, while somewhat brief, includes boldly highlighted topics along with related subtopics for easy access. In short, this is a wonderful book, thoughtfully constructed, offering valuable information in a sensitive, compassionate, while professional, manner.

Where To Find/Buy:
Bookstores and libraries.

General Overview

★★★

WHAT EVERY BABY KNOWS

Description:

This resource takes the reader through the lives of five families. The book is divided into five major sections, each of which reflect the family histories and then delve into each family's core. Part I is about the Cotton family (who have twins) with information concerning their quiet child/active child, a section about sibling rivalry, and discipline within this family. Part II focuses on the Mazza family, their separation and divorce, and the sleep problems they have had with their child. Part III is about the Considine family, questions they have about their child's crying, the feelings of their middle child, and concerns about a non-walking child. Part IV follows the Sheehan-Weber family with issues involving early learning, stressful situations, and self-esteem. The final section, Part V, is about the Schwartz family, their new baby, and their expectations. Part VI outlines the family systems theory underlying the work of Brazelton's Child Development Unit and the link between the five families in this book and the "brand of behavioral pediatrics" developed in the Unit's program.

Evaluation:

This book contains some very valuable, timeless information. It is a well-written book, with clear, concise information set in a question-answer format making it a very enjoyable reading experience. The content is thorough and does a fine job of yielding to the old textbook-type format without being aloof. Parents are given the rare opportunity of following five families through their parenting struggles, enabling the reader to more closely identify and relate to specific questions they may share with the sample families. Brazelton provides sensitive answers with appropriate developmental background information. He carefully dissects each family's issues and concerns, then allows the reader to share in his follow-up when he revisits them and sees "where they are now." There are many black and white photographs throughout this resource which help to illustrate the subject matter; content is well-supported by research with a clear bibliography and index concluding the guide. Add this book to your family library for professional advice on parenting with a personal flavor.

Where To Find/Buy:

Bookstores and libraries.

Overall Rating
★★★
Unique approach; although written some time ago, basic information still prevails

Design, Ease Of Use
★★★★
Clear and concise; question-answer format makes for untiring reading; consistent format

1–4 Stars

Author:
T. Berry Brazelton, MD

Dr. Brazelton, one of the most-renowned pediatricians, is a Professor of Pediatrics at Harvard Medical School, as well as chief of the Child Development Unit at Boston Children's Hospital. He is also a political advocate for families and has a TV show.

Publisher:
Ballantine Books
(Random House)

Edition:
1987

Price:
$11.00

Pages:
272

ISBN:
0345344553

Media:
Book

Principal Subject:
Your Newborn

Newborn Subject:
General Overview

VI. Your Newborn

★★★

Overall Rating
★★★
Comprehensive, balanced, supportive; needs updating re: SIDS, immunizations, etc.

Design, Ease Of Use
★★★
Easy to read, easy to reference; unclear as to why sections are numbered

1–4 Stars

Author:
Benjamin Spock, MD, and Michael B. Rothenberg, MD

Benjamin Spock, M.D., practiced pediatrics in New York City from 1933 to 1947. Then he became a medical teacher and researcher. Michael B. Rothenberg, M.D., is a pediatrician and child psychiatrist who had combined these two fields in his work since 1957.

Publisher:
Pocket Books
(Simon & Schuster)

Edition:
6th (1992)

Price:
$7.99

Pages:
832

ISBN:
0671760602

Media:
Book

Principal Subject:
Your Newborn

Newborn Subject:
General Overview

General Overview

DR. SPOCK'S BABY AND CHILD CARE
The One Essential Parenting Book

Description:

Dr. Spock and Dr. Rothenberg together have created a sixth edition of the well-known Dr. Spock Baby and Child Care Book. This 832 page book is written in short numbered sections of about a page each. Each numbered entry covers a single aspect of child care. Sections are grouped into subject categories such as: the role of the parents, equipment and clothing, medical and nursing care, infant feeding, breastfeeding, bottlefeeding, daily care, problems of infancy, managing young children, age related issues (from birth to adolescence), child development, illness, special situations, and many more subjects. Although information is provided from the perspective of the authors, two persons with documented authority and experience on the subject, it is written in a first person format. The clear intent of this book is to provide factual and supportive information for first-time parents so they can handle the huge learning curve they need to climb in order to become well-informed parents.

Evaluation:

Spock's reassuring voice may be just the one a new parent needs to hear in order to claim some personal control over a new and occasionally anxious situation. Parents face a world offering various opinions on what a parent should or should not do, what is good and what is not good for the child. This book attempts to provide a balanced and experienced perspective in a positive and succinct way. The scope of this book is massive; every possible topic appears to be touched on at least briefly. The style of writing is authoritative, yet done in a gentle and inviting manner, allowing the reader to reflect on all possible options and not feel that it must be done "the Dr. Spock way." For the most part, the organization of the book is clear and easily referenced. While not the kind of book one sits down to read straight through, each section is written in an interesting and factual way. Some sections definitely need updating due to latest findings (SIDS, immunizations, etc.); other sections reflect the author's opinion (sometimes inconsistent with current scientific fact), but generally the book seems fresh and relevant whether your child is six days or six years old.

Where To Find/Buy:

Bookstores and libraries.

General Overview

KIDSOURCE ONLINE

Description:

This online community, created by a group of parents with varied backgrounds, aims to find "the best of the healthcare and education information . . . and deliver it . . . in new and innovative ways. . . ." General options on the site's homepage offer various articles under the headings of "Education," "Health," "Recreation," "Parenting," "Guide to Best Software," "New Products," and more. Specific options address four age groups—newborns, toddlers, preschoolers, and K–12. Within these categories are subtopic headings that lead to links on topics such as safety, specific areas (education, health, growth & development, parenting, etc.), online forums, websites, and other related areas. Also listed within these categories are articles categorized by what's new, recent recalls, and product information. Brief descriptions of these articles are offered. Most of the articles within this website are ranked using a five star system, with five stars being "best, in depth and most helpful overall." A list of articles is then presented, along with a brief synopsis of the article's contents and its rating; generally, articles average two to three pages.

Evaluation:

This well-organized site hosts unusual contributors—the U.S. Department of Education, child-related organizations (child abuse consortia, etc.) and associations (learning disabilities), among others. The articles' succinct nature, positive tone, and friendly voice easily can be handled by any busy parent. Rating the articles presents yet another convenient way to ease up on the plethora of articles that face a parent interested in getting some new information and advice. Graphics are absent from the site intentionally, say the creators, because "most of (the) visiting parents do not have time to wait for extensive graphics to download"; the site will upgrade its design as parents upgrade their systems. The general discussion forums are well-organized and titled. Unfortunately, the age specific forums were cumbersome, simply consisting of a running list of titles; subject groupings would be more helpful. This site is a good informational site; other sites, however, provide better opportunities for discussions and chats with other parents.

Where To Find/Buy:

On the Internet at the URL: http://www.kidsource.com/

Overall Rating

★★★

Unusual contributors, succinct articles make research an easy and interesting task

Design, Ease Of Use

★★★

Graphics are absent; articles are cross-referenced and rated according to a 5 star system

---

1–4 Stars

Media:
Internet

Principal Subject:
Your Newborn

Newborn Subject:
General Overview

VI. Your Newborn

General Overview

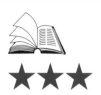

OUR BABIES, OURSELVES
How Biology And Culture Shape The Way We Parent

Overall Rating
★★★
Well-researched, intriguing look at the emerging field of ethnopediatrics

Design, Ease Of Use
★★★
Attractive; information is dense yet well-written and readable

1–4 Stars

Author:
Meredith F. Small

Small is a professor of anthropology at Cornell University. She is author of *Female Choices: Sexual Behavior of Female Primates* and *What's Love Got to Do with It? The Evolution of Human Mating.*

Publisher:
Anchor Books (Bantam Doubleday Dell Publishing Group)

Edition:
1998

Price:
$24.95

Pages:
292

ISBN:
0385482574

Media:
Book

Principal Subject:
Your Newborn

Newborn Subject:
General Overview

Description:

Our Babies, Ourselves is presented as "the first book to explore to what extent the way we parent our infants is based on our biological needs and to what extent it is based on culture—and the startling consequences ignoring nature's imperatives can have on the well-being of our children." Small's 292 page book is laid out in seven chapters: "The Evolution of Babies"; "The Anthropology of Parenting" (description of the concept of ethnopediatrics); "Other Parents, Other Ways" (comparisons of various societies and how their societal impacts and is impacted by parenting styles); "A Reasonable Sleep" (an examination of infant sleep patterns and sleep locations); "Crybaby" (description of "infant state" including crying, temperament, etc.); "Food for Thought" (breastfeeding, bottlefeeding); and "Unpacking the Caretaking Package" (how to navigate the parenting choices available and "weigh a series of trade-offs"). A center section of photographs illustrates varying cultural baby-rearing styles. Also included are extensive note, reference, and index sections.

Evaluation:

Small combines her years of experience in cultural anthropology with the new science of ethnopediatrics to study "why we parent our children the way that we do." By comparing parenting styles across cultural boundaries, from the most primitive to the most sophisticated, Small seeks to cut through cultural ethnocentricity to find out which baby-rearing practices offer the most benefits to infants and their newly formed families. "Each culture, and often each family, offers advice and directives on the right and wrong way to raise and care for infants, from feeding, interaction, and emotional support to mandating what is normal in terms of infant sleeping, crying, and more. Yet scientists are finding that . . . the right way to parent our children is often based on nothing more than cultural tradition—and may even run counter to a baby's biological needs." Small concludes that cultural practices such as nestling a child to sleep with her parents, allowing her to feed on demand, and spending most of his time in tactile contact with his mother and others are examples of cultural choices that actually benefit a baby's physical health and psychological development. The text is a bit dense, but it packs within it quite a lot of interesting knowledge.

Where To Find/Buy:
Bookstores and libraries.

General Overview

YOUR AMAZING NEWBORN

★★★

Description:

Authors Marshall and Phyllis Klaus combine their years of experience in the field of newborn development with 120 photographs of babies less than two weeks old to present information on how babies and those who love them bond in the first days of life. This 113 page book is presented in 10 chapters, including: "Before Birth: Dawning Awareness;" "The First Minutes;" "Waking to the World;" "Newborn Sight"; "Newborn Hearing"; "Touch, Taste and Smell"; "Motions and Rhythms"; "Expressions and Emotions"; "The Newly Adopted Baby"; and "The Newborn Family." The black and white photographs range from fetal images to newborns up to two weeks of age. The photos are used to illustrate ways babies and their families instinctively move toward and within "an intimate and reciprocal choreography." Also included is an authors' preface, a notes section, and an index.

Evaluation:

Make no mistake here: the eyes have it. Or, in the case of these tiny newborns, their entire cherubic faces. *Your Amazing Newborn* uses more than 100 black and white photos of babies less than two weeks old to illustrate how newborns and their families find one another and naturally bond, when allowed the instinctual closeness they crave. The Klaus' expertise in the field allows them to present the most up-to-date findings on how newborns develop. While the photos will draw your attention first, you'll come back for the information contained within the text itself. Readers will view images of a newborn less than one hour old crawling unassisted to the mother's breast, recognizing the parents' voices, and shutting out unwanted sights and sounds. Experience here the first gaze, the first reach, the first spark of recognition "that ignites a lifetime bond." This is a priceless book for all who love innocence and breathtaking inner wisdom of a newborn. It would also make a delightful gift for prospective parents.

Where To Find/Buy:

Bookstores and libraries.

Overall Rating
★★★
Beautiful book that inspires awe at the miracle of a newborn

Design, Ease Of Use
★★★
Effective combination of text and black and white photographs

1–4 Stars

Author:
Marshall H. Klaus, MD, and Phyllis H. Klaus, CSW, MFCC

Klaus, neonatologist and researcher, teaches pediatrics at the University of California, San Francisco, School of Medicine, and is author of several works in that field. Klaus teaches and practices psychotherapy at the Erikson Institute in Santa Rosa.

Publisher:
Perseus Books

Edition:
1998

Price:
$20.00

Pages:
113

ISBN:
0738200131

Media:
Book

Principal Subject:
Your Newborn

Newborn Subject:
General Overview

VI. Your Newborn

★★★

Overall Rating
★★★

Focuses more on caring for the older baby through age five; some info on newborn care

Design, Ease Of Use
★★★

Compact print difficult to read; consistent format; numerous color photos and charts

1–4 Stars

Author:
Penelope Leach

Leach, with a Ph.D. in psychology, is a Fellow of the British Psychological Society and a founding member of the UK branch of the World Association for Infant Mental Health. She is a leading authority and advocate in the field of child development and care.

Publisher:
Alfred A. Knopf
(Random House)

Edition:
3rd (1997)

Price:
$20.00

Pages:
559

ISBN:
0375700005

Media:
Book

Principal Subject:
Your Newborn

Newborn Subject:
General Overview

General Overview

YOUR BABY & CHILD
From Birth To Age Five

Description:

This third revised edition of Leach's book incorporates the "latest research and thinking on child development and learning, and reflects the realities of today's . . . new approaches to parenting." Leach is also known for her TV series under the same title—"Your Baby & Child." This 559 page resource is divided up into five sections which include information on newborns, babies in their first six months, older babies (from six months to one year), toddlers (one year to two and a half), and young children (from two and a half to five years). Each section includes characteristics for each age group, such as feeding/eating and growing, teeth and teething, everyday care, excreting, sleeping, and crying and comforting. Some sections also contain material on the senses, muscles, eyesight and hearing, listening and speaking skills, and playing and learning/thinking skills. The book is written in a text format with italic side bar headings, full color illustrations, charts, and highlighted question and answer sections. An index concludes the book.

Evaluation:

If parents want a book that covers nearly every aspect of childcare in terms of an older baby's development through the age of five, they should choose this one. This resource provides parents and caregivers with the information they need to truly understand and enhance their child's growth. However, parents of newborns will find their questions answered but in a rather clinical manner; advice on breastfeeding is adequate but not definitive, and is sometimes derogatory. For example, in describing benefits of bottlefeeding, Leach states that it "let[s] you off the intense (and sometimes uncomfortable) physical and emotional involvement with your baby that establishing breast-feeding requires." Different to this version is the absence of a medical section. Instead, it has been replaced by tinted text sections offering parent's point of views on various subjects. While not necessarily reflecting the author's opinion, these opinions may open up debate issues as parents strengthen their beliefs—for example, "any toddler who bites . . . should be bitten . . . back." New questions have been added along with notes on hazards and safety guidelines. This book's advice sometimes reflects the author's perspective, but on the whole it is well-researched.

Where To Find/Buy:
Bookstores and libraries.

General Overview

BABY MANEUVERS

Description:

The author, a veteran traveler prior to being a parent, aims to provide reassurance and information to parents about the logistics of toting supplies and traveling anywhere with young children. Fourteen chapters make up this 224 page guide which is divided into three main parts to gradually ease parents into maneuvering around with their child—The Crawling Maneuvers (chapters 2–4), The Walking Maneuvers (chapters 5–10), and Advanced Baby Maneuvers (chapters 11–14). Chapter topics include dealing with: bodily functions on the road (breastfeeding, diapers, etc.), eating out, day trips (errands, grocery store, zoo, etc.), types of travel (by foot, car, boat, train, bus), what to pack in a day pack, air travel, types of vacation lodgings, outdoor adventures, traveling alone with a child, work travel with a baby, and overseas travel. Each chapter begins with bulleted points that summarize what will be covered. A page-by-page listing of the book's contents is included in the table of contents. Two appendices (odds and ends, resources) and an index complete the book. Lutz's tips are included throughout in colored block insets.

Evaluation:

No other book deals quite as thoroughly with this subject as this one, almost exhaustingly, does. Whether parents are beginning "baby maneuvers" or already feel confident with baby on outings, they will be sure to find advice in this book that they've never come across before. The author's tone is very friendly; her humor is delightful and sure to receive a knowing glance from her audience—"the supermarket can be fun, or a trip through a chamber of horrors." A principal problem with this book, however, is that it is often difficult for the reader to maneuver through its content. Each chapter is broken into too many subheadings causing one to oftentimes become confused and/or exhausted. All that aside, this guide would make an unusual baby shower gift or perhaps a wonderful read prior to a family's first vacation together.

Where To Find/Buy:

Bookstores and libraries.

★★★

Overall Rating
★★★
Advice from a seasoned traveler on how to parent a child while on the road with them

Design, Ease Of Use
★★
Humorous and engaging, but numerous subheadings within chapters halt navigation

1–4 Stars

Author:
Ericka Lutz

Lutz writes fiction and non-fiction and travels extensively with her daughter, now four years old. Her writings have been published in books, magazines, and periodicals nationwide including *Parents' Press, Chicago Baby,* and the anthology, "Child of Mine."

Publisher:
Alpha Books (Macmillan General Reference/Simon and Schuster Macmillan)

Edition:
1997

Price:
$14.95

Pages:
224

ISBN:
0028617320

Media:
Book

Principal Subject:
Your Newborn

Newborn Subject:
General Overview

★★★

Overall Rating
★★★
Author's approach presents facts, disputes myths, so parents can be decision-makers

Design, Ease Of Use
★★
Vague table of contents; good headings within book; book's size & weight cumbersome

1–4 Stars

Author:
Marianne Egeland Neifert, MD, with Anne Price and Nancy Dana

Neifert is an award-winning pediatrician, professor of pediatrics, and mother of five children.

Publisher:
Signet
(Dutton Signet/Penguin Books)

Edition:
1986

Price:
$6.99

Pages:
529

ISBN:
0451163117

Media:
Book

Principal Subject:
Your Newborn

Newborn Subject:
General Overview

General Overview

DR. MOM
A Guide To Baby And Child Care

Description:

Neifert coined the name "Dr. Mom" because she believes strongly in "the importance of nurturing new parents, in order to bring to blossom their long-term competency." Her 529 page book is divided into 17 chapters. The first three focus on preparation for parenthood from making the decision to giving birth to outfitting the nursery. Chapters 4–6 center on newborn and infant care. Children's development (birth to age five) is discussed in Chapter 7. Chapter 9 offers 10 pages of information on "toilet learning." Chapter 8—"The Challenge of Parenting" addresses discipline choices, while Chapter 10 focuses on understanding various behaviors (tantrums, biting, pacifiers, etc.). The next 3 chapters offer information on caring for a sick child, dealing with illnesses and disorders (80 pages), and what to do in an emergency. The pros, the cons, and feedback on "contemporary concerns" (sexual abuse, kidnapping, the family bed, breastfeeding in public, etc.) are presented in Chapter 14. The last three chapters deal with parenting styles and family strategies (nonsexist, working parents, single families, divorce, etc.).

Evaluation:

Neifert does a fine job of commingling her personal experiences as the mother of five with her professional aspiration to nurture new parents by "acknowledging their good intentions and sound intuition . . . supplying them with factual information . . . (so that they can) meet their children's needs. . . ." Throughout her book, she grants parents the privilege of making their own decisions on parenting issues. Some resources do a better job dealing with topics such as toilet training/learning, discipline, and behavior. Neifert's book does a better job at examining the various sides of "hot" issues today such as the family bed, nursing in public places, and more. Some information is outdated due to the book's copyright so, as always, parents should check with their baby's doctor before making certain decisions. The book's size is awkward; hopefully future editions will be a larger format with fewer pages making it easier to hold and read. The section on illnesses/disorders is well-done and comparable to that found in better resources. Not recommended for use on its own, this book would be a welcome companion to another more inclusive resource.

Where To Find/Buy:

Bookstores, libraries, or order direct by contacting Penguin USA at P.O. Box 999, Dept. #17109, Bergenfield, NJ 07621.

General Overview

PARENT'S OWNER'S MANUAL: NEWBORN
Volume I: A Child Care Series

Description:

Creative Outlook's goal is to "ease your transition into parenting and enhance your comfort level in this new role." To that end, they have broken this 55 minute videotape into various segments: baby furniture (essentials), different ways of holding and picking up a baby, what to do when baby cries, using a pacifier, swaddling, feeding (breastfeeding, bottlefeeding), burping, diapering (pros and cons of cloth/disposables, how-tos), buying the layette (safety and comfort constraints), dressing, bathing (sponge bath, infant bath), sleeping (how-tos, sleep positions), nail trimming, "the medicine box" (essential supplies, medical aids), playtime, and packing the diaper bag for outings. Each segment includes live footage taken of parents as they illustrate the narrator's dialogue. In many cases, numbered highlights appear on the screen to isolate main points. Freeze frame techniques are also used to capture highlights in various segments.

Evaluation:

Parents who are visual learners and work best with live hands-on instructions may appreciate this tape. Others will do better to invest their money in other resources that offer more in-depth information about the same topics. Although this tape's intent is applaudable, once parents have seen it a few times, they'll wonder why they invested time and money in it at all. This tape's primary value would be in its use for new parents-to-be perhaps as a follow up for a parenting class on newborn care. For home use, however, its possibilities are limited. Viewers will also note subtle biases: the discrepancy between the details given for bottlefeeding compared to those for breastfeeding, advice to increase response time to baby's cries, and advice on training a baby to sleep on its own. Additionally, sleep positions described do not reflect new SIDS research. Parents will find that this videotape is not a complete "owner's manual" but is better used as a catalyst for seeking other sources offering more in-depth information and advice.

Where To Find/Buy:

Bookstores, libraries, videotape dealers, or order direct by calling (800) 97-KIDS-1.

Overall Rating
★★
Best used for parenting classes to introduce newborn care; incomplete for home use

Design, Ease Of Use
★★★
Well-organized and laid-out with numbered highlights on screen, segment headings

---

1–4 Stars

Publisher:
Creative Outlook

Edition:
1995

Price:
$29.98

Media:
Videotape

Principal Subject:
Your Newborn

Newborn Subject:
General Overview

VI. Your Newborn

★★

Overall Rating
★★

A massive amount of information conveyed in a question and answer format

Design, Ease Of Use
★★★

Easy to reference, easy to read

1–4 Stars

Author:
Arlene Eisenberg, Heidi E. Murkoff, Sandee E. Hathaway, BSN.

Arlene Eisenberg, Heidi E. Murkoff, and Sandee e. Hathaway, B.S.N. are the authors of the bestselling "What To Expect" series.

Publisher:
Workman Publishing

Edition:
2nd (1996)

Price:
$22.00

Pages:
671

ISBN:
1563058766

Media:
Book

Principal Subject:
Your Newborn

Newborn Subject:
General Overview

VI. Your Newborn

General Overview

WHAT TO EXPECT THE FIRST YEAR
The Comprehensive Guide That Clearly Explains Everything Parents Need To Know About The First Year With A New Baby

Description:
What to Expect the First Year is arranged in a textbook-like fashion. The Table of Contents illustrates the details to be found in this 671 page book, with an outline type format on what is to be found within. Part One addresses the infant's first year. The facts on such topics as bottle vs. breastfeeding, along with recommended equipment for either, is coupled with the emotional concerns of impending parenthood. Each chapter covers issues for each month of the baby's life. What the baby may be doing, what to expect from the monthly checkup, feeding issues, normal parental concerns for this stage, and "what it's important to know" are included. Part Two—"Of Special Concern"—addresses special interest areas (summer clothing and winter concerns), common baby illnesses, first aid, adoption, and more. Supportive information is also provided on babies with problems, including references on the most common birth disorders. The last five chapters in this part deal with emotional and lifestyle adjustments. Part Three is a collection of recipes and common home remedies as well as a table on common childhood illnesses.

Evaluation:
Reading this book is like reading a user friendly encyclopedia. Throughout, it sounds like advice from an experienced mother/nurse down the street who can be counted on to know exactly what to expect from the baby at whatever stage of his/her development and how to do whatever needs to be done. It's light on illustrations, but made readable by frequent sub-heading breaks in the two-column text which insert questions and answers on child care issues. One example of this is the question on vegetarian diet, with a parent questioning whether a strict vegetarian diet provides enough nutrition. The answers are given in bulleted paragraphs, each with a different possible solution to the question depending on the age of the infant. This approach is used throughout the book. As a general reference this book is comprehensive; its information is mainstream with a friendly supportive tone and generous safety and medical tips.

Where To Find/Buy:
Bookstores and libraries.

General Overview

BABY: AN OWNER'S MANUAL

★★

Description:

This book was written by an experienced pediatrician, and a first-time mother. This book consists of "some fast answers to questions we know you're going to ask, addressing the issues that are common to virtually all new parents." It is intended to be used as a source of quick, accessible information, easy "to grab in the middle of the night." Although there is no table of contents, questions and answers are arranged in roughly chronological groupings, from taking the baby home from the hospital to bottle- and breast-feeding, setting up a feeding schedule, diaper rash, colic, and crying spells. The book progresses to questions dealing with choosing a day care, weight gain, teething, starting on solid foods, fevers and colds, child proofing your house, discipline, and maintaining balance in your own life.

Evaluation:

This pediatrician takes a decidedly and unapologetically old-fashioned approach to baby-rearing. The advice given is sensible, succinct, and often humorous, obviously drawing on his experience in answering questions of anxious mothers ("Question: Can his umbilical cord come untied? Answer: I have this vision of an umbilical cord coming untied and a baby flying around the room backward, deflating like a balloon . . ."). Dr. Zukow, a self-described "parent advocate," believes that parents who "get back into their routines as quickly as possible are generally rewarded with more easy-going and independent kids as they grow." Thus, parents will find advice about setting up feeding schedules, getting your baby to sleep through the night, and so forth. Also stressed is the parents' right to make choices, unpressured by current trends (such as deciding whether to use bottle or breastfeed). Altogether, this resource will be helpful to those who subscribe to Zukow's parenting style.

Where To Find/Buy:

Bookstores and libraries.

Overall Rating
★★
Advice and support with a light, often humorous touch

Design, Ease Of Use
★★
No table of contents, roughly listed chronologically; index helps; easy Q & A format

1–4 Stars

Author:
Bud Zukow, MD and Nancy Sayles Kaneshiro

Zukow is Chairman Emeritus of the Dept. of Pediatrics at Encino/Tarzana Regional Medical Center in Tarzana, CA., where he is also in private practice. He is the author of a previous book on parenting. Kaneshiro is the mother of Ian, a patient of Dr. Zukow's.

Publisher:
Kensington Books

Edition:
1996

Price:
$14.00

Pages:
226

ISBN:
1575660555

Media:
Book

Principal Subject:
Your Newborn

Newborn Subject:
General Overview

VI. Your Newborn

★★

Overall Rating
★★
Information dry but adequate; Brazelton fans most likely will be disappointed here

Design, Ease Of Use
★★
Navigation design is average

1–4 Stars

Publisher:
Procter & Gamble

Media:
Internet

Principal Subject:
Your Newborn

Newborn Subject:
General Overview

General Overview

PAMPERS PARENTING INSTITUTE
Expert Advice For Caring Parents

Description:

This site is also dubbed "Total Baby Care: Newborn to Toddler." The homepage focuses on five main areas: "House Call," "Well Baby," "Healthy Baby Skin," "Pampers Diapers," and "Ask our Experts." T. Berry Brazelton, a pediatrician, offers advice, encouragement, and information about your child's development in "House Call." You may select your baby's age (newborn, three weeks, six weeks, etc., to three years.) and interest area (feeding, sleeping, communication, cognitive, motor skills, etc.). "Well Baby" includes a comprehensive encyclopedia of child care information provided by Suzanne Dixon, M.D, a pediatrician; various ages again can be selected along with interest areas. Caring for your baby's skin, from cord care to rashes and sunburn, is the focus of "Healthy Baby Skin," written by Alfred Lane, M.D., a pediatric dermatologist. Diapering and product information is included in "Pampers Diapers." "Ask our Experts" is just what the title implies—a list of frequently asked questions and their answers on topics such as development, behavior, sleep, feeding, and health. Visitors can submit questions and receive replies by email.

Evaluation:

For those who enjoy T. Berry Brazelton and his perspectives, this site likely will prove disappointing. The information included within his segment is dry and barely covers the subject matter. His advice reads like "sound bites," lacking the usual warmth and compassion evidenced by "What Every Baby Knows," his television program. The site asks the visitor to select the child's age and choose an interest area; information is displayed and can then be browsed or printed. The developmental information in "Well Baby" is well laid out and easily can be read in a sitting. The information offered in this section is general in nature and offers guidelines to babycare in the various age groups. For instance, a sample menu is offered in the "feeding" section, according to age. The "House Call" section of the site answers questions and addresses problems regarding the same topics and age groups as "Well Baby." Together, the two sections of this website complement each other; one offers general information and the other answers specific questions about specific issues. Overall, this site is best when combined with other sources.

Where To Find/Buy:

On the Internet at the URL: http://www.totalbabycare.com/

General Overview

PARENTING OF BABIES AND TODDLERS
Your Mining Co. Guide

Description:

An at-home mother who studied child development, psychology, and other areas developed this site—one of The Mining Co.'s family of websites—to offer support and information on the issues facing parents of toddlers and babies. The homepage offers "Net Links" on various topics such as: answers from experts, baby care, baby's first year, child health and nutrition, early learning, etc. Topics are listed alphabetically. Each topic is a compilation of other resources' highlights (mainly print references), or a connection to other websites, or both; a one sentence summary of each resource is provided so parents will know the gist of what is included. The site's homepage also includes articles "In The Spotlight" consisting of the creator/author's newest features; drug addicted babies, crib to bed transition and one-income living were among topics spotlighted at the time of our visit. A chat room, bulletin boards and a newsletter are also provided. General topics are listed to one side of the page for reference. Feature articles are centered on the page, and the alphabetical listing of the articles is accessed on the right side of the page.

Evaluation:

Once parents get to the information offered here, they'll find that the site does an acceptable job of presenting the major points concerning most parenting issues. Unfortunately, the source of the information at times is unclear and the visitor can only be confused at times regarding what he/she is reading—is it the creator's opinion, recaps from other sites, or references to other printed resources? This needs to be made more clear. Also, the online newsletter can only be accessed through a subscription, although past issues are readily available. The topics in those issues, however, should be indexed for easy search. The layout of this website is simple and effective. Easy navigation on the homepage consists of a list of general topics that are addressed. The available articles are alphabetized, but could be categorized. Despite the easy navigation, the content of the information tends to leave one wanting more information. Parents need to check out more solid resources.

Where To Find/Buy:

On the Internet at the URL: http://babyparenting.miningco.com

Overall Rating
★★
Summary information from other references, websites; unclear as to the source at times

Design, Ease Of Use
★★
Improved site design, but can sometimes get lost, no site map; concise info is rather dry

1–4 Stars

Media:
Internet

Principal Subject:
Your Newborn

Newborn Subject:
General Overview

Overall Rating

★

Good for a chat, making a card or getting a recipe; information is dry, largely unusable

Design, Ease Of Use

★★

Categories are mostly vague; no site map is available; graphics slow down navigation

1–4 Stars

Media:
Internet

Principal Subject:
Your Newborn

Newborn Subject:
General Overview

THE BABYNET

Description:

Here you'll find 31 category selections, plus contests and links to catalogues. Several options revolve around baby products, stores, and manufacturers. Alphabetical lists give contact information (phone, address). Another option contains an extensive list of product recall notices. At this site, one can create a birth announcement and greeting card, or participate in games and contests. Baby shower ideas are provided, along with rhymes and songs to sing with your baby. BabyNet offers chat rooms and bulletin board forums; topics for the bulletin board include parenting forums, "expectant clubs" (choose the month you're due), and labor and pregnancy issues. The department "Tender Loving Care" offers information on the following: prenatal care (pregnancy, Chinese birth chart), newborn care (breastfeeding, why babies cry), health issues (ear infections), help for parents (product recalls, safety issues, babysitting) and more.

Evaluation:

This site contains a little of everything, but not a lot of anything. It is true that most of its options offer visitors some lighthearted material, which tired parents certainly will enjoy. One can come here to chat, make a card, print out a recipe, even enter a contest. But it contains little more than that. The information packed into "Tender Loving Care" is cumbersome and dry, with few graphics to help one digest information. Titles to some of the departments are vague or misleading. For example, "Freebies" leads one to believe it is a resource for finding free or discounted product information; it actually is a solicitation to enter a contest. Also, it is difficult to know what you are jumping into when entering the department "Splash"; visitors, it turns out, are invited to tell their stories about where they were when their water broke. Extensive links to child-related products, stores, and manufacturers are the sole unexpected delight, but also lend a feeling of commercialism to this site. Parents with the time to follow the links will find unusual and delightful baby and child items. Where else would you find heart-shaped adhesive bandages? Still, those whose primary purpose for visiting isn't shopping will find their online time more wisely spent elsewhere.

Where To Find/Buy:

On the Internet at the URL: http://www.thebabynet.com

General Overview

ATTACHMENT & BONDING

Description:

This website states that it is a "support and information forum for full time moms or dads parenting in ways that promote attachment between parent and child." The homepage simply is a registration for a visitor to sign onto an e-mail mailing list. When a member posts an email message, it goes to the 300 other members of the email list. The site lists topics that are open for discussion: gentle pregnancy and birth, breastfeeding, delaying solids, extended breastfeeding, child-led weaning, family bed, baby-wearing and more. Topics not supported also are listed, such as: forced weaning, sleep training, spanking, etc. The site states that it does not endorse any particular medical approach, but instead supports attachment and bonding. Members subscribing to the SAH-AP (stay-at-home—attached parent) list are invited to voice concerns, ask questions and share the joys of being a stay-at-home parent. The method of subscribing is explained at the site, along with a description of what one will receive. The site offers links to another sites for information on FAQs and other resources.

Evaluation:

As an experiment, one of the reviewers for this book subscribed to this website's list. She immediately began receiving an endless stream of email (over 300!) before she got off the list. Email "conversations" ranged from "what do you look like?" to "do swings in parks promote detachment?" to "what do I bring for treats to my La Leche League meeting?" In our effort to unsubscribe from the mailing list, we contacted the webmaster/creator at the email address given if "you have any questions or problems." After several weeks we still had not been contacted by the webmaster/creator. If one wants to eavesdrop or partake in casual conversation with other stay-at-home parents, there are other parenting sites that support attachment parenting and offer more directed/moderated forums.

Where To Find/Buy:

On the Internet at the URL: http://www.kjsl.com/sah-ap

Overall Rating

★

Offers only email connections for stay-at-home, attachment parenting moms and dads

Design, Ease Of Use

★

Once you're connected, you're barraged with email; email offers no clues as to topics

1–4 Stars

Media:
Internet

Principal Subject:
Your Newborn

Newborn Subject:
General Overview

Overall Rating

★

This site lacks interest and purpose

Design, Ease Of Use

★

Amateurish layout is distracting, as are the typos; no graphics except for the logo

1–4 Stars

Media:
Internet

Principal Subject:
Your Newborn

Newborn Subject:
General Overview

THE BABY AND CHILD PLACE

Description:

Various options are presented at this site's homepage. Pertinent topics are entitled: "Passionate About Parenting," "On the Fire," "Net Nurse," "Your Section: Parents' Articles and Comments," along with online baby pictures. Visitors may view photos or submit their own baby's picture. "Passionate About Parenting" is a new feature to this site in which an author writes weekly on a given topic. One recent example is "Quality and Quantity," a half page of advice to parents about giving time to their child, written by the editor/publisher of *Nurturing Magazine*. "On the Fire" offers one the chance to submit questions and responses, or read responses to questions already posed to the site; currently seven questions are listed. "Net Nurse" offers advice about common questions parents might have concerning their child, such as "What is that stuff in my baby's eyes?" written by a nurse with a disclaimer to seek medical attention if symptoms arise. "Your Section . . ." includes advice and suggestions by parents on various subjects ranging from eating dinner to discipline to teething.

Evaluation:

This site dreams of being a place "where parents can go to find everything they want to help care for their children." That dream has not, as yet, been accomplished. Due to its amateurish layout and content, visitors to this site will spend far more time figuring out where they're going and what they're reading than the resulting material is worth. Even if the site improves its design in the future, there isn't much content to hold it together. This site desperately needs direction, purpose, and an underlying premise. Parents want sincere answers, not pat responses (on how to have a "healthy, happy and active baby": "while your baby is asleep for about 3–4 hours, you have all this time for yourself . . ."). Parents want helpful advice, not cliches ("One of the most important ways to be a good parent is to be there . . ."). In summary, parents will want to spend their precious time with other resources.

Where To Find/Buy:

On the Internet at the URL: http://www.babyplace.com/

Baby Care

BABYSENSE
A Practical And Supportive Guide To Baby Care

 Recommended For:
Your Newborn

Description:

In its 2nd edition, this well-known guide to baby care includes updated information about breast- vs. bottle-feeding, child care, the adjustment to motherhood, and more. In the introduction, the author states, "I spent a lot of time . . . working out solutions to problems that had been worked out before by countless other parents." The book's basis is that "parents are the ultimate experts" on baby care. Written for the first-time mother separated from extended family networks, this guide includes common-sense advice her mother would give her in a warm, personable tone. The first section of six discusses newborns, feeding (breast, bottle, solids), and such "comfort" matters as interpreting the baby's crying, colic, sleep, bathing, and clothing. The next two parts discuss coping with motherhood and childcare. The last section contains a hodgepodge of "practical matters," from traveling with your baby to childproofing your house, health care, and "playing and learning." Interspersed throughout are anecdotes and tips from real mothers, forming, as the author puts it, "the backbone of the material in this book."

Evaluation:

New mothers looking for a single book offering excellent information about baby care with warmth and support will appreciate this resource. It is wonderfully written, presenting practical how-tos clearly and effectively. It offers both breadth and depth, running the gamut of baby care issues from getting to know one's newborn to a recipe for home-made playdough. Recent SIDS findings are not included, so information on newborn sleeping positions is inaccurate; also, some breastfeeding guidance is outdated. Most readers will appreciate the author's belief that parents are the real experts on their baby's care, avoiding professional opinions that leave parents feeling "inadequate and imperiled." You'll find lots of helpful tips from real mothers, as well as a memorable account of the author's own 12-hour day with her firstborn. Useful drawings show everything from positions to nurse and burp babies to the safest ways to hold a baby during bath time. In an age when a first-time mother may not have someone to show her how to swaddle a baby or reassure her when she feels she's reached the end of her tether, this book makes a heroic attempt to give both practical advice and a sense of community to mothers.

Where To Find/Buy:

Bookstores and libraries.

★★★

Overall Rating
★★★
An excellent, sensitive, and "human" guide to baby care; needs updating regarding SIDS

Design, Ease Of Use
★★★★
Wide pages, personable tone makes reading enjoyable; many chapters use Q & A format

1–4 Stars

Author:
Frances Wells Burck

Frances Wells Burck is the author of another book on parenting, *Mothers Talking: Sharing the Secret.* She lives outside New York City with her husband and three daughters.

Publisher:
St. Martin's Press

Edition:
2nd (1991)

Price:
$16.95

Pages:
313

ISBN:
0312050569

Media:
Book

Principal Subject:
Your Newborn

Newborn Subject:
Baby Care

★★★

Overall Rating
★★★
Concise, sensitive "operations manual" for arriving home with the new baby

Design, Ease Of Use
★★★
Well drawn illustrations, helpful charts and index

1–4 Stars

Author:
Linda Todd, MPH

Linda Todd, M.P.H. is coordinator of prenatal education at Fairview Riverside Medical Center in Minneapolis. She has been a faculty member for the International Childbirth Education Association's workshops and is the author of *Labor and Birth: A Guide for You.*

Publisher:
Harvard Common Press

Edition:
1993

Price:
$6.95

Pages:
134

ISBN:
1558320547

Media:
Book

Principal Subject:
Your Newborn

Newborn Subject:
Baby Care

Baby Care

YOU AND YOUR NEWBORN BABY
A Guide to the First Months after Birth

 Recommended For:
Your Newborn

Description:

Written by a childbirth educator with 25 years of experience, this book reflects a growing desire on the part of participants in her childbirth classes to focus on what is one to expect after the birth. Consequently, it offers ideas on things one can do to make the time after birth easier. The book consists of three major parts: "The Newborn Mother," "The Newborn Baby" and "The Newborn Family." The "Newborn Mother" part addresses questions about how the mother can take care of herself physically and emotionally before and after the birth. "The Newborn Baby" part focuses on health care of the baby, her/his development of sensory and motor skills, and basics regarding feeding, bathing and diapering. The final part, "The Newborn Family," encourages the family to keep their relationships strong with the birth of a new family member. Special attention is given in this section to the "postpartum father" and to other children in the family.

Evaluation:

In the United States, where nearly 99% of women give birth in hospitals, the time that a mother and her baby remain in the hospital after the birth continues to shrink. In fact, by the year 2000, discharge from the hospital within 24 hours of the birth will probably become the norm. Such a continuing trend challenges the family of the newborn as they alone face the postpartum experience, cut off from trained personnel who, in many other countries, are there to teach parenting skills, assess the mother's and baby's health, and provide moral support. This book, then, is meant to fill in that gap. Its tone is that of a well educated, sensitive, reassuring professional who is vicariously there to help the family who feels so happy, but also overwhelmed and disorientated, as they walk into their home with a new child. Along with its encouraging and sensitive tone, the book is filled with well drawn illustrations regarding breastfeeding, diaper changing, swaddling, etc. If one is desperately searching for a no-panic "operations manual" to substitute for the caretaker who will not be there, this short, easy to read book may fit the bill.

Where To Find/Buy:

Bookstores and libraries.

Baby Care

BABYCARE FOR BEGINNERS

★ ★

Description:

This 96 page book's spiral-bound, cardboard-stand format allows it to open upright on a changing surface, table, or bath leaving parents' hands free as they take care of their baby. Offering numerous step-by-step color photographs on each page with additional information on the flipside (once it's standing upright), this baby care guide is divided into 10 parts of how-tos with an additional 4 page illustrated first aid section (choking, CPR, etc.), a detailed table of contents, and an index. Instructional tips and photographs for taking care of baby include: handling, carrying, soothing, feeding, diaper changing, dressing, sleeping, cleaning/bathing, daily care routines, and signs of illness. Photographs within the ten parts include specific instructions for breastfeeding (positioning, pumping/expressing), bottlefeeding (sterilizing, mixing, feeding), getting baby into a sling or other type of carrier, cutting nails, brushing teeth, cleaning a girl, cleaning a boy, and more.

Evaluation:

New parents who have very little access to others' help and hands will appreciate this book's format and how-to instructions. Although some topics are treated lightly (signs of illness, amusing your baby, soothing your crying baby, etc.) and some suggestions are not advised for safety reasons (carrot sticks for an infant), most of the photographs are detailed enough to guarantee parents confidence and success. The format and information in this baby care guide will be most helpful for parents of newborns but less so for parents of older babies. These parents will need to look to other resources for additional information and suggestions surrounding the topics of feeding solids, playing with their baby, bathing in the tub, etc. Although the user of this resource may enjoy a format which frees up an extra set of hands while conducting certain baby care tasks, other resources can be easily found which also address the how-tos of newborn care along with tips for continued care throughout their first year.

Where To Find/Buy:

Bookstores and libraries.

Overall Rating
★★
Offering step-by-step photos to help parents learn to take care of their newborn baby

Design, Ease Of Use
★★★★
Large color photographs, bold headings; vertical standing format, spiral bound

1–4 Stars

Author:
Dr. Frances Williams

Publisher:
Carroll & Brown Limited (Harper Perennial/ HarperCollins Publishers)

Edition:
1996

Price:
$16.95

Pages:
96

ISBN:
0062731041

Media:
Book

Principal Subject:
Your Newborn

Newborn Subject:
Baby Care

VI. Your Newborn

★ ★

Overall Rating
★★
Excellent advice, but geared more toward parents of toddlers and preschoolers

Design, Ease Of Use
★★★★
Detailed table of contents introduces a clearly written, bulleted, and highlighted text

1–4 Stars

Author:
Vicki Lansky

Vicki Lansky has authored over 25 books, and is well-known for her column in *Family Circle* magazine and *Sesame Street Parents' Guide* Magazine. She has also appeared on national TV shows like "Donahue," "Oprah," and "Today."

Publisher:
Meadowbrook Press
(Simon & Schuster)

Edition:
3rd (1992)

Price:
$8.00

Pages:
186

ISBN:
0671792059

Media:
Book

Principal Subject:
Your Newborn

Newborn Subject:
Baby Care

VI. Your Newborn

Baby Care

PRACTICAL PARENTING TIPS
Over 1,500 Helpful Hints For The First Five Years

Description:

This 186 page resource, in its third edition, is separated into eight major sections. The first section, "New Baby Care," includes information on such topics as Cesarean deliveries, what to do if your baby cries, diapering, and working moms. The second section focuses on the "basics" in caring for your child. Some topics that are discussed here include feeding, clothing, and sleeping issues for babies, toddlers, and young children. Section 3 deals with hygiene and health. Cleanliness, dental care, first aid, encouraging good habits, illnesses, and toilet training are a few of the topics addressed. Section 4 focuses on childproofing and safety. Section 5 offers advice and suggestions on manners, tantrums, sibling rivalry, kicking habits, fears, and developing self-esteem. Family heritage and traveling with family are addressed in sections 6 and 7. The final section, 8, includes seasonal fun for both inside and outdoors, arts and crafts, encouraging reading, and preparing a child for school. An index is also provided.

Evaluation:

This book is more a rescue guide than simply a guide with helpful hints. With over 1,500 ideas for making a parent's life easier, here is a cure-all for everything from how to remove gum from hair to advice such as draping a towel over the top of the bathroom door to keep your child from locking himself inside. This guide covers a wide variety of topics in a progressive and logical manner. However, it focuses primarily on taking care of older children, principally preschoolers. Included in the book's hints are the best shared experiences, recipes, and tips from other parents. Bold subheadings and bulleted sections make this resource easy and quick to use. The author uses a relaxed, comfortable writing style while offering a variety of suggestions from which parents may choose. Comical illustrations add to the book's humor. The author has taken care to make sure that new ideas (400) have been incorporated in this revised edition and that former material has been updated to accommodate current lifestyles and parenting information. Parents of older children will find this book is worth buying, however, parents of newborns looking for tips and suggestions on baby care will find other resources better suit their needs.

Where To Find/Buy:

Bookstores and libraries, or order direct by calling (800) 2232 or (612) 930-1100. FAX orders may be placed by calling (612) 930-1940.

Baby Care

YOUR NEWBORN BABY WITH JOAN LUNDEN
Everything You Need To Know

Description:

Narrated by *Good Morning America*'s Joan Lunden and featuring her family pediatrician, Dr. Jeffrey Brown, this 60 minute videotape outlines topics concerning newborn infant care. Eleven segments are introduced by cartoon vignettes with a corresponding icon in the lower right hand corner also displayed on the videotape jacket. These icons are designed to be used with search/scan features of VCRs to locate information. Topics included in the discussions are: choosing your baby's doctor, decisions to think about before birth (breastfeeding, rooming-in, circumcision, etc.), preparing for baby (equipment, layette, packing for the hospital), "the magic moment" (hospital birth), newborn appearances and senses, feeding your baby (breastfeeding, bottlefeeding), diapering and caring for baby's bottom, bathing, how to deal with baby's cries, what to expect for baby's sleep, and when to call your baby's doctor. The guidelines in this 1985 videotape are based on recommendations from the American Academy of Pediatrics.

Evaluation:

Parents viewing this videotape will have the uncanny sense they are viewing episodes from *Good Morning America*. Produced in an interview format either with prospective mothers, the featured pediatrician, or parents of newborns, Lunden interjects her personal experiences along with professional advice. These short, concise segments may appeal to some, but most new parents will find the topics are treated too lightly to be of much value. Some sections are done well including the segments on the how-tos of breastfeeding (endorsed by La Leche League), when to call your doctor, and how to prepare for baby's arrival (includes what to pack for the hospital). However, due to the video's outdated copyright, some advice is currently considered to be unacceptable practice (putting a baby to sleep on their stomach), unnecessary (sterilizing bottles with a sterilizing device), or missing (how to deal with colic). The tape has an attractive sticker price, but parents will find their money better spent on more useful and up-to-date resources.

Where To Find/Buy:

Bookstores, libraries, videotape dealers, or order direct by calling Library Video Company at (800) 843-3620, through FAX at (610) 645-4040, or online at libraryvideo.com.

Overall Rating
★
Info far too concise to be of much practical use; some info currently not recommended

Design, Ease Of Use
★★★★
Short interview-type vignettes; icons for accessibility; recaps at end of each segment

1–4 Stars

Publisher:
J2 Communications/Ripps Communication

Edition:
1985

Price:
$9.98

Media:
Videotape

Principal Subject:
Your Newborn

Newborn Subject:
Baby Care

VI. Your Newborn

★★★★

Overall Rating
★★★★
Complete, supportive & affirming guide sure to be a companion to every nursing mother

Design, Ease Of Use
★★★★
A guide with style; user friendly and intelligently formatted; numerous color photos

1–4 Stars

Author:
Sheila Kitzinger

Sheila Kitzinger, a childbirth educator, has written over 16 books on pregnancy, birth, and childcare.

Publisher:
Dorling Kindersley (Alfred A. Knopf/Random House)

Edition:
(6th) 1997

Price:
$20.00

Pages:
160

ISBN:
0679724338

Media:
Book

Principal Subject:
Your Newborn

Newborn Subject:
Breastfeeding

Breastfeeding

BREASTFEEDING YOUR BABY

 Recommended For:
Your Newborn

Description:
There are eight major sections in this 160 page book. The first section outlines the benefits of breastfeeding, how pregnancy can change your breast shape, and problem-solving tips for various breast types (large, small, inverted nipple, breast surgery). The second section discusses the first days of breastfeeding including topics such as nursing positions, latching on, sucking rhythms, nursing at night, and clothing suggestions for mother and baby. The physiological process of breastfeeding is addressed in the next section along with suggestions on how to take care of yourself to ensure a good milk supply, and more. Section Four offers help for possible problems, such as engorgement, sore and cracked nipples, mastitis, and other deterrents to nursing. The next four sections highlight: learning about your baby's needs (the sleepy baby, the excited baby, etc.), the baby with special needs (jaundice, handicaps, etc.), the family's dynamics (baby, siblings, parents), and "security and adventure" (older baby, sex, traveling, weaning, and returning to work). A reference section, support organization contact information, and an index are given.

Evaluation:
This is clearly a beautiful, well-written book. Numerous color and black and white photographs are provided on virtually every page with clear, concise captions that fully explain and illustrate each topic. Step-by-step instructions, bulleted notations, and bold subheadings also add to this book's ease of use. This guide does an excellent job of covering all aspects of breastfeeding in a progressive, matter-of-fact format. Not just concerned with the basics and how-tos, this resource also covers other issues, such as time management, what to do if you are thinking of giving up breastfeeding, how to deal with babies with special needs, how to nurse the older baby, and more. Topics are presented knowledgeably, with constant reassurance and advice on the most frequently encountered aspects of breastfeeding. Additional resources will be needed to support nursing mothers planning to return to work; minimal advice is given here. But for those women who want a companion to support them in their decision to breastfeed, this is the book that will guide them each step of the way.

Where To Find/Buy:
Bookstores and libraries.

Breastfeeding

DR. MOM'S GUIDE TO BREASTFEEDING

 Recommended For:
Your Newborn

Description:

This 470 page book begins with an introduction by Neifert where she tells of her long (20 year) history of breastfeeding experience, and research. In the remainder of the book, Neifert sets out to offer "a blueprint for attaining your breastfeeding goals, a practical guide to help you achieve the success you desire and deserve so you can one day look back on your breastfeeding experience with infinite pride and satisfaction." First, the reader is educated about the choice to breastfeed: "Why Breastfeed?" "Preparation for Breastfeeding—Before the Baby Arrives," and "How Milk Is Made and Released." Then, there is a broad overview of the breastfeeding experience with special attention to techniques, what to expect (including myths and facts), nutrition, problems with insufficient milk, and special situations (returning to work, twins, etc.). In the last chapter, weaning is described, both literally and emotionally; additional information is provided on nursing the older baby. At the back of the book, there is an index and a seven page "Breastfeeding Resource List."

Evaluation:

Neifert's introduction captures the reader's trust. Readers will benefit from Neifert's attitude, knowledge, and experience. Her dual role as both a breastfeeding mom and a professional breastfeeding expert is conveyed throughout the text. The factual teachings in this book strongly encourage the choice to breastfeed, while the compassionate delivery offers further support for that choice. Throughout her research and work, breastfeeding problems that must be solved, instead become problems that can be prevented. Although breastfeeding is a natural process, the possible obstacles to breastfeeding are so numerous (originating from a mother, an infant, and/or their cultural environment) and as such are outlined here. However, Neifert acknowledges both the benefits and possible challenges to breastfeeding, offering new mothers a prevailing "I can do it" attitude. Consequently, inexperienced and experienced breastfeeding mothers will benefit from the information contained in this book. This comprehensive book is worth reading from cover to cover and may be easily revisited due to its helpful organizational elements.

Where To Find/Buy:

Bookstores and libraries.

Overall Rating
★★★★
Honest, informative, supportive evaluation and practice of breastfeeding

Design, Ease Of Use
★★★★
Well organized, easily referenced with bold print and index, clearly communicated

1–4 Stars

Author:
Marianne Neifert, MD

A pediatrician and lactation specialist (20+ years experience), Neifert lectures to health professionals nationwide about breastfeeding, serves on the Health Advisory Council of La Leche League International, and started one of the first U.S. breastfeeding referral centers.

Publisher:
Plume (Penguin Putnam)

Edition:
1998

Price:
$14.95

Pages:
470

ISBN:
0452279909

Media:
Book

Principal Subject:
Your Newborn

Newborn Subject:
Breastfeeding

★★★★

Overall Rating
★★★★
An excellent resource on breastfeeding

Design, Ease Of Use
★★★★
Easy to read; conversational and humorous writing style

1–4 Stars

Author:
Janet Tamaro

Janet Tamaro became a certified lactation educator after her first daughter was born. She is a television correspondent, reporter, and author. She has worked for ABC News, Fox, and KingWorld Productions.

Publisher:
Adams Media

Edition:
2nd (1998)

Price:
$10.95

Pages:
304

ISBN:
1580620418

Media:
Book

Principal Subject:
Your Newborn

Newborn Subject:
Breastfeeding

Breastfeeding

SO THAT'S WHAT THEY'RE FOR!
Breastfeeding Basics

 Recommended For:
Your Newborn

Description:

This 15-chapter book on breastfeeding basics is divided into three parts: "The Learning Curve," "Mine Didn't Come with a Manual," and "Everything Else You Wanted to Know but were Too Tired to Ask." Tamaro taps from a large pool of breastfeeding-related resources, as documented in her list of references. She also uses many breastfeeding anecdotes from her own life, as well as from many others she has interviewed. The book begins in Part One with background on social influences on breastfeeding and the debate between breastfeeding and formula feeding. Part Two launches into how to prepare for baby and breastfeeding, and the how-tos and early days and weeks of breastfeeding. Topics include nursing apparel, your stay at the hospital, the anatomy of the breast, and common questions and mistakes. Part Three addresses the many breastfeeding-related concerns after mom has become a pro at breastfeeding. Among the many subjects discussed are starting baby on solids, air travel, mom's diet and exercise, breast pumps, storing breastmilk, returning to work, and sex after baby. The book is lightly illustrated. Related resources are provided at the back of the book.

Evaluation:

Taking a humorous approach, this resource offers all the fundamentals on why and how to breastfeed along with discussing physiological and social problems. Many anecdotes are provided, adding light entertainment value. These diversions are a nice complement to merely offering factual information, giving readers added humor at a time when many new tired parents struggle to laugh. Tamaro's breastfeeding-related tales range from teaching a mother gorilla how to breastfeed to a father who squirted an elderly man with his wife's breastmilk in an airport. Her writing style is casual and conversational, as she interlaces personal stories as well as others' stories with facts. A well-rounded list of related resources includes contact information for lactation consultants, pump manufacturers, drug information, and milk banks. Tamaro also presents information on some subjects other resources ignore or treat lightly, such as breastfeeding multiples, adoptive children, babies with Down syndrome, and more; a chapter is dedicated to helping fathers feel involved. This informative guide is easy and fast reading, and well worth having on your bookshelf.

Where To Find/Buy:

Bookstores, libraries, or order direct by calling (800) 872-5627, or in Massachusetts call (781) 767-8100.

Breastfeeding

NURSING MOTHER, WORKING MOTHER
The Essential Guide For Breastfeeding And Staying Close To Your Baby After You Return To Work

★★★★

 Terrific Resource For:
Nursing mothers who want to continue breastfeeding when they return to work

 Recommended For:
Your Newborn

Description:

This 184 page book extends a section of the author's book, *Nursing Your Baby*. Divided into seven chapters, this guide focuses on the needs of the woman who wishes to continue breastfeeding when she returns to work. Pryor's preface and Chapter 1 offer a treatise on the importance of forming an attached relationship between baby and mother; beliefs of current society are challenged here (encouraging the baby to be "independent," i.e., letting baby cry it out, sleep separately, not room-in after birth, etc.). She then details why breastfeeding is important for both mother and baby along with "breastfeeding basics." The next three chapters are dedicated to enjoying maternity leave and adjusting to baby, getting ready to go back to work (getting necessary supplies/equipment, reconnecting with coworkers, finding care), and returning to work (dealing with fatigue, pumping and storing milk at work, business travel, baby's illness, and more). Chapter 7 is a plea to help change negative attitudes in the workplace concerning motherhood. Resources, a sample proposal for a pumping space at work, and an index are given.

Evaluation:

If read from cover to cover, this guide offers working women answers to just about every breastfeeding question they can think of, except how to choose childcare. Parents will need to look to other resources for that information. Sometimes distracting, but always interesting, are Pryor's strong opinions, mostly backed by research. The message she threads throughout the book is that women need to take more initiative about their role in the workplace as they tackle new motherhood. She believes that women and children suffer because women feel they must ignore motherhood while working and vice versa. To that end, she has included numerous strategies and offers welcome tips for those who choose to go back to work and continue breastfeeding. The chapter on "Your Return to the Outside World" is especially useful offering advice from how to deal with leakage at work, to taking baby on business trips, to what to do when baby gets sick. No other guide is available that focuses solely on this subject. Every prospective mother who plans to breastfeed and eventually return to work needs to read this resource before her child is born.

Where To Find/Buy:

Bookstores and libraries.

Overall Rating
★★★★
Full explanations of how to continue breastfeeding upon returning to work

Design, Ease Of Use
★★
More details in table of contents would help; flows well but must be read cover to cover

1–4 Stars

Author:
Gale Pryor

Pryor, a graduate of Cornell University, is the co-author with her mother, Karen, of the highly respected *Nursing Your Baby*. She lives outside of Boston with her husband and her two children, both of whom she breastfed while working full-time.

Publisher:
The Harvard Common Press

Edition:
1997

Price:
$9.95

Pages:
184

ISBN:
1558321179

Media:
Book

Principal Subject:
Your Newborn

Newborn Subject:
Breastfeeding

★★★

Overall Rating
★★★
A sensitive and instructive guide to successful breastfeeding

Design, Ease Of Use
★★★★
Well written, with numerous and very helpful photos and drawings

1–4 Stars

Author:
Mary Renfrew, Chloe Fisher, and Suzanne Arms

Renfrew is a midwife who earned a doctorate for her research in breastfeeding. Fisher has over 30 years' experience as a community midwife. Arms has been a teacher, mother, and photographer, as well as an author of other books on women, childbirth, and adoption. Maggie Conroy is an artist and illustrator, with experience also as an art therapist.

Publisher:
Celestial Arts Publishing

Edition:
1990

Price:
$14.95

Pages:
225

ISBN:
0890875715

Media:
Book

Principal Subject:
Your Newborn

Newborn Subject:
Breastfeeding

Breastfeeding

BESTFEEDING
Getting Breastfeeding Right For You

Description:

This guide to breastfeeding, accompanied by photos and drawings, presents the "mechanics" of breastfeeding and cultural and emotional issues. The authors state that "breastfeeding is not always easy for women who live in societies where it is hidden, and we don't get a chance to learn how to do it." Thus, this book focuses on convincing mothers that breastfeeding is really "bestfeeding," and gives ways to overcome cultural/social resistance and emotional/physical obstacles. The first part offers a rationale for breastfeeding. The next three parts deal with: becoming familiar with positioning, posture, support, and latching on; learning to express and store breast milk, diet; what to do for babies with special needs; how to deal with too much or little milk flow, sore nipples, and fussy/dissatisfied babies. Cultural factors are discussed, including a look at harmful "modern myths." Closing sections include case studies of women with specific problems, and a "storyboard" detailing the basics of breastfeeding in English and Spanish with drawings. Also included are lists of other resources (groups, books) offering help and support.

Evaluation:

If you are considering or have chosen to breastfeed, this is one of many good resources to help you. This book includes a strong message about the importance and superiority of breastfeeding, and it will help women overcome many of the problems that arise when they make the effort to breastfeed their babies. It focuses on the mechanics of positioning (of both mother and baby) which is often the real source of a myriad of problems from sore nipples to too much or little milk flow to a fussy baby. Invaluable illustrations and photos show correct and incorrect positions, and how a baby should properly latch on to the breast. This book also focuses on the emotional aspects of breastfeeding since successful breastfeeding depends on a relaxed, confident mother as well. Overall this is an excellent guide for mothers who plan to breastfeed.

Where To Find/Buy:

Bookstores and libraries, or order direct by calling (800) 841-BOOK.

Breastfeeding

BREASTFEEDING
Pure & Simple

Description:

This 6-chapter, 116-page book discusses the "whys" and "hows" of breastfeeding. Included in Chapter 1 are background information, benefits of breastfeeding, and a short section about La Leche League. Chapter 2 discusses preparation, including breast and nipple care, selecting a health care provider for baby, and lifestyle changes after baby comes. Chapter 3 highlights topics such as breastfeeding the newborn, breastfeeding positions, frequency, and breastfeeding after a Caesarean. How to deal with breastfeeding difficulties is covered in Chapter 4. Advice is offered about sore nipples, sleepy babies, breast infections, and more. Chapter 5 describes the growth of a baby and daily life with a breastfed baby. Also outlined are ways to return to normal life, deal with social criticism, and ways mothers and fathers can take care of themselves (diet, drugs, smoking, medications) and deal with new feelings. Chapter 6, "Looking Ahead," focuses on babies' changing behavior as they get teeth, eat solid food, and grow; also discussed are how to return to work, breastfeed, supplement, and wean. A list of resources is also provided.

Evaluation:

Breastfeeding Pure & Simple is a very good information source for mothers who plan to breastfeed or are in the early days of breastfeeding. It does well in filling the needs and allaying the concerns of parents new to breastfeeding. It also provides encouragement to those who may have had problems or are in doubt about breastfeeding. This book answers common questions that parents-to-be and new parents may have about breastfeeding. The book progresses in an easy-to-follow, logical order: from getting ready before baby is born, to breastfeeding the new baby, and various aspects of life after breastfeeding has been established (parents' sex life, going out with baby, and more). This resource is also good to have on hand if problems related to breastfeeding arise. For example, help is given on what to do if baby is not nursing well, what to do in the event of a breast infection, and how to handle baby's biting while nursing. Also given is good advice on how to express and store breast milk which is useful for mothers returning to work. This book is succinct and concise, but no information is provided for those mothers having multiple births or breastfeeding an older and younger baby.

Where To Find/Buy:
Bookstores and libraries.

Overall Rating
★★★
Contains much of the necessary basic information for breastfeeding

Design, Ease Of Use
★★★★
Logical order and easy reading; succinct and concise; includes resource list and photos

1–4 Stars

Author:
Gwen Gotsch

Gotsch has written and edited numerous books, articles, and pamphlets on breastfeeding and parenting. She was also editor of "Breastfeeding Abstracts," La Leche League's newsletter for health professionals, and she is an accredited LLLI Leader.

Publisher:
La Leche League International

Edition:
1993

Price:
$8.95

Pages:
116

ISBN:
0912500425

Media:
Book

Principal Subject:
Your Newborn

Newborn Subject:
Breastfeeding

VI. Your Newborn

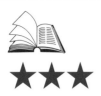

★★★

Overall Rating
★★★
An informed guide to diet and nutrition for nursing mothers, with healthy recipes

Design, Ease Of Use
★★★★
Well laid-out, easy to work through

1–4 Stars

Author:
Eileen Behan, RD

Eileen Behan, R.D., is a member of the American Dietetic Association, a registered dietitian, and a mother of two. She is the author of another book on child nutrition, and works currently as a nutrition consultant for individual families.

Publisher:
Villard Books
(Random House)

Edition:
1992

Price:
$11.00

Pages:
235

ISBN:
0679733558

Media:
Book

Principal Subject:
Your Newborn

Newborn Subject:
Breastfeeding

VI. Your Newborn

Breastfeeding

EAT WELL, LOSE WEIGHT WHILE BREASTFEEDING
The Complete Nutrition Book For Nursing Mothers . . .

Description:

Drawing from her experience as a dietitian and as a mother, the author wrote this book to help other mothers learn about healthy ways to eat and lose weight as they breastfeed. The first chapter discusses the benefits of breastfeeding for infants. Chapters 2–4 describe how a mother's body makes milk, and the specific foods, vitamins, and minerals her body needs. Safe, healthy weight loss and caloric requirements for lactating mothers are discussed next. A simple and safe meal plan for losing weight is included in chapter 6, including a one week sample menu for breastfeeding mothers. Chapter 7 discusses the benefits of exercise, as well as suggestions about safe conditioning. The next two chapters focus on real and mythical dangers in the foods you eat (spicy food, caffeine, alcohol, etc.) and complications (allergies, colic, lactose intolerance, vegetarian diets, anemia, high blood pressure, etc.). Chapter 10 consists of healthy, easy recipes for breakfast, lunch, dinner, and dessert. The last chapter includes answers to common questions that breastfeeding mothers may have.

Evaluation:

Diet and nutrition are significant concerns during a woman's pregnancy. However, few books focus on the months after birth when a breastfeeding mother either has difficulty losing weight or is concerned about eating well for her baby's sake. As the author points out, it is important for mothers to focus first and foremost on themselves and their babies, remembering that weight loss is not as important as "a safe and satisfying nursing experience." However, as many mothers find that the weight isn't coming off while they are breastfeeding, the simple suggestions in this book should help them slim down safely. Newer information is included about foods traditionally not recommended for nursing mothers either because the foods were found to be distasteful or dangerous as it passed into the breastmilk and consequently to the baby. For example, new studies show that garlic may actually make breastmilk more flavorful to babies; on the other hand, studies have found that foil-wrapped wines may be a source of lead. The recipes included are healthful and easy to prepare—something useful for busy health-conscious nursing mothers.

Where To Find/Buy:

Bookstores and libraries.

Breastfeeding

BREASTFEEDING AND NATURAL CHILD SPACING
How Natural Mothering Spaces Babies

★★★

Description:

This 208 page, 17 chapter book is built around "complete" and "total" breastfeeding as a means of natural infertility and way to space babies naturally. That is, a strict adherence must be made to giving no water, juice, solid foods, or pacifier to a baby during the first six months at least. Many other details on "complete" and "total" breastfeeding are given. "Natural mothering" (in general, freely responding to baby's needs) is also a theme of this book. In addition to describing how breastfeeding can be used to space babies, the basics on breastfeeding (why, how, frequency, benefits of), and much more are also discussed. Chapters include "Your Baby's Sucking Needs," "New Light on Night Feedings," "Stepping Out with Baby," "Weaning and the Return of Fertility," "The First Six Months," "Nursing the Older Child," "Sex and the Lactating Mother," "Personal Experiences," and "Natural Family Planning." Two appendices ("A Postscript to Husbands" and "Personal Research"), an index, and a "Mini-catalog" listing related resources are provided at the back of the book.

Evaluation:

If the reader can get over some of the relatively dated feel of Kippley's style, advice, and even the book's physical design, the reward will be much solid and substantive information. *Breastfeeding And Natural Child Spacing* covers a well-rounded, wide range of topics related to breastfeeding and "total breastfeeding." Many personal experiences of the author and others give diversified viewpoints. The author uses many of these personal experiences, through their successes and failures, to help fully illustrate the strict definition of "total breastfeeding." In Chapter 13, "Disappointments with Ecological Breastfeeding," Kippley also gives fair treatment to the alternative view of breastfeeding as a means of natural infertility. This is a complete book on educating couples on how to space babies through breastfeeding. However, if a parent is interested only in breastfeeding for its nutritional and emotional value for their baby or needs basic information on breastfeeding, this is still a worthwhile book to read.

Where To Find/Buy:

Bookstores, libraries, order direct by calling (800) 745-1184, in Ohio call (513) 471-2000, or FAX at (513) 557-2449.

Overall Rating
★★★
Complete book on spacing children naturally; contains good general breastfeeding info

Design, Ease Of Use
★★★
The writing is clear and easy to understand; graphics would be nice addition

1–4 Stars

Author:
Sheila Kippley

Sheila Kippley became interested in breastfeeding following the birth of her first child. She started a La Leche League group in Canada and, as a result of many questions she received about breastfeeding and its relationship to child spacing, she began collecting material to help mothers and eventually wrote *Breastfeeding And Natural Child Spacing*. In 1971 she and her husband founded The Couple to Couple League, which helps couples learn the art of natural family planning.

Publisher:
The Couple to Couple League International

Edition:
2nd (1989)

Pages:
208

ISBN:
0960103686

Media:
Book

Principal Subject:
Your Newborn

Newborn Subject:
Breastfeeding

★★★

Overall Rating
★★★
An experienced, relaxed and personal support resource for breastfeeding

Design, Ease Of Use
★★★
Clear, easy to read; inserts are poorly positioned and occasionally confusing

1–4 Stars

Author:
Janis Graham

Janis Graham is the author of *Your Pregnancy Companion*. She also writes articles on health and fitness that have been published by *Family Circle, Self, McCall's* and *Working Mother*.

Publisher:
Pocket Books
(Simon & Schuster)

Edition:
1993

Price:
$10.00

Pages:
211

ISBN:
0671749633

Media:
Book

Principal Subject:
Your Newborn

Newborn Subject:
Breastfeeding

Breastfeeding

BREASTFEEDING SECRETS & SOLUTIONS
Fast, Reliable Answers To The Questions Mothers Really Ask

Description:
This 211 page book takes the experienced mother approach to provide a modern woman's perspective on the issues and challenges a first-time mother will encounter when choosing to breastfeed her baby. Common questions that occur during pregnancy are fielded first, then each successive stage is addressed, from how to hold the baby for comfort and healthy posture, to how to prevent soreness, diet and nutrition information, milk supply concerns, and food allergies. The later chapters of the book deal with related issues including those of a working mother maintaining a breastfeeding schedule, concerns about food supplements, and solid foods and weaning. The author also summarizes family and behavioral issues that can occur with older babies and second children. The author cites resources such as the American Association of Pediatrics, La Leche League International and the International Childbirth Education Association. Additional resources are listed for women with special needs such as mothers of multiples, mothers of babies with Down Syndrome, cleft lips and/or palates, and mothers of adopted babies.

Evaluation:
This is a useful book on preparing to breastfeed, and is supportive of the practice regardless of lifestyle. The writing style is clear, relaxed, and personal. Information is presented informally and made relevant by a light intermingling of personal experience. The author is a mother herself (still in the process of nursing her second child), which gives the book an informed, balanced and experienced perspective. She avoids sermonizing and assists mothers with choosing the best course through the maze of "Dos & Don'ts" that are offered by well-meaning relatives, friends, and conservative medical professionals. Of use to the first-time mother in particular, the book is still useful during additional breastfeeding experiences due to its insightful and informative approach to the problems, issues and concerns that can arise from differences between one child and the next. To the woman who is not surrounded by other mothers who can share their experience, this book will be a welcome companion.

Where To Find/Buy:
Bookstores and libraries.

Breastfeeding

MILK, MONEY, AND MADNESS
The Culture And Politics Of Breastfeeding

★★★

Description:

The aim of this book, written by a science writer and a former advisor to UNICEF and WHO, is to "bring alive the history, the culture, the biology, and the politics of breastfeeding so women can appreciate the contribution of breastfeeding to the survival of our species." As the authors state, this is not a how-to book but rather a why-to book. They also do not intend the book to be a "tirade" against formula but instead to balance the scales, "to make informed choice a reality." Within the 256 pages of this 3 section, 6 chapter book, you'll be exposed to breastfeeding beliefs and practices around the world past and present, a comparison of breastmilk with formula/artificial feeding, and the relationships between formula manufacturers/promoters, politics, and economics throughout the years. Seven appendices offer the following information: organizations working to promote breastfeeding, reading and resource lists, infant formula recalls (1982–1994), boycott information (Nestle and American Home Products), breastfeeding legislation (as of June 1995), and more.

Evaluation:

Not for the faint-of-heart, this book doesn't mince words. Intimidating at first due to the amount of information, data, and historical accounts contained within, this book nonetheless packs a powerful punch you can't avoid. The authors' expose of formula manufacturers' tactics to push their products upon the medical profession, arguments used to convince lower economic groups and developing countries to not breastfeed, and the rates of infant mortality, especially in the U.S., as a result will leave you angry. Although pregnant women, unsure of whether or not they should breastfeed, will be better able to make informed decisions after reading this book, breastfeeding mothers will also find it useful as they deal with criticism for continuing to breastfeed after society's "approved" nursing period. We recommend this book primarily for professionals and hospitals who are bombarded with enticing freebies from formula manufacturers, yet must struggle to offer an unbiased opinion to new or prospective mothers. You'll be frightened but you'll become enlightened.

Where To Find/Buy:

Bookstores and libraries.

Overall Rating
★★★
Excellent "why-to"—best for medical professionals & those who need supportive data

Design, Ease Of Use
★★★
Table of contents lists all chapter contents, good graphics, reads much like a textbook

1–4 Stars

Author:
Naomi Baumslag, MD, MPH and Dia L. Michels

Baumslag is Clinical Professor of Pediatrics at Georgetown University Medical School in Washington, D.C. and president of the Women's International Public Health Network (Bethesda, MD). Michels is a science writer. Both are published authors and frequent lecturers.

Publisher:
Bergin & Garvey

Edition:
1995

Price:
$26.95

Pages:
256

ISBN:
0897894073

Media:
Book

Principal Subject:
Your Newborn

Newborn Subject:
Breastfeeding

VI. Your Newborn

Overall Rating
★★★
Original content, a welcomed "Lighter Side" offers humorous relief to nursing moms

Design, Ease Of Use
★★
Beautiful images; site map would help since info can seem scattered, unorganized

1–4 Stars

Media:
Internet

Principal Subject:
Your Newborn

Newborn Subject:
Breastfeeding

Breastfeeding

BREASTFEEDING.COM
The #1 Site For Breastfeeding Information, Support And Attitude

Description:

The purpose of this site is to "support breastfeeding women and to provide information on nursing to anyone (including fathers) who want to know more." Sections listed on the homepage include: "All About," "Lighter Side," "Advocacy," "Reading," "Help Me," "Shopping," and a directory of lactation consultants. "All About" lists many articles that address how a prospective mother can prepare for nursing prior to the birth of her child, information on why a mother should breastfeed, positioning, and common myths and their realities. "The Lighter Side" takes a humorous look at breastfeeding by offering a gallery of cartoons and photos, funny stories, and a comic history of breastfeeding. Articles on the infant food industry, legislation, breastfeeding in public, and many more topics are included in the "Advocacy" section. "The Reading Room" is a place to purchase breastfeeding and parenting books, find online articles, and links to magazines and journals. A shopping area is also included at this site.

Evaluation:

This site is a joyous, exciting, and fun promotion of breastfeeding for expectant and nursing parents. Many photos and illustrations are used to identify articles, without cluttering the layout. The video clips and art gallery are not to be missed. One of the most exciting and novel parts of this website is the Lighter Side which takes a humorous look at breastfeeding, without ridicule, stating, "No matter what the trouble, the day goes easier with a little humor." Essays include, "Pumping at 35,000 feet," "Bird's eye view," "Stop the exploitation of dairy cows," and "Express Yourself." Another bonus of this site is its inclusion of beautiful photos and artwork depicting breastfeeding images, provided throughout the site, but especially contained within the Art Gallery. Actual information may seem scattered and unorganized; be sure to link with the article titles contained within "All About." This section—and its intended purpose—would be better served if it were retitled; visitors may be misled thinking this section defines the website's mission and background. Overall though, this site provides definite value to prospective mothers and those who are currently nursing.

Where To Find/Buy:

On the Internet at the URL: http://www.breastfeeding.com/

Breastfeeding

THE NURSING MOTHER'S COMPANION

★★★

Description:

Huggins', a maternity and newborn nurse and founder of a breastfeeding clinic, has written this book "to provide mothers with a practical guide for easy reference throughout the nursing period." The seven chapters of her 240 page guide focus on breastfeeding and deal with the following topics: preparation during pregnancy, the first week, special mothers (mothers with diabetes/epilepsy/herpes/thyroid conditions, nursing after breast surgery, nursing an adopted baby, and more), and special babies (premature, twins, birth defect, etc.); four chapters specifically focus on baby's needs the first two months, from two to six months, and needs of the older baby and toddler. Following each of these special chapters are "survival guides." The cover page of each of these guides lists its contents. These sections are intended to be a "quick yet thorough reference for almost any problem you or your baby may encounter. . . ." The end of the book includes three appendices listing resources for nursing mothers, charts to determine baby's milk needs during the first six weeks, and a listing of drugs and whether or not they are safe while breastfeeding your baby.

Evaluation:

Mothers-to-be and nursing mothers will find this reference guide useful, practical and up-to-date. Of special interest are the sections on dealing with "special mothers" and "special babies"—situations not often covered in many breastfeeding guides. Also of use are the survival guides, helpful for busy mothers who need suggestions quickly. The appendices of resources and drug effects is something every hospital should give mothers upon their departure. Chapters focusing on nursing the older baby and toddler offer many reassurances in dealing with disapproval from others. The only unnecessary item is the appendix for determining the baby's milk needs. Breast milk can only be measured if it's expressed into a bottle. Since bottles are not suggested until AFTER six weeks (due to nipple confusion), this section seems unclear. A helpful resource, the chapters focusing on preparing during pregnancy and breastfeeding the first week are good, and old advice about breast preparation is dispelled—"nipple 'toughening' maneuvers . . . brisk rubbing," etc.

Where To Find/Buy:

Bookstores and libraries.

Overall Rating
★★★
Terrific for the beginning nurser, may be intimidating for the unsure mother-to-be

Design, Ease Of Use
★★
Table of contents dense; each chapter lists contents separately on chapter cover page

1–4 Stars

Author:
Kathleen Huggins, RN, MS

Huggins's has been a maternity and newborn nurse and is founder of a breasfeeding clinic and telephone counseling service.

Publisher:
Harvard Common Press

Edition:
3rd (1995)

Price:
$11.95

Pages:
240

ISBN:
1558321055

Media:
Book

Principal Subject:
Your Newborn

Newborn Subject:
Breastfeeding

VI. Your Newborn

★★★

Overall Rating
★★★
Great tips on integrating breastfeeding into your life, including working moms

Design, Ease Of Use
★★
Small type, rather dense style; more illustrations would help breastfeeding discussion

1–4 Stars

Author:
Karen Pryor and Gale Pryor

Karen Pryor is a writer and a biologist specializing in behavior and learning. Her daughter, Gale Pryor, is a freelance writer and collaborated on this while nursing her own first child and working full-time.

Publisher:
Simon & Schuster (Pocket Books)

Edition:
3rd (1991)

Price:
$6.99

Pages:
416

ISBN:
0671745484

Media:
Book

Principal Subject:
Your Newborn

Newborn Subject:
Breastfeeding

Breastfeeding

NURSING YOUR BABY

Description:
Written by a mother-daughter writing team, this 416 page book's 3rd edition includes updated information "reflecting changes since the sixties." Part 1 discusses the facts behind human lactation. Included in this part are descriptions of how the breasts function, how the baby functions (body and behavior), the positive benefits of human milk, how breastfeeding strengthens the mother-baby bond, and the "politics of breastfeeding" (lack of support, the marketing of formula to medical professionals, etc.). In part 2, a "mother-to-mother, month-by-month practical guide" is provided for breastfeeding newborns to toddlers. You'll find tips on selecting a hospital and doctor (obstetrician, pediatrician) that support breastfeeding. You'll find suggestions on first and subsequent nursings including positioning, relaxation tips, dealing with home stresses, and problem-solving; "confidence builders" are also included for dealing with others' criticisms. The final two chapters focus on breastfeeding for working mothers (24 pages) and nursing an older baby. An appendix lists sources of breastfeeding information and supplies.

Evaluation:
The only complaint we find with this resource on breastfeeding is the way the information is presented. The table of contents at times is vague, the headings within the chapters impersonal, the writing style dense, the type compact, and not enough illustrations (we counted 6 total). But, if you're ambitious and can wade through it, this is a great book on breastfeeding at a great price. Especially useful are the week-to-week and then month-by-month advice that reflect the changes you and your baby go through. No other book addresses the evolution of the breastfeeding relationship quite so thoroughly. We also appreciated the effort that went into the section for "The Working Mother: How Breastfeeding Can Help." Practical input such as getting yourself and your baby ready to go back to work (from four weeks onward), how to express, pump, and store milk, realistic points to consider (fatigue, stress, leaking, etc.), and more are highlighted. The book's strong supportive dialog, its discussion of how breastfeeding changes as your baby develops, and its suggestions for working mothers makes this book a good choice for women considering breastfeeding.

Where To Find/Buy:
Bookstores and libraries.

Breastfeeding

PROMOM, INC.
Promotion Of Mother's Milk, Inc.

Description:
This website, now encompassing a former website known as "The Breastfeeding Advocacy Page," contains information on two aspects of breastfeeding. The first is the educational component of how and why to breastfeed. Included in this category is a list of ten things expectant parents should know about breastfeeding, 101 reasons to breastfeed, along with tips on how to return to work and continue breastfeeding. Other issues include taking medication while breastfeeding, the risks of breastfeeding, breastfeeding a toddler, monitoring milk intake, and others. The second aspect of the website is the advocacy of breastfeeding in the United States. Website authors are "dedicated to seeing breastfeeding become the number one choice of infant nourishment in the U.S." This site addresses the remaining cultural taboos concerning breastfeeding. Links to resources regarding laws that protect public breastfeeding are included. Other advocacy topics include the importance of breastfeeding, why breastfeeding rates are low, and how to support breastfeeding as an individual, employer, or organization. The "Interactive" link takes visitors to message boards, chat rooms and opportunities to sign up for a mailing list.

Evaluation:
The message of this website is straightforward—breastfeeding is the best thing one can do for one's child and oneself, and support systems abound to make it easier. Surprisingly, actual how-to information is scarce at this website. However, mothers can find links and contact information here for help with breastfeeding. The site's format could be better organized to reflect its two focuses—dealing with the how-tos and promoting advocacy in support of breastfeeding. "Features" offers articles on reasons to breastfeed, opportunities to become an activist in support of breastfeeding in our society, and various essays. The articles detailing a perceived cultural prejudice against breastfeeding may be useful in arousing some parents to take action; a number of letters to companies and media outlets taking various advocacy positions are included. There is a lack of graphics at this website which would do much to soften the text's edges. Parents searching for basic information on breastfeeding will use this site primarily as a jumping-off point to other collections of links. For parents who have experienced the frustration of breastfeeding in American society and want to do something about it, this site is the place to go.

Where To Find/Buy:
On the Internet at the URL: http://www.promom.org/

Overall Rating
★★★
Great website for advocacy of breastfeeding, less useful for actual how-to information

Design, Ease Of Use
★★
Straightforward navigation, information is minimal, graphics would be an added asset

1–4 Stars

Media:
Internet

Principal Subject:
Your Newborn

Newborn Subject:
Breastfeeding

★★★

Overall Rating
★★★
A great deal of information, much of it conveyed through anecdotes

Design, Ease Of Use
★★
Clear, well-illustrated, and organized; anecdotal sidebars distract from text

1–4 Stars

Author:
La Leche League International

La Leche League International started 35 years ago when seven women, committed to breastfeeding at a time when most babies were bottlefed, met to provide information and encouragement to breastfeeding mothers. Currently there are 3000+ groups worldwide.

Publisher:
Penguin Books USA (Plume)

Edition:
5th (1991)

Price:
$13.95

Pages:
446

ISBN:
0452266238

Media:
Book

Principal Subject:
Your Newborn

Newborn Subject:
Breastfeeding

Breastfeeding

THE WOMANLY ART OF BREASTFEEDING
La Leche League International

Description:

The Womanly Art of Breastfeeding is an acknowledgment of the 9,000+ active Leaders in the U.S., Canada, and 43 other countries who contributed to this work. This 446 page book begins with "Planning to Breastfeed" with a chapter each focusing on the "whys" of breastfeeding, the "hows" of planning before birth, and ways to gather support networks. Part 2, "The Early Months," covers ways to adapt to breastfeeding, stating that it is 10 percent technique and 90 percent attitude. Many basic issues on child and mother care are addressed, like latching-on, engorgement, the family bed, breastfeeding in public, and more. Part 3 discusses issues related to "Going Back to Work," and part 4 addresses "Life as a Family" with tips on how fathers can get involved, how to manage home duties, other children, etc. Part 5, "As Your Baby Grows," addresses solid food, weaning, and discipline as "loving guidance." Part 6 discusses "special situations" (C-sections, multiple births, premature babies, etc.) and how to breastfeed. Part 7 highlights advantages of "why breast is best" and Part 8 commemorates LLL's 35th anniversary.

Evaluation:

This book contains useful information and is touted as the "bible of breast feeding." Although this revised edition includes updated information about the benefits of breastfeeding, some extension of the section for working mothers would enhance the book. The sixteen pages that are included on how to juggle breastfeeding and working seems far too light a treatment of the topic. The reality for most women is that they do return to work; more logistical tips, information on their rights on the job, resources that are available, and information on skills that could help combine work and breastfeeding would be useful. For the first-time mother all the anecdotes may provide the support she needs; to others they distract from the facts buried in the text. But, for most women with busy lives this book will seem to drag on and on. There are other resources on the market which address the same issues in a more succinct fashion.

Where To Find/Buy:

Bookstores and libraries.

Breastfeeding

MEDELA
Welcome To Breastfeeding Solutions And Medela, Inc.

Description:

Medela "has been providing superior-quality breastpumps and breastfeeding accessories to nursing mothers" since 1979. The homepage features the benefits of breastfeeding, how to breastfeed, choosing a breastpump, common problems and solutions, working and breastfeeding, board certified lactation consultants, and related links. A list of company products, prices, and where resources can be purchased is also available. "How To Breastfeed" offers an article written by Dr. William Sears and Martha Sears, R.N., detailing techniques and positions, complete with blackline drawings and color photographs. Information about collecting, storing, and freezing milk also is provided, along with information on how to use various breastpumps. "Problems and Solutions" offers remedies for various breastfeeding problems (breast engorgement, breast infections, sore nipples, flat/inverted nipples, and more). "Working and Breastfeeding" focuses on creating employer awareness of a nursing mother's needs and desires, selecting a caregiver who supports the desire to breastfeed, and helpful hints for combining work and breastfeeding.

Evaluation:

Good, basic information can be found here to get a mother through most problems and questions she'll encounter concerning breastfeeding. Some visitors, however, will find themselves annoyed at the constant thread of commercialism apparent at this site. Its mission is clear—to sell Medela products. While the information is pertinent and ample to steer mothers through the difficulties of breastfeeding, many will find the product promotion intrusive. For example, "How to Breastfeed" offers the message "to help make breastfeeding an easy and pleasant process, Medela offers a variety of resources to give you expert instruction and helpful information." On the other hand, if a woman already uses and/or likes Medela products and/or she can ignore the "propaganda," she will obtain good information here on breastfeeding.

Where To Find/Buy:

On the Internet at the URL: http://www.medela.com/

Overall Rating
★★
Good information, but a strong commercial tone promoting this company's products

Design, Ease Of Use
★★★
Well-organized site layout with color photos, blackline drawings

1–4 Stars

Publisher:
Medela, Inc.

Media:
Internet

Principal Subject:
Your Newborn

Newborn Subject:
Breastfeeding

Overall Rating
★★
Disappointingly meager information from a well-respected breastfeeding advocacy group

Design, Ease Of Use
★★
Difficult to find the real information; no graphics, no illustrations

1–4 Stars

Publisher:
La Leche League International

Media:
Internet

Principal Subject:
Your Newborn

Newborn Subject:
Breastfeeding

Breastfeeding

LA LECHE LEAGUE INTERNATIONAL

Description:
La Leche League International (LLLI), "an international, nonprofit, nonsectarian organization dedicated to providing education, information, support, and encouragement to women who want to breastfeed," offers many features at their homepage. Pertinent to new moms' needs are the topics of "Breastfeeding Information from LLLI Periodicals," "Frequently Asked Questions about Breastfeeding," and "Breastfeeding Help Form." Also available are LLLI's conference, meetings, and chatroom schedules. LLLI's periodicals contain selected breastfeeding topics including 100+ articles dealing with subjects such as "Breastfeeding Multiple Babies and Tandem Breastfeeding," "Common Breastfeeding Concerns," "Working and Breastfeeding," and more. Each subject area lists how many articles can be found within it. Answers to "Frequently Asked Questions" are found within general topic headings (varying from newborn needs to special situations—nursing an adopted baby, tandem nursing, etc.). Breastfeeding support is available through LLLI's online help form; answers to questions will be sent by email "within one week."

Evaluation:
La Leche League's reputation and proactive stance in the breastfeeding arena are well-known. One would then visit this site with great expectation that this is the site for all there is to know about breastfeeding. Those expectations would be too high. This site is not the be-all and end-all regarding breastfeeding. To illustrate: in the article "Preparing to Breastfeed," the only advice given to an expectant mother is to attend a local La Leche League meeting prior to childbirth. That's it. New moms may find their questions answered within the "FAQ" section, although this area lacks the graphics necessary to illustrate key points; for example, in answering the question of how to position a baby at one's breast, it is difficult to translate words into actions without visual aids. The online help forum is useful unless one needs immediate advice. In summary, La Leche League meetings generally are excellent sites for obtaining information about breastfeeding; the website, however, is not, and one needs to check other sites for information and help.

Where To Find/Buy:
On the Internet at the URL: http://www.lalecheleague.org/

CHILD CARE THAT WORKS
A Parent's Guide To Finding Quality Child Care

★★★★

 Terrific Resource For:
Describing the pros and cons of various childcare options

 Recommended For:
Your Newborn

Description:
Divided into 6 parts with 19 chapters, this 355 page book highlights various options and considerations to "help you locate and organize child care arrangements that satisfy you and support the healthy development of your child during your absence." Part 1 offers an overview of the available options using several examples to illustrate the look and feel of quality care. Six chapters are included in Part 2 and deal separately with various types of care (family and group family child care, center care, part-day programs, care in your home, school-age child care, and "creative alternatives"), how to find them, and what to look for. Possible emotional reactions to child care, both from the standpoint of the child and the parent, are illustrated in Part 3. Part 4 outlines various ways to build a partnership with a caregiver and Part 5 focuses on how much to pay for a caregiver's services as well as tax information. In Part 6, the authors invite readers to become advocates and work toward improving child care conditions. Appendices (9) are provided including organization and referral agency contacts, checklists and child care forms, and more.

Evaluation:
The strength in this book lies in its continual thread of support for those parents who must choose child care for their children. Unlike many books on this topic, it combines an emotional and informational approach when discussing the various choices available. In terms of the emotional side, it refutes the myths parents generate internally when they must place their child in the care of others and their feelings of guilt and anxiety in doing so. Also, many of the other resources on this subject mention, but don't devote much effort to, the importance of building a partnership with a caregiver. This one does a nice job of this. Careproviders get equal time here; although parents may complain about the high rate for quality care, the effects of low compensation for a careprovider's services unfairly leads them to a lower quality of life. The sample forms this resource provides are also a plus. Parents looking for a book on quality care will find this to be a quality book.

Where To Find/Buy:
Bookstores and libraries.

Overall Rating
★★★★
Presents a reassuring but informative study of the various child care options

Design, Ease Of Use
★★★
Needs bolder headings, there's a tendency to get lost; excellent checklists & forms given

1–4 Stars

Author:
Eva Cochran and Mon Cochran

Mon Cochran is a member of the governing board of NAEYC and was a professor of early child development and family studies at Cornell University for 25 years. Eva Cochran is a former director of the Day Care and Child Development Council in New York.

Publisher:
Houghton Mifflin

Edition:
1997

Price:
$14.00

Pages:
355

ISBN:
0395822874

Media:
Book

Principal Subject:
Your Newborn

Newborn Subject:
Choosing A Caregiver

Overall Rating
★★★★
Good information presented in a step-by-step format with many helpful employee forms

Design, Ease Of Use
★★★
Descriptive chapter titles, an index would also help; blocks of highlighted text useful

1–4 Stars

Author:
Cora Hilton Thomas

Cora Hilton Thomas is the founder and owner of Mother's Helpmates, a childcare placement agency. The mother of three, she lives and works in Brandon, Florida.

Publisher:
Avon Books
(Hearst Corporation)

Edition:
1995

Price:
$10.00

Pages:
154

ISBN:
0380782286

Media:
Book

Principal Subject:
Your Newborn

Newborn Subject:
Choosing A Caregiver

Choosing A Caregiver

THE COMPLETE NANNY GUIDE
Solutions To Parents' Questions About Hiring And Keeping An In-Home Caregiver

 Terrific Resource For:
Choosing a nanny as caregiver of your baby

 Recommended For:
Your Newborn

Description:
This 154 page guide, written by the founder of a child care agency, seeks to help parents find and keep a reliable nanny. It provides "all the information you need to hire in-home help and will save you the labor and cost of enlisting a child care placement agency." The book contains 12 chapters. Subjects discussed include in-home care vs. daycare; finding the right kind of person; costs; conducting interviews and screening applicants; keeping a nanny; filing taxes, Social Security, and payroll programs; using a placement agency; and current laws. In addition, chapter 11 deals with finding a nanny for children with special needs. There are seven appendices. These contain a listing of U.S. nanny training schools, sample employment applications, checklists for screening applicants, a criminal background release form, tax and government forms, and more. A listing of childcare placement agencies and services in the United States is also given. There is no index.

Evaluation:
This is a well researched book with good, sound, up-to-date information. The author's experiences from owning a placement agency adds strength to this book. She offers a detailed outline of the standard procedures a nanny placement agency uses when screening household help for families. Her suggestions on securing and keeping a nanny along with her presentation of hard facts and laws on hiring in-home help makes this book credible. Questions are answered succinctly in a progressive, logical manner. Additional sources of information for parents are noted where appropriate in each chapter. Using this book as a guide, parents will be able to successfully sort out the best way to obtain childcare for their specific family's needs. Unique to this resource is the wealth of forms provided by the author. This affords parents the opportunity to familiarize themselves with these forms before beginning the hiring process. Parents looking to add a nanny to their family will find this guide to be very informative and necessary.

Where To Find/Buy:
Bookstores and libraries.

Choosing A Caregiver

HOW TO HIRE A NANNY
A Complete Step By Step Guide For Parents

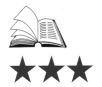

★★★

Description:

This step-by-step 96 page guidebook presents a progressive plan to hiring a nanny. The table of contents includes six sections. Section one discusses how to define the job or the nanny's role. This also includes fundamental issues (safety, health, discipline, etc.) as well as specific tasks (housekeeping, cleanup, etc.) and responsibilities (meals, bathing, etc.); worksheets are included. Section two involves costs. Salary vs. hourly wages, benefits, and filing state and federal employer tax forms are just some of the topics addressed. "Finding the Right Nanny," in section three, highlights the pros and cons of using an agency, how to interview, network, extend an offer, and more. Sections 4 and 5 focus on the management issue of having a nanny and the changes in family priorities, respectively. Self-explanatory examples are included throughout the book, such as examples of phone interviews, reference interviews, employment applications, and writing a classified advertisement. There is no index.

Evaluation:

Logically ordered and concise, this reference offers an easy-to-follow plan for parents interested in hiring a nanny. Clearly written and appropriately detailed, this book guides you through the process of searching for, interviewing, hiring, and keeping a nanny. It also offers input on responsibilities your nanny will undoubtedly do, and how to understand current tax and employee regulations without feeling overwhelmed; a useful table is provided of "what to do" and "when to do it." Parents will find that this succinct resource provides a summary list of required activities so that finding the right nanny will be a relatively pain-free experience. For serious but busy parents, this book will be a big timesaver, arming them with all of the right tools to help in their decision. Although there is no index, the table of contents aptly serves as a competent compass to help parents find answers to their specific questions. This book is a handy resource and well worth the buy.

Where To Find/Buy:

Bookstores and libraries.

Overall Rating
★★★
A true resource to guide busy parents; comprehensive and complete

Design, Ease Of Use
★★
Smooth, progressive flow; numerous worksheets to focus parents; no index provided

1–4 Stars

Author:
Elaine S. Pelletier

Elaine S. Pelletier is a business professional, wife, and mother of two children.

Publisher:
André & Lanier

Edition:
1994

Price:
$9.95

Pages:
96

ISBN:
0963557572

Media:
Book

Principal Subject:
Your Newborn

Newborn Subject:
Choosing A Caregiver

★★★

Overall Rating
★★★
Informative resource coupling research studies with suggestions on finding quality care

Design, Ease Of Use
★
Broad, non-specific table of contents; not easily read or cross-referenced

1–4 Stars

Author:
Susan B. Dynerman

Susan B. Dynerman, a journalist and speech writer, has previously worked in corporate communications as an executive. She and her husband live in Washington, D.C. with their two sons.

Publisher:
Peterson's

Edition:
1994

Price:
$19.95

Pages:
372

ISBN:
1560793341

Media:
Book

Principal Subject:
Your Newborn

Newborn Subject:
Choosing A Caregiver

Choosing A Caregiver

ARE OUR KIDS ALL RIGHT?
Answers To The Tough Questions About Child Care Today

Description:

This 372 page guide consists of two main parts with ten chapters. Part One offers results from various research studies. Topics discussed include: the problems associated with the various types of childcare available, the day care debate (day care vs. mother care, day care and behavior problems, etc.), parental attachment, the realities of parental/family leave, and how a parent's work life affects the lives of their children. Part Two—"Growing Children: A Practical Guide"—focuses on childcare and how it affects babies' development, how to choose the right care for children, how to meet the needs of young children, and what to consider when seeking care for school-age children; interview questions and problem checklists are also given. Each chapter concludes with a summary of the material presented. A "Notes" section is included offering a chapter-by-chapter cross-reference. A 14 page bibliography is included along with an index.

Evaluation:

This guide exposes the many pitfalls of our current childcare system and attempts to allay parental fears by offering answers to their questions based on research studies. This book neatly cites child development research and examines several issues that are controversial depending on one's point of view—the correlation between how much parents work and its effect on their children, the effect of childcare on children at various ages, and the correlation of good/bad childcare and school/life performance. The book concludes with pointedly making the statement that the present system of childcare in America today is abominable and change should be a priority. While a rather depressing dissertation, this interesting book should prove useful in opening adults' eyes for the betterment of our children. While not easy reading and not well-organized, this guide should be reviewed by all parents facing the childcare situation before they give birth to their child.

Where To Find/Buy:

Bookstores and libraries.

Choosing A Caregiver

CHILD CARE
A Parent's Guide

★★

Description:

There are seven chapters in this 173 page book focusing on finding "the best child care." Chapter 1 offers the author's early childhood memories along with a "Self-Test" the results of which are to be used by parents as they narrow down their childcare choices. Chapters 2 and 3 offer suggestions on how to find the appropriate childcare for children based on their age and needs. Chapters 4 and 5 discuss in-home care and family day care centers. Also provided are interview questions and ways to make the transition. Alternatives to childcare are addressed in Chapter 7. Chapters 8, 9, 10, and 11 offer an "action plan" for finding childcare (a step-by-step check-off list), an overview of employer-sponsored childcare options, ways to cope with guilt, and the long-term consequences of child care. A resource listing, day care center regulations by state, and an index complete the book. There are many sample charts, question and answer examples, and a bibliography for each chapter.

Evaluation:

This guide offers practical advice on finding and evaluating a nanny, a day care center, or an in-home care provider. Using a personal approach, the author provides basic suggestions and alternatives for parents looking for quality childcare. "Homework" assignments, given at the end of some chapters, help parents to discover needs specific to their own child's personalities. Good information is provided within this resource including things to look for in a care facility, questions to ask prospective caregivers, and a list of emergency instructions. This guide presents both the advantages and disadvantages of the various programs based on children's age and development needs. The book is weak, however, at helping children make the transition; one paragraph is devoted to this purpose whereas a chapter is devoted to the parents' transition. Well-written and easy to understand, this is a good first approach book for families considering day care for their children. Other resources will answer more in-depth questions.

Where To Find/Buy:

Bookstores and libraries.

Overall Rating
★★
Good practical advice outlining the advantages and disadvantages of various options

Design, Ease Of Use
★★
Topics easy to find but not detailed in table of contents; some tables might need updating

1–4 Stars

Author:
Sonja Flating

Sonja Flating, a child care consultant, is a member of the Child Care Coalition in Sacramento, CA. This coalition is an organization that studies child care and works with real estate developers in incorporating child care into their master planning.

Publisher:
Facts On File

Edition:
1991

Price:
$24.95

Pages:
173

ISBN:
0816022321

Media:
Book

Principal Subject:
Your Newborn

Newborn Subject:
Choosing A Caregiver

VI. Your Newborn

★★

Overall Rating
★★
Treatise on the crisis in the childcare system with proposals for societal changes

Design, Ease Of Use
★★
Heavy textbook style; author and subject index, with an adequate table of contents

1–4 Stars

Author:
Edward F. Zigler and Mary E. Lang

Zigler, designer of the Head Start Program, Sterling Professor of Psychology and Director of the Bush Center in Child Development and Social Policy at Yale University, has earned many awards for his contributions. Lang specializes in child and family policy issues.

Publisher:
The Free Press (Macmillan)

Edition:
1991

Price:
$27.95

Pages:
271

ISBN:
0029358213

Media:
Book

Principal Subject:
Your Newborn

Newborn Subject:
Choosing A Caregiver

Choosing A Caregiver

CHILD CARE CHOICES
Balancing The Needs Of Children, Families, And Society

Description:

Written by the architect of the Head Start program and a specialist in child and family policy issues, this 271 page book observes the childcare situation from a society's viewpoint. It explores the economic issues of childcare as well as the quality of care given and the obligations of a democratic society to provide families with "real choices" for raising responsible children. This text contains ten chapters. Chapters 1 and 2 examine the childcare system with information on working mothers, a child's environment, and the various types of childcare available. Chapters 3–7 focus on ways to meet a family's childcare needs and how to find quality care for infants, toddlers, school-age children, and children with special needs. Chapter 8 addresses how companies are tackling the childcare issue. Chapter 9 outlines a unified system of childcare for the 21st century. Chapter 10 details a child allowance trust fund to create childcare options for families of infants and toddlers. There is an extensive reference section, followed by an author index and a subject index.

Evaluation:

Although this book delves deeply into the challenges and solutions of our current day childcare system, many new insights and ideas have come to pass since this book was copyrighted. This text is not about how to find and keep good childcare help. It is about understanding the system, so that society can offer parents good supportive childcare choices that best suits their family's needs and parenting goals. This book does a great job in gathering all of the information about the childcare system and what it will take to change the system to address the issues most worrisome to parents of today. The book offers well-presented proposals for revamping our present system to improve the quality and quantity of day care services. These proposals are aimed at the educational system, the corporate environment, the family, and the child and health care systems (specifically social security). This resource is more of a treatise for policy changes than a "how-to" guide; parents will need to compare present-day policies of the childcare system, however, to determine the accurateness of this text.

Where To Find/Buy:

Bookstores and libraries.

Choosing A Caregiver

WORKING AND CARING

★★

Description:

Dr. Brazelton, in the beginning of this book, describes the conflicts working mothers face when torn between their beliefs in women's rights to experience the satisfaction of working, and their love and intense attachment to their babies. Here, he tries to address a woman's feeling of being split apart and ways to heal them. This is done by pointing out that the ambivalence a woman feels toward returning to her job generates new energy as she discovers new abilities. The big questions are when to return to work, how to share the care, and how to handle the development hurdles of normal childhood when caring for children is not your only job—issues that confront all parents, whatever their circumstances. By following the lives of three families (working professionals, a single parent, and a couple in which the father must be away for long stretches of time) through the first year of their new baby's life, he illustrates the challenges these families faced, and how these families managed to adjust. The center of his advice is to save some energy at the end of the day for the family's physical and emotional needs.

Evaluation:

In this book, Brazelton does a credible job of emphasizing that it is not just women's dilemma about how to combine work and home life. "The problem in a working family is that no one is there all the time to care for the children." To reflect men's changing roles in terms of fathering, men also need to take steps to further their nurturing abilities, say the author. The main problems of this book center on its presentation. It tends to ramble between the narratives on the families and Brazelton's interjected, sometimes distracting, comments. The type used in printing this book is also a negative, i.e. its too small for easy reading, leaving one feeling cramped. Also, the book needs to be updated regarding the facts and statistics quoted concerning working parents. And so, while this book is filled with experienced insights on the issues involved with returning to work after having a baby, there are other better books on the market today.

Where To Find/Buy:

Bookstores and libraries.

Overall Rating
★★
Too outdated to be of much use to busy parents trying to combine work and home life

Design, Ease Of Use
★★
Difficult to read, unclear on helpful solutions, rambling text

1–4 Stars

Author:
T. Berry Brazelton, MD

T. Berry Brazelton, M.D. is Associate Professor of Pediatrics at Harvard Medical School and Chief of the Child Development Unit at the Boston Children's Hospital Medical Center. Dr. Brazelton is considered a leading authority on child development.

Publisher:
Addison-Wesley Publishing (A Merloyd Lawrence Book)

Edition:
2nd (1985)

Price:
$13.00

Pages:
197

ISBN:
0201632713

Media:
Book

Principal Subject:
Your Newborn

Newborn Subject:
Choosing A Caregiver

VI. Your Newborn

Overall Rating

★

Addresses the many ways of returning to work, but light treatment of childcare options

Design, Ease Of Use

★★★

Bulleted and blocks of highlights; great parent quotes; light on forms, checklists, etc.

1–4 Stars

Author:

Teresa Wilson

Wilson, a postnatal counselor for the National Childbirth Trust (NCT), has written about pregnancy and early childhood issues, and has been a full-time, stay-at-home mother, worked part time, and worked full time.

Publisher:

Fisher Books

Edition:

1997

Price:

$12.95

Pages:

180

ISBN:

1555611265

Media:

Book

Principal Subject:

Your Newborn

Newborn Subject:

Choosing A Caregiver

Choosing A Caregiver

YOUR BABY & YOUR WORK
Balancing Your Life

Description:

The author of this 180 page guide states that her aim is to "reflect the many ways of working that now exist and the kinds of childcare you can choose." Including numerous quotes from working parents, the book is divided into 11 chapters with a conclusion, list of resources, and an index. The author explores issues such as why women return to work, how they feel about returning, how they balance their work and home life, how mothers and fathers juggle their roles as a family, and more. Six chapters discuss the various types of childcare available—family daycare homes, preschools, workplace childcare centers, nannies, au pairs, informal childcare (neighbors, friends, relatives), after-school options, and other support care (postpartum doulas, mother's helper). Each chapter lists the benefits derived from that kind of care, the problems, how to find quality care, and more. Also presented are viewpoints from the childcare providers about the benefits and problems for each of these childcare options. The final chapter focuses on how mothers can continue to breastfeed when they return to work.

Evaluation:

Parents using this book will get great advice on how to assuage their feelings of guilt about returning to work but they will get less direct advice on how to get childcare. The author includes numerous parent anecdotes to illustrate her points, the main one being that being a working parent is a challenge, a balancing act in which women and men work to resolve all their family's needs while enjoying a role in the workplace. Wilson states that if parents understand all of their options for both work-related and child-related issues, then they can strike this balance more successfully, hence the reason for this book. The issues related to returning to work are treated in-depth here, but less so are the issues related to childcare. Parents will get an overview of each option but nothing in detail. Interview questions, for example, are given for hiring a nanny, but none for the other available options. Many other resources include various checklists, forms for checking references, forms for applicants, etc. that help busy parents stay organized and prepared. Parents can use this resource to assuage feelings of guilt but they may well want to use other resources for finding quality childcare.

Where To Find/Buy:

Bookstores and libraries.

Choosing A Caregiver

CHILDCARE KIT
How To Recruit, Screen And Monitor Baby-Sitters And Caregivers

Description:
This larger-sized 63 page book contains three major sections. The section following the Introduction contains information to help parents create their own personal childcare kit, definitions of some terms, and current childcare prices. The next section focuses on "outside-the-home childcare" and discusses safety inspections, how to check a caregiver's references, some suggested questions to ask potential prospects, and more. The rest of the guide deals with childcare in the home including topics of how to find care whether for baby-sitting, full-time, or occasional care. Examples of interview questions, applications, reference check forms, checklists, agreements, and an orientation list for the home are given. Also provided are forms for daily schedules, safety expectations (outside play, infant and toddler equipment, etc.), medical release info, discipline statements, allergy/special diet information, and more Black and white line drawings are repeated throughout this resource. There is no index.

Evaluation:
This book, based on the author's personal experience as owner of a daycare operation and referral business, offers numerous generic forms that parents may find useful, but it provides little value in helping parents decide upon a caregiver. Overall, the guide seems hurried and incomplete. The redundancy and often misplaced clip-art style art is distracting at times—why is there a picture of a fire fighter in the section concerning observation of a daycare? These drawings could have been omitted. Many of the sample questions are droll and uninspiring—"What are your interests and/or hobbies?" "How will you entertain my children while I am absent?"—Perhaps resulting in an uninspiring caretaker. Other books offer similar forms with more homework done in their development. The content contained in this resource is very basic and hardly worth the price. Parents should look to other resources with better scope, more depth, and thorough content to help them make this important decision.

Where To Find/Buy:
Bookstores and libraries, or order direct from Childcare Publications, 49 Evergreen Estates, Sudbury, Ontario, Canada P3G 1B3.

Overall Rating
★
Short, elementary, and concise information on how to find good childcare

Design, Ease Of Use
★
Resource contains no index; relies heavily on marginal table of contents

1–4 Stars

Author:
Faye D. Campeau
Faye D. Campeau has personal and professional experience, both as a parent, caregiver, and an owner/operator of a childcare referral service.

Publisher:
Childcare Publications

Edition:
1995

Price:
$9.95

Pages:
63

ISBN:
1895292573

Media:
Book

Principal Subject:
Your Newborn

Newborn Subject:
Choosing A Caregiver

VI. Your Newborn

Overall Rating

★

Too much negative element to help you approach this process positively

Design, Ease Of Use

★

What? No index? You'll need help to find your way through this one

1–4 Stars

Author:
P. Michele Raffin

P. Michele Raffin is the coauthor of a previous book and has four children.

Publisher:
Berkley Books
(Berkley Publishing Group)

Edition:
1996

Price:
$12.00

Pages:
276

ISBN:
0425151336

Media:
Book

Principal Subject:
Your Newborn

Newborn Subject:
Choosing A Caregiver

Choosing A Caregiver

GOOD NANNY BOOK (THE)
How To Find, Hire, And Keep The Perfect Nanny For Your Child

Description:

How to find, hire, and keep a nanny for your child is explained in this 276 page, 8 chapter book. Chapter 1 focuses on whether or not a nanny is needed. Chapter 2—"Visualizing a Nanny from Heaven"—discusses realistic expectations. Chapters 3 and 4 offer suggestions on how to find a nanny and how to select a nanny, respectively. How to prescreen applicants, interview them, check their references, devise an application, and more are highlighted. Chapter 5 presents an array of nannies from "heaven" and "hell"; various scenarios are illustrated along with questions to use to match a nanny's personalities with your family's needs. Chapters 6, 7, and 8 give information on setting up your home for a nanny, managing an employee, and living with a nanny. The Epilogue includes testimonials from parents and children on the good nannies in their lives, and from nannies who speak about their jobs. Three appendices offer a list of in-home childcare definitions, a sample work agreement, and childrearing tips. There is no index.

Evaluation:

Most of this book is about the author's own experiences with nannies. At first glance, much of the book seems to offer sound advice and suggestions. But, the parent anecdotes, while interesting, are often a bit overdone and lengthy, perhaps used to fill in space to pad the book's real content. Although these real life situations lend an interesting point of view, the book still tends to be the author's biased singular opinion in many cases, often with far too much negativity. Her judgements about good and bad nannies are somewhat harsh and prejudicial ("Make sure if you hire a Queen Bee that she gets her own phone and is financially responsible for it."); these suppositions are not always based on performance, but rather personality types. This resource would have fared better moving in a positive direction with the subject matter. Focusing on strategies to find a good nanny and letting the "down" side go, would have been a better approach. There are other, better, resources.

Where To Find/Buy:
Bookstores and libraries.

Crying And Sleeping

CRYING BABY, SLEEPLESS NIGHTS

 Recommended For:
Your Newborn

Description:

Written by a "recognized authority on crying babies," this 162 page book details the meaning and importance of a baby's cries. The first of 11 chapters explains "Baby Crying Basics," including a quick reference chart listing different types of cries (16), descriptions, and what to do. Chapter 2 follows with techniques for dealing with a baby's cries (motions, sounds, touch, etc.). Chapters 3 and 5 debunk the myths of babies sleeping through the night; included is evidence that contradicts those researchers who insist that babies should be trained to sleep using various behavior mod techniques. How to successfully feed your baby is the topic of Chapter 4 with the focus on breastfeeding. Descriptions of possible causes of colic and ways to help a baby with colic are highlighted in Chapters 6 and 7. The effects of various diseases and drugs on a baby are presented in Chapter 8 along with advice on how to find a good match between you and a doctor for your baby. Chapter 9 deals with crying in older babies and toddlers. The book finishes with tips for parents on handling stress in Chapters 10 and 11.

Evaluation:

Sleepless nights, a crying baby—these are things that either bring out the best or worst in a parent. In an era of parenting in which babies are being trained at an early age to "cry it out," Chapters 3 and 5 are especially enlightening. Sleep trainers who insist that the baby's cries should not interrupt the parents' sleep offer, as the author suggests, "seductive promises" that can easily convince them to buy into their methodology. A reading of these chapters, however, can only leave them cautious about "magic cures" which not only cause them to override the baby's normal communication signals but also shame them into believing that they are being manipulated by the baby. On the contrary, this book offers insights as to why the baby needs to cry and why the parental role is to heed that cry. And it does so in a way filled with support and helpful techniques which can only be reassuring and comforting to any sleep-starved parent.

Where To Find/Buy:

Bookstores and libraries.

★★★★

Overall Rating
★★★★
Parent support and insight based on studies of thousands of infants

Design, Ease Of Use
★★★★
Checklists, quick reference charts to summarize points, parental anecdotes in margins

1–4 Stars

Author:
Sandy Jones
Sandy Jones, a recognized authority on crying babies, has written six books and has published numerous articles in major magazines.

Publisher:
Harvard Common Press

Edition:
2nd (1992)

Price:
$10.95

Pages:
162

ISBN:
1558320458

Media:
Book

Principal Subject:
Your Newborn

Newborn Subject:
Crying & Sleeping

★★★★

Overall Rating
★★★★
Comforting explanations of why babies are colicky; tips for how to soothe them

Design, Ease Of Use
★★★
Well-organized table of contents with subheadings; small dense text due to book's size

1–4 Stars

Author:
William Sears, MD

Sears, "one of America's most renowned pediatricians," has been in practice for 20 years and authored 10 books. Currently, he's a clinical assistant professor of pediatrics at USC School of Medicine.

Publisher:
Penguin Books (Signet Books)

Edition:
1989

Price:
$5.99

Pages:
192

ISBN:
0451163273

Media:
Book

Principal Subject:
Your Newborn

Newborn Subject:
Crying & Sleeping

Crying And Sleeping

THE FUSSY BABY
How To Bring Out The Best In Your High-Need Child

 Recommended For:
Your Newborn

Description:
"A fussy baby can bring out the best and the worst in a parent. This book is designed to bring out the best," says Sears in his introduction. Various words are used to describe fussy babies throughout this 192 page book—colicky, fussy, high need. The underlying premise of this book, along with Sears' other books, is attachment parenting. The first two chapters of this 14 chapter guide highlight characteristics of high need babies along with explanations as to why they fuss. The next seven chapters focus on taking care of your baby. Topics focus on the early weeks of baby care, a detailed chapter on baby's cries, possible reasons for babies being colicky, and soothing, feeding, fathering, and taking care of your baby at night. Chapter 10 concentrates on avoiding mother burnout. Chapter 11 refutes the argument to let babies "cry it out" by describing the "shutdown syndrome;" patient anecdotes are used for illustration. Sears' attitudes toward disciplining high need children along with "the pay-off" or benefits of attachment parenting are the focus of chapters 12 and 13. Chapter 14 is a case history of a family with a high need child.

Evaluation:
If the reader is open to the concept of attachment parenting and is the parent of a "colicky" baby, this resource is a "must read." Although some of the book's content is duplicated in Sears' *The Baby Book*, this book includes more detail. The following sections are especially enlightening: Chapter 11, describing "shutdown syndrome" or the result of babies crying it out; Chapter 12, focusing on disciplining the high need child; and Chapter 13, for those who worry that attachment parenting will lead to a dependent child. Sears, along with his other books, supplies the reader with numerous anecdotes from other family situations; these examples can only comfort a parent who is struggling with a child that others describe as difficult. Sprinkled throughout this book, particularly in chapters 5–9, are tips and tricks for soothing your baby. Sears states that "being fussy and demanding has survival benefits for these babies. If they didn't fuss, their needs might not be met." Parents of high need babies, then, will find this resource valuable, both for meeting the needs of the baby and their own.

Where To Find/Buy:
Bookstores and libraries.

Crying And Sleeping

THE FAMILY BED
An Age Old Concept In Child Rearing

★★★

Description:

The author, the mother of two children and a former La Leche League counselor, wrote this book from her experience with her daughter who would not sleep alone, and after discovering that many parents solved this problem by "... Tak(ing) the child to bed ..." This book explores the benefits of allowing babies and older children to sleep with their parents, and the modern "taboo" against the practice. The first five chapters discuss current beliefs and attitudes towards shared sleeping, why and how parents began allowing their children to sleep with them, concerns and fears about it, and the psychological importance to the child. The next two chapters include a history of shared family sleep from medieval times onwards, and observations of sleep arrangements in various cultures throughout the world. Chapters 8–10 discuss the needs of the infant and older child, how siblings fit into the picture, and marital relations. The last three chapters discuss special circumstances (hospitalization, adopted children), nighttime parenting (discipline) as a continuum of daytime parenting, and the benefits of the family bed.

Evaluation:

Of the many ways in which modern society alienates its members, putting a baby to sleep in a separate room, some argue, may be one of the most subtle. As we learn from this book, the concept of shared sleep is hardly new—families have been sharing beds since the beginning of time. Many of the "scientific" reasons of why shared sleeping is so bad are discredited here, and experts and parents alike have been looking twice at the practice. Sharing sleep, the author argues, is practical (no more getting up in the middle of the night to breastfeed) and psychologically beneficial (babies and young children may feel more secure); it also ends the difficulty of putting a child to bed—when they are secure enough to sleep by themselves, they will. Especially interesting is the "brief history" of family sleeping, and the gradual rise of "sterile child rearing" that reached its zenith in the 1940s. Parents interested in or curious about the idea of the shared family bed will find this a persuasive and informative read.

Where To Find/Buy:

Bookstores and libraries.

Overall Rating
★★★
Persuasively presents the practical and psychological benefits of shared family sleep

Design, Ease Of Use
★★★★
Extremely well written and researched

1–4 Stars

Author:
Tine Thevenin

The author began this book as a research report before it grew into a book manuscript. She was born in the Netherlands, and is the mother of two children. She has also been a counselor for La Leche League.

Publisher:
Avery Publishing Group

Edition:
1987

Price:
$9.95

Pages:
159

ISBN:
0895293579

Media:
Book

Principal Subject:
Your Newborn

Newborn Subject:
Crying & Sleeping

VI. Your Newborn

★★★

Overall Rating
★★★
Rationale and tips for finding a "sensitive solution to your baby's sleepless nights"

Design, Ease Of Use
★★★★
All subtopics listed under chapter headings in table of contents; useful photographs

1–4 Stars

Author:
William Sears, MD

Sears, "one of America's most renowned pediatricians," has been in practice for 20 years and authored 10 books. Currently, he's a clinical assistant professor of pediatrics at USC School of Medicine.

Publisher:
Penguin Books USA (Plume)

Edition:
1987

Price:
$11.95

Pages:
203

ISBN:
0452264073

Media:
Book

Principal Subject:
Your Newborn

Newborn Subject:
Crying & Sleeping

Crying And Sleeping

NIGHTTIME PARENTING
How To Get Your Baby And Child To Sleep

Description:

Sears has written this guide to answer the question, "Should I let my child cry it out at night, or console my crying child?" His goal, in this 203 page, 17 chapter book, is "to help parents and children achieve sleep harmony" . . . "lessening your child's night-waking and increasing your ability to cope." Sears draws on both his experience as a father of 8 and from returns of a questionnaire sent to patients. The foundation of the book, as with all of Sears' books, lays in the tenets of attachment parenting (where babies and caregivers best form a secure relationship by being very connected to each other's cues); chapter 1 explains this in detail. Other chapter topics deal with the difference between baby and adult sleep, where baby should sleep, dealing with night-waking, food that helps sleep, nighttime fathering, demands of the high need child, SIDS, sleep disorders, nap times, single nighttime parenting, and more. Sears asserts throughout his book the importance of babies and young children "sharing sleep" with their parents; in other words, sleeping in the parents' bed.

Evaluation:

Does Sears answer the question, "Should I let my child cry it out at night?" You bet. His points are well-made, using both research findings and anecdotes from parents. Everyone agrees that a baby's cries are a baby's language. However, as Sears asserts, "if the baby's cries fall on deaf ears, he is less motivated to cry" . . ."the baby loses trust that the caregiver will respond." One can always find arguments to defend any parenting style; parents and advisors to parents should read all the viewpoints and choose one that resonates with them. Sears' book represents a point of view that some parents will strongly embrace and others will just as strongly reject, research or no research. A weakness of this book, however, is that some areas need updating. For example, since 1987 (its copyright date), new research has come to light regarding SIDS, including the pros and cons of sleeping with your baby. Also, special situations, such as working mothers, need some extended suggestions and support, especially since this is the norm for many households.

Where To Find/Buy:

Bookstores and libraries.

Crying And Sleeping

BABY MASSAGE
A Practical Guide To Massage And Movement For Babies And Infants

★★★

Description:

This reference consists of four chapters detailing the benefits of baby massage. Chapter One talks about the importance of touch and explaining the healing potential of massage. Chapter Two includes general information about massage (supplies needed (oils), when not to do it, etc.) along with the specific benefits of baby massage; also included is a massage technique for newborn infants as well as a full body routine for infants two months and up. In Chapter Three parents will find how movement and flexibility exercises combined with massage can help children through the developmental stages of sitting, crawling and walking. The final section, Chapter Four, highlights how massage can help children with special needs, as well as how it can be used to assist with a few of the most common childhood illnesses, such as constipation, wind, colic, and congestion. There is an index and worldwide "Useful Addresses" for mother-to-mother support groups, childbirth education information, breastfeeding, and more.

Evaluation:

For readers whose interest lies in this subject, this 128 page book will surely leave you satisfied. With more than 100 beautifully detailed full color photographs and line drawings, readers unfamiliar with massage techniques will come away from this book confident and charged to try the author's "soothing caresses." This is a well-written, easy-to-read guide extolling the virtues of touch between infant and parent. The information is based upon the author's ten years of experience as a physical therapist attending hundreds of mothers and babies. The book is meant to be read cover to cover. The author is careful to stress gentleness, patience, and consistency. The how-to instructions are clear and concise; a novice will have no trouble picking up the author's suggestions on how to calm an infant or encourage their flexibility and strength as they begin more movements. Parents eager to try new ways to work with a fussy baby or capitalize on the bonding period will no doubt find a treasure trove of tips here.

Where To Find/Buy:

Bookstores and libraries.

Overall Rating
★★★
Unique approach with emphasis on the nurturing qualities of a gentle touch for babies

Design, Ease Of Use
★★★
Table of contents vague, but index makes for easy navigation; beautifully illustrated

1–4 Stars

Author:
Peter Walker

Peter Walker is a physical therapist with over fifteen years of experience in working with children, parents, and parents-to-be. He offers baby massage workshops to midwives and other health-care professionals throughout the United Kingdom.

Publisher:
St. Martin's Griffin (St. Martin's Press)

Edition:
1995

Price:
$16.95

Pages:
128

ISBN:
0312145454

Media:
Book

Principal Subject:
Your Newborn

Newborn Subject:
Crying & Sleeping

VI. Your Newborn

★★★

Overall Rating
★★★
Useful for cross-examining the various methods available for teaching children to sleep

Design, Ease Of Use
★
No index, minimal table of contents makes searching for specific methods impossible

1–4 Stars

Author:
Tamara Eberlein
Eberlein has written over 200 articles on parenting, health, and psychology. Her work has appeared in magazines such as *Redbook, Good Housekeeping, Family Circle,* and more. She is a graduate of the Georgetown University School of Languages and Linguistics.

Publisher:
Pocket Books
(Simon & Schuster)

Edition:
1996

Price:
$5.99

Pages:
214

ISBN:
0671880381

Media:
Book

Principal Subject:
Your Newborn

Newborn Subject:
Crying & Sleeping

Crying And Sleeping

SLEEP
How To Teach Your Child To Sleep Like A Baby

Description:

This six chapter, 214 page book aims to answer the question "How can I get my child to sleep through the night?" Based on "in-depth interviews with more than two dozen of today's leading experts in sleep research, pediatric medicine, and child psychology," the author has also conducted a "thorough" review of the research that has been done; the "experts" are listed in the Acknowledgments and literature reviewed is cited in the Resources section. Chapter One reviews children's sleep patterns and problems. Then Chapter Two describes ways to deal with "bedtime battles" while Chapter Three offers techniques for managing "middle-of-the-night awakenings." Chapter Four focuses on what to do to help children who have nighttime fears. "Where should your child sleep?" is the topic of Chapter Five outlining pros and cons of various sleep locations (family bed, bassinet, crib, big bed, etc.). "Special Situations" are addressed in Chapter Six and include circumstances that interfere with a child's sleep (siblings, twins, babysitter, travel, divorce, preemies, sleep disorders, etc.). No index is given.

Evaluation:

This book's intention is admirable given the amount of discussion today focusing on sleep issues and how many experts can't agree on how to handle sleep problems. Supplying parents with information on all the different methods that are available allows parents to compare methods and make their decision based on their family's needs. To this goal, organization elements in this book would have made this search more rewarding. Yet, there are no details in the table of contents and there is no index. Instead, parents will need to read the entire text, write down names and page numbers of methods, and jot down notes because there are no other ways to relocate the information. The author does highlight various sections within the chapters with titles such as "The Beat-Him-To-The-Punch Approach" or "The Reassuring Approach," but this offers little real help. A comparison chart that contrasts such things as amount of parental involvement or absence, the length of time needed to resolve sleep problems, etc. would be more helpful along with cross-references to page numbers. Parents should use this as a start but keep their paper and pen handy.

Where To Find/Buy:

Bookstores, libraries, or order direct by contacting Mail Order Department, Simon & Schuster, 200 Old Tappan Road, Old Tappan, NJ 07675.

Crying And Sleeping

GETTING YOUR CHILD TO SLEEP . . . AND BACK TO SLEEP
Tips For Parents Of Infants, Toddlers, And Preschoolers

★★

Description:

The ten chapters of this 131 page guide highlight many of the facets of children's sleep. Chapter One discusses a baby's sleep patterns during the first six months while Chapter Two offers tips on developing bedtime routines for a baby. Chapters Three and Four focus on how to deal with baby's cries and colic. Chapter Five offers tips for getting a "night waker" back to sleep. Whether or not to allow a baby or child to share the parents' bed is the topic of Chapter Six. Helping parents cope with loss of sleep is Lansky's focus in Chapter Seven. "Naptime" how-tos and suggestions for older children are discussed in Chapter Eight, while Chapter Nine discusses "reasonable bedtime routines" for older children. The last chapter offers strategies for helping children handle their nighttime fears, bad dreams, and night terrors. A one page index concludes the book as well as a list of other resources. Each chapter contains bulleted tips, blocked insets of highlighted advice and parental quotes, and sometimes organizational contacts or products.

Evaluation:

Lansky has provided an overview here of all prevailing theories on how to deal with sleep issues from having baby "cry it out" to sleep arrangements in "the family bed." Although she presents the pros and cons of these sleep issues, most often Lansky's opinion is center stage following her line of reasoning that she had "made peace with the fact that sleep as [she] had known it was no longer to be part of [her] life" and "it was somehow okay." While this may not bide well with those who want sleep training methods to teach their baby to sleep, Lansky, does, however, offer strategies and support to overcome the tiredness plaguing many parents in the early months and years. She balances her opinions with quotes from parents who have tried the reverse of Lansky's suggestions and also had success. While not a definitive guide, Lansky's guide gives parents a plan for dealing with sleep issues. Parents will get practical tips ("play a radio, with an automatic shut-off timing feature . . .") and support ("learn to make jokes about your lack of sleep"). They can then look to other resources if necessary for additional support or how-tos.

Where To Find/Buy:

Bookstores, libraries, or order direct by calling (612) 475-3527 or (800) 255-3379.

Overall Rating

★★

Good overview of sleep issues, pros and cons of various methods, and practical tips

Design, Ease Of Use

★★★★

Easily read with bulleted tips, inset blocks of advice and parental quotes; succinct

1–4 Stars

Author:

Vicki Lansky

Lansky is a mother and author. She can also be read regularly in *Sesame Street's Parent Guide* section and in *Family Circle* where she writes the "HELP!" column.

Publisher:
The Book Peddlers

Edition:
2nd (1991)

Price:
$6.95

Pages:
131

ISBN:
0916773191

Media:
Book

Principal Subject:
Your Newborn

Newborn Subject:
Crying & Sleeping

VI. Your Newborn

Crying And Sleeping

HELPING YOUR CHILD SLEEP THROUGH THE NIGHT
A Guide For Parents Of Children From Infancy To Age Five

Overall Rating
★

Considers child's developmental issues, but backed up only by personal research

Design, Ease Of Use
★★★★

Well-organized, concrete steps presented for each age; each chapter stands on its own

1–4 Stars

Author:
Joanne Cuthbertson and Susie Schevill

Cuthbertson and Schevill are both mothers and married to pediatricians.

Publisher:
Main Street Books (Doubleday/Bantam Doubleday Dell)

Edition:
1985

Price:
$11.95

Pages:
246

ISBN:
0385192509

Media:
Book

Principal Subject:
Your Newborn

Newborn Subject:
Crying & Sleeping

Description:
Written by two mothers, this 246 page resource is "devoted to showing you how to establish and maintain good sleeping habits for your children." An introduction outlines various elements of sleep including the "science of sleep" (bio rhythms, physiology), security objects, possible locations of sleep, bedtime rituals, and more. The remaining five chapters highlight the authors' sleep training methods, advice, and discussions of sleep disruptions (in light of habits, development, and specific situations) for various age groups: from birth to 4 months, 5 to 9 months, 10 to 18 months, 18 months to 3 years, and 3 years to 5 years. Each chapter is designed to stand on its own. It is suggested, however, that parents, read the introduction prior to turning to the chapter that corresponds to their child's age. A Q & A segment is included at the end of each chapter. A bibliography, suggested bedtime books for children, and an index conclude the resource.

Evaluation:
Of the various sleep training methods that exist, this resource considers reasons for sleep interruptions along with the child's developmental stage. The main problem we found, however, with this method is that it has not been tested by large controlled studies. It is based on the authors' reading and experience with their own children and friends' children. One concern in particular we had involves training a 3 day old newborn. It is suggested that after the newborn receives their "focal feeding" (at about 11 pm), upon waking later they should be comforted to sleep, and if need be, offered a bottle of water (or glucose water), and then placed in bed. This "stretching" the time between feedings is the heart of the authors' method. Many pediatricians, though, advise newborns be fed on demand. Nursing mothers are also advised not to use a bottle for several weeks due to nipple confusion on the part of the infant. And what if the baby, who, research states, is naturally inclined to be drawn to sweet tastes, decides the glucose water is a fine substitution for milk? Look to other more sound resources for help in getting your child to sleep.

Where To Find/Buy:
Bookstores and libraries.

Crying And Sleeping

SOLVE YOUR CHILD'S SLEEP PROBLEMS

Description:

This 250 page book addresses the issues of sleeplessness and how it affects the parents as well as the child. Ferber states that "when your child's sleep patterns cause a definite problem for you or for him, then he has a sleep problem." Throughout the book, he describes the tired, frustrated, and angry responses of parents with a young child who will not settle into the normal routines of the family. Ferber then offers reassurance to parents that these problems have nothing to do with poor parenting, nor is it a "stage" that must be waited out. Instead, he describes problematic "sleep associations" (nursing or bottle, rocking, holding, cuddling, music) that a parent must "begin to correct" from infancy onward. He advocates scheduled daytime feedings (both nursing and bottles) and naptimes, no nighttime feedings, his "progressive waiting" program (not heeding child's waking cries for specific time intervals), and "door-closing" techniques (holding door closed from the outside until child returns to and stays in bed). Ferber states that sleeping alone is necessary to teach an infant or child to see himself as an independent individual.

Evaluation:

Charts, graphs, recording worksheets, programmed steps, and tables are integral parts of Ferber's solution to "sleep problems." These strategies help distract the reader from the inherent problems present in Ferber's argument for sleep training. On one hand, he states that pediatricians "recommend that you try to follow your infant's cues." Then Ferber suggests that a baby should learn to "self-comfort" himself without rocking, touching, bottles, nursing, or pacifiers; that this fundamental assumption is best for infants is disputed by many. He also describes the importance of our natural circadian rhythms—"if your child's circadian rhythms are disrupted, her sleep-wake patterns deteriorate." Then he devotes the rest of his book to explain how to ignore an infant's nighttime "wants," and how to change these circadian rhythms by scheduling a baby's sleeping pattern so it more clearly mirrors an adult's. Doing so, he believes will help adults and babies sleep through the night. The detail throughout the book is dense. This book dictates steps, and offers warnings and threats ("Take the steps necessary to correct [sleep problems]. If you do not, it may persist for months, even years."). Look for resources more soundly based on infant development.

Where To Find/Buy:

Bookstores and libraries.

Overall Rating

★

Dry description of how to regulate children's sleep habits, full of contradictions

Design, Ease Of Use

★★

Dense text, reliance on charts, graphs, tables; must be read cover-to-cover

---

1–4 Stars

Author:

Richard Ferber, MD

Ferber, an authority in the field of children's sleep problems, directs the Sleep Lab and the Center for Pediatric Sleep Disorders at Children's Hospital in Boston. He also teaches at Harvard Medical School and is a pediatrician.

Publisher:

Fireside (Simon & Schuster)

Edition:

1985

Price:

$12.00

Pages:

250

ISBN:

0671620991

Media:

Book

Principal Subject:

Your Newborn

Newborn Subject:

Crying & Sleeping

VI. Your Newborn

Overall Rating

★

Detached technique not well-grounded in recommended child care advice

Design, Ease Of Use

★

Difficult to find direct tips or strategies; few graphics

1–4 Stars

Author:
Gary Ezzo and Robert Bucknam, MD

Publisher:
Multnomah Publishers

Edition:
2nd (1998)

Price:
$9.99

Pages:
223

ISBN:
1576734597

Media:
Book

Principal Subject:
Your Newborn

Newborn Subject:
Crying & Sleeping

Crying And Sleeping

ON BECOMING BABYWISE, BOOK ONE
Learn How Over 500,000 Babies Were Trained To Sleep Through The Night The Natural Way

Description:

The author states in his preface that his book is "more than an infant-management concept; it is a mind-set for responsible parenthood." Chapter 1 describes the importance of establishing and maintaining a family, as opposed to being "child-centered or mother-centered." A historic overview of "feeding philosophies" is presented in Chapter 2, along with the "The Babywise Alternative" or "parent-directed feeding" (PDF) which is described as a "24 hour infant-management strategy designed to help moms connect with their babies and their babies connect with them." Throughout the remainder of the book, Ezzo compares and contrasts PDF with "hyperscheduling on one extreme and attachment parenting at the other" in his discussions of babies' sleep, feedings, waketime, naptime, parental response to babies' cries, and more. He presents statistical findings from a number of studies, "including the ones we commissioned in our pursuit of establishing *Babywise* norms for sleep, weight gain, and average length of time our mothers breast-fed their babies." A new chapter to this revised edition discusses PDF as it relates to multiple births; Ezzo also offers pointers for "starting late."

Evaluation:

This book offers another strategy for "teaching good sleep habits" starting from day one of a newborn's life. Ezzo suggests parents observe and tune in to their newborn's inherent feeding and sleeping schedule. He then offers his "flexible schedule" which then dictates when they should eat, when they should sleep, when they can play; nursing mothers are admonished to "stabilize [their] lactation." Readers should note, however, that the author has no medical background or apparent credentials to speak on this subject. Numerous physicians and lactation consultants have written to decry Ezzo's methods, his own original church has distanced themselves from his stance, and his work is almost in direct contradiction to the American Academy of Pediatrics' statement on breastfeeding. In addition, a number of "failure to thrive" cases in babies have been linked to this method. Throughout, Ezzo speaks in an uncompassionate detached tone. At one point, he likens a mother's emotional response to a baby's cries as "set[ting] the stage for child abuse." He offers much misinformation and advice dangerous to a baby's health. Parents should check other resources that better address their needs while ensuring their baby's well-being.

Where To Find/Buy:
Bookstores and libraries.

Equipment And Supplies

BABY BARGAINS SECRETS

 Recommended For:
Your Newborn

Description:

This 9" x 4-1/4" resource contains 333 pages of information on how to find bargains as parents prepare for a new baby. There are twelve chapters in this book's second edition. Chapter 1 discusses how a baby will monetarily change your life. Chapters 2, 3 and 4 contain information on nursery necessities (furniture, bedding, layette). Chapter 5 includes information on maternity/nursing clothes and equipment for feeding baby. Chapter 6 addresses things around the house: baby monitors, toys, bath, food, high chairs, swings, and more. Chapter 7 discusses car seats, strollers, and carriers. Chapter 8 suggests ways for affordable baby proofing. Chapters 9, 10, and 11 offer the "best gifts for baby," "etcetera" (books, Internet websites, and choosing child care), and lists of mail-order catalogs grouped by subject matter with contact information. In Chapter 12, the authors compare typical savings parents can attain if they use the book's suggestions. Child product sources and safety requirements of Canada are included in the appendix.

Evaluation:

This revised second edition includes more brand name reviews, e-mail suggestions from readers, an added section on playpens, baby bottles, formula, and money-saving advice. All of the information and prices have been updated. Overwhelmed at first, parents will need to take some time because this resource covers a great many items. The reviews in the book are based upon the authors' experiences and those of parents interviewed. Reviews of selected manufacturers are rated on a star system from a Four Star rating ("Excellent-our top pick!") down to a One Star rating ("Poor—yuck! could stand some major improvement"). There is no advertising in the book, crediting the authors' intent to not accept money to "buy" favorable reviews, thus also insuring objectivity. Helpful "Smart Shopper Tips," "Wastes of Money," "Money Saving Secrets," and more are included throughout the book. Parents willing to do a bit of homework will find this resource offers the best bargains for anything their baby will need.

Where To Find/Buy:

Bookstores and libraries, or order direct by calling (303) 442-8792 or (800) 888-0385.

Overall Rating
★★★★
Lots of helpful tips and useful information "guaranteed" to save parents at least $250

Design, Ease Of Use
★★★★
Intimidating at first but a 13 page index & a detailed table of contents make access easy

1–4 Stars

Author:
Denise Fields and Alan Fields

Denise and Alan Fields are consumer advocates who have been featured on *Oprah, The Today Show, Good Morning America,* and *Dateline NBC.* Their previous books include *Bridal Bargains, The Bridal Gown Guide* and *Your New House.*

Publisher:
Windsor Peak Press

Edition:
2nd (1998)

Price:
$13.95

Pages:
333

ISBN:
1889392006

Media:
Book

Principal Subject:
Your Newborn

Newborn Subject:
Equipment & Supplies

VI. Your Newborn

★★★★

Overall Rating
★★★★
An expert assessment of the most (and least) necessary baby products

Design, Ease Of Use
★★★★
Succinct, highly usable, with helpful page "tabs"; appendices offer contact info, etc.

1–4 Stars

Author:
Ari Lipper and Joanna Lipper

Ari Lipper manages Albee's, a baby products store in New York City, where he and his wife, Joanna, also live.

Publisher:
Dell Publishing
(Bantam Doubleday Dell)

Edition:
1997

Price:
$9.95

Pages:
215

ISBN:
0440507847

Media:
Book

Principal Subject:
Your Newborn

Newborn Subject:
Equipment & Supplies

Equipment And Supplies

BABY STUFF
A No-Nonsense Shopping Guide For Every Parent's Lifestyle

 Recommended For:
Your Newborn

Description:
"Reading this book should give you a good understanding of the products that are out there, how they work, which ones are necessities, and which ones are best for you to consider based on your lifestyle," is how the author introduces his 215-page guide to baby products. Drawing on his familiarity with baby-related items, Lipper gives a run-down of "must haves" (necessities), "might wants" (items to consider based on your budget), and "totally optional" products (frills). The products are divided into 6 main subject areas: the Nursery, the Layette, Carriages and Strollers, Getting Around, Food, and Safety, easily located by both a table of contents and page tabs. Each section describes the products, rates them, tells how long your baby may need them, what their "borrowability" is (and advice in case you do borrow an item), safety issues, and how to fit them into your budget (brand names, prices, where to buy). Also included are sections on where to shop to get the best value, borrowing tips, and nannies. Three appendices give timetables for products, brand names and prices, and a list of manufacturers' telephone numbers.

Evaluation:
In the buying fever that often arrives even before baby does, parents hoping to purchase the best possible products for their baby find themselves unprepared for the expense and overwhelming array of baby items all of which tout themselves as "necessities." Ari and Joanna Lipper's book should prove to be a steady and expert guide to the world of baby products. Its no-nonsense evaluations of each baby item allow parents to purchase the necessities (the crib, diaper pail, clothing, thermometer, stroller, car seat, high chair, etc.), weigh and consider desirable items (bassinet, changing table, baby monitor, portable crib, etc.), and take a look at the "frills" (comforter, pram, jogging stroller, hip carrier/backpack, etc.). There is help here for every parent's budget: well-made, reasonably priced items are recommended and some pricier items are justly critiqued ("A crib is a crib. No matter if you pay $200 or $600 . . ."). In this age of consumerism, this book will save parents time, money, and frustration while showing them how to purchase the best products for their baby.

Where To Find/Buy:
Bookstores and libraries.

Equipment And Supplies

IBABY.COM
All Your Baby Needs

 Recommended For:
Your Newborn

Description:

This website is almost exclusively an online shopping source for baby items. The homepage offers several ways to shop, including going to the various departments (categories of similar items), gifts for babies (a list of gifts for a baby, with links to those products that they sell), best buys (lists of links to the best selling items), and a product search. In addition to the shopping opportunities, a baby registry is available to expectant parents who want to provide gift ideas for a baby shower. This registry can be edited/updated by the parent, or the site automatically updates the registry as purchases are made. To aid in planning for purchases for a new baby, the site also offers a new parent checklist that includes items and quantity of items needed to prepare for a newborn. To find a specific item, a visitor can access the product search function of the site. To use the site, a visitor first must register by submitting mailing information; an account number and password then is issued. Individual items are listed, with an illustration, product information, price, size, and color, if applicable.

Evaluation:

One would expect an online shopping website to be overdone with sales pitches. However, we were amazed at the simple yet effective layout of this source. The departments are well-organized and offer a variety of ways to access products, depending on the customer's needs, without cluttering up the page. Similar to a traditional store, this site offers sale items and best buys. All products include colorful descriptions, in-stock status, price, and product number. Simply click the corresponding button to add the item to your "shopping cart." The online baby registry is a great time saver for anyone who cares to shop online. The new parent checklist is a helpful organizational tool, even if it is a bit dictatorial. For example, it recommends that 16 to 24 outlet plugs be purchased instead of suggesting the customer count his or her outlets. The product recall list is too confusing to be useful, unfortunately. Given the still prevalent concern about security, this site should add more information about its security measures. For ease of use, this site is topnotch. One caution: this site does not appear to make any evaluations or comparisons about the products offered; judgements must be made using other tools.

Where To Find/Buy:

On the Internet at the URL: http://www3.ibaby.com/

Overall Rating
★★★
Useful tools to use when shopping for baby; good information on individual products

Design, Ease Of Use
★★★★
Excellent format, variety of ways to access the products

1–4 Stars

Media:
Internet

Principal Subject:
Your Newborn

Newborn Subject:
Equipment & Supplies

Overall Rating
★★
A generally useful list of practical and monetary concerns during your baby's first year

Design, Ease Of Use
★★
Eclectic gathering of topics with some uneven treatment; "necessity checklist" a plus

1–4 Stars

Author:
Anne K. Blocker, RD

The author has taught prenatal nutrition and counseled on gestational diabetes, maternal nutrition, infant feeding, and breastfeeding for over 10 years. She is also the mother of three children.

Publisher:
Chronimed Publishing

Edition:
1997

Price:
$12.95

Pages:
295

ISBN:
1565610903

Media:
Book

Principal Subject:
Your Newborn

Newborn Subject:
Equipment & Supplies

Equipment And Supplies

BABY BASICS (PRINT)
A Guide For New Parents

Description:
To quote: "It's common knowledge that babies cost a bundle. That's . . . what this book is all about—keeping the bundle from becoming the national debt by simplifying baby care." This is a guide to the practicalities of baby care. The 15 chapters of this 295 page book focus on identifying one's options, ways to save family money, and understanding health and safety issues for such areas as medical care, health insurance, traveling with baby, and babyproofing one's home. Other chapters focus on other investments such as choosing maternity clothes, buying nursery furniture, selecting baby clothes, diapers, and toys. Additional tips are offered in areas such as feeding the baby, choosing child care, weighing decisions about returning to work, and investing in one's future (financial matters). Each chapter introduces its topic which is accompanied by a "necessity checklist" of things to do/buy, and includes tips on safe use, what to consider when buying an item, smart shopping tips, and "budget helpers," as well as a list of further reading, catalog resources, support groups and organizations, and more.

Evaluation:
The author provides a rather eclectic array of topics related to baby care in her book, all of which seem to revolve around issues of decision-making, finance and budgeting, and safety. Reading through this book should give one a grasp of many of the practical aspects involving raising a baby. What it lacks is overall coherence. Is this book about safety or budgeting or health/nutrition? At times the book makes up for this lack of coherence with a good chapter, e.g. "Baby's Basic Wardrobe," a chapter which provides in-depth information about buying clothing a few sizes ahead to save money as your baby grows, safety tips such as avoiding drawstrings and arm/leg bands, laundry tips, etc. Also useful are the chapters on travel safety, baby proofing your home, and child care. But other chapters, such as those on feeding and health, really include only the basics and do not offer the depth of advice that other resources do. Overall this book might best be used to introduce some practical concerns and identify those that need to be researched further with the help of other resources.

Where To Find/Buy:
Bookstores and libraries, or order direct by calling (800) 338-2232.

Equipment And Supplies

GUIDE TO BABY PRODUCTS
Buy The Best For Your Baby

Description:

This 326 page guidebook is targeted to all consumers of baby products. Beginning with the statement that there is no guaranteed safety for a product made for children, the book then looks at the range of products currently sold in American markets and the availability of safety information on each product. Not all products are rated, but ratings are included when available. Topics covered include: backpacks/soft carriers, various infant beds, bathing accessories, bottlefeeding equipment, breastfeeding accessories, changing tables, child safety seats, clothing and footwear, baby foods, gates, hazard reduction/childproofing products, high chairs/booster seats, infant seats, monitors, nursery decor/accessories, playpens, strollers, swings, toilet-learning aids, toys, and walkers. Information is arranged alphabetically and with occasional photographs. Each section begins with information and advice on what to look for, rules on how to use some products, and a list of recalled products. Items selected for testing were based on information obtained from manufacturers. Manufacturers' contact information and an index are included.

Evaluation:

Though the book is subtitled "Buy the Best for Your Baby," too little information was provided in most cases for a "best" evaluation. The introduction was somewhat disorganized and illogical. Is the assumption here that the consumer wants to buy the safest product for the least money? Or is safety the primary rating factor? Information on how products are rated and who is responsible for the rating should be presented more clearly—did the same parents who tested the products also rate them? The product listings contain maker and model, description, design info, and special features, but often there is no safety rating specific to that product, making evaluation difficult. It is unclear as to whether omission from these lists means the products were found unsafe or simply not supplied by the manufacturer. The text in these listings is small and hard to read. Photographs would be an added plus but there are too few to really be helpful. There is certainly a need for books like this one to facilitate consumers wading through the overwhelming mass of baby products, but this one falls short.

Where To Find/Buy:

Bookstores and libraries.

Overall Rating
★★
Offers products that meet authors' or Consumers Union's safety standards

Design, Ease Of Use
★
Listing information is too small and lacks overall ratings; listing criteria unclear

1–4 Stars

Author:
Sandy Jones and Werner Freitag

Sandy Jones is a well-known expert on baby products and safety, and is the author of many books and articles for parents. Werner Freitag is a project leader at Consumers Union, where he has worked for over 30 years. He has helped draft baby product safety standards.

Publisher:
Consumer Reports Books

Edition:
5th (1996)

Price:
$14.95

Pages:
326

ISBN:
0890438544

Media:
Book

Principal Subject:
Your Newborn

Newborn Subject:
Equipment & Supplies

Overall Rating
★
Entertaining but not really informative

Design, Ease Of Use
★★
Some useful tips and amusing color illustrations

1–4 Stars

Author:
Matthew Bennett

Publisher:
Meadowbrook Press

Edition:
1992

Price:
$10.00

ISBN:
0671867776

Media:
Book

Principal Subject:
Your Newborn

Newborn Subject:
Equipment & Supplies

Equipment And Supplies

THE BABY JOURNAL
Your Weekly Guide To Baby's First Year

Description:

The companion book to *The Maternal Journal*, this resource "is designed to provide you with an enriched experience of your baby's first year of life." Accompanied by color illustrations, *The Baby Journal* provides developmental milestones, facts, tips, and selected information about one's baby from his/her first month through the fourteenth. Presented in a wall-calendar style, it also has a little space (about 1" x 1") for making notes on about the baby from day to day. Special highlighted tips (roughly half a page) include information on giving massage to one's baby, skin care, bathtime, getting more sleep for the parent and the baby, exercise tips for mothers, introducing solid foods, babyproofing one's home, emergencies/first aid, playtime, weaning, choosing toys, avoiding gender stereotypes when choosing toys, and interacting with one's child.

Evaluation:

As this "journal" aims more at entertainment than information, an introduction warns the reader that it is "by no means intended to be a comprehensive encyclopedia of all existing data on raising children . . ." With that in mind, potential consumers must weigh this book's value against the more extensive information the same money would purchase in another resource. Advice offered here is really on the slim side. Additionally, there is hardly any space for mothers to actually write notes or journal entries, an activity that many parents may find useful and cathartic. The illustrations are amusing, and it makes a colorful wall-hanging. But parents should save their dollars and buy either a real journal with adequate space, a good book on baby care, or even a nature/art calendar that your baby will enjoy looking at too.

Where To Find/Buy:

Bookstores and libraries, or order direct by calling (800) 338-2232.

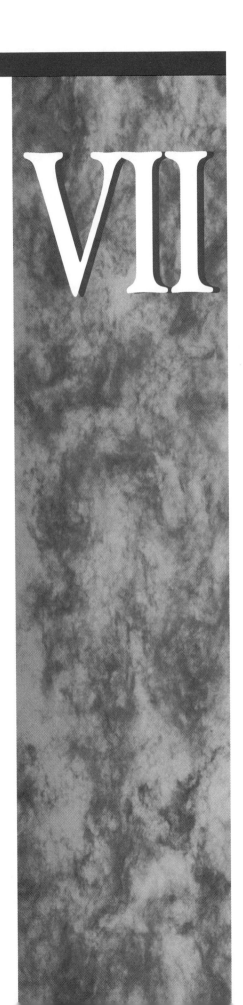

SOLUTIONS
FOR INFERTILITY

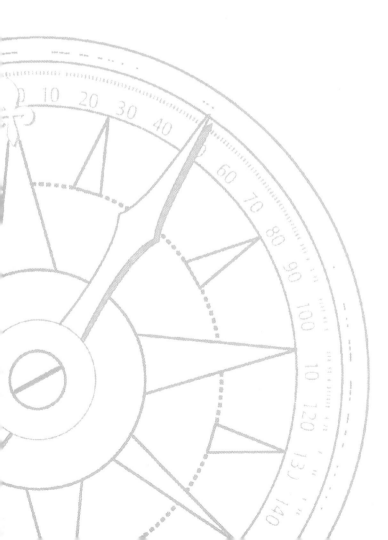

INTRODUCTION

Many couples in their thirties and forties share a common concern—after all these years of compulsive contraception, will we be able to have a child? Couples at any age may have trouble conceiving, however this difficulty increases with the age of the couple and with any aggravating factors that may exist.

Most healthy couples in their twenties will conceive within about six unprotected menstrual cycles. Using a fertility-awareness method can help couples know when they are most likely to conceive. For a woman with a regular, 28-day cycle, her most fertile time will be days 12–14 after the first day of her last menstrual period. Having intercourse every 36–48 hours during the fertile part of the menstrual cycle offers the best chance for conception to occur. Using additional information, such as cervical mucus observation or an ovulation prediction kit, can also help determine the best time to conceive. About 85 percent of couples should conceive within one year, and another 7 percent in the second year, so the true infertility rate is only about 7 percent overall. However, older couples or couples with other contributing conditions comprise the majority of those infertile couples.

Couples in their twenties who are trying to get pregnant but have not conceived within one year, or couples in their thirties and forties who have not conceived within six months, should consider having an evaluation done to determine the cause of their inability to conceive. This evaluation will likely include full physical exams of both partners, analysis of a man's semen for adequate sperm count and function, blood tests for hormone levels, testing to assure that a woman's fallopian tubes are open, and tests to be sure she is ovulating normally. A family physician or gynecologist can perform most of these initial tests. Sometimes the answer will be obvious and the solution will be relatively simple. Keep in mind that about 40 percent of infertility problems can be traced to the woman, about 20 percent to the man, and about 40 percent may include factors from both partners.

Female infertility usually involves irregular ovulation, blocked fallopian tubes, and/or endometriosis. Irregular ovulation can often be treated with clomiphene citrate (Clomid), an oral medication which induces ovulation. A woman takes this medicine during days five through nine of her menstrual cycle, and usually ovulates about day 14. Clomiphene raises a woman's hormone levels as well, so it also causes side effects such as bloating and sore breasts. It has also been associated with an increased risk of ovarian cysts and cancer, so ultrasounds of the ovaries should be done for any woman who uses clomiphene for more than a month or two. Clomiphene increases the possibility of having twins from about 1/80 to about 1/20, but it doesn't usually lead to a higher number of multiple births. Problems with the fallopian tubes or presence of endometriosis may require surgery.

Male infertility is usually due to a decreased sperm count or abnormalities of the sperm's function. The testes function most effectively at 96 degrees Fahrenheit (36 centigrade), which is somewhat lower than the general body temperature. Consequently, men who are trying to conceive should avoid hot tubs or hot baths—20 minutes in the hot tub can decrease sperm count for up to four months! Wearing boxer shorts instead of briefs, and avoiding tight pants can also help keep the temperature down and encourage sperm production. Sometimes, a man has a dilated vein in the scrotum called a varicocele; this condition can also raise the temperature of the scrotum and may require surgery. If a man's sperm count is too low for conception, the couple may wish to consider using donor sperm for artificial insemination. Donors are carefully screened for genetic and infectious disease. However, it is recommended that only semen that has been frozen for six months should be used to allow time for re-screening of the donor for both HIV and hepatitis before insemination.

If these relatively straightforward interventions do not lead to conception, a couple may choose to pursue evaluation and treatment at a fertility center. Unfortunately, most medical insurance policies do not cover infertility, and some of the techniques can be very expensive. This transition point is a good time to examine your feelings and your relationship before proceeding. The technology associated with assisted conception becomes more sophisticated almost daily, and there is certainly hope for many infertile couples. However, news of septuplets and octuplets notwithstanding, none of the high-tech methods result in high rates of successful pregnancy. And the emotional and financial costs associated with the newest reproductive technology can be quite high.

The high-tech interventions for dealing with infertility problems are a bit of an "alphabet soup" of acronyms. "IUI" stands for intrauterine insemination, in which washed and concentrated sperm are placed directly into a woman's uterus at the time she is ovulating. This technique can help with male infertility or if there is a problem with the cervical mucus. "GIFT" and "ZIFT" involve the collection of eggs from a woman, using a needle inserted into her pelvis with ultrasound guidance, then implanting either eggs and sperm or an early embryo into her fallopian tubes. This treatment generally serves patients who have blocked tubes with or without associated male infertility problems. One of the newer techniques, "ICSI" (intra-cytoplasmic sperm injection) involves taking eggs from a woman and injecting an individual healthy sperm into each egg. This can be used for extreme cases of male infertility, or when other techniques have failed. All of these techniques use high-powered ovulation-inducing drugs that can potentially lead to triplets or higher order births. And each of these techniques can be done with the couple's own eggs and sperm, or with donor eggs or sperm if needed.

Infertility can be devastating, and the evaluation and treatment involved can lead to an emotional roller coaster. If you are facing infertility, focus on your relationship, explore your feelings about adoption, and discuss how you feel about remaining child-free. This will help you set reasonable limits on your efforts to conceive.

To help focus your search for information, advice, and support, we have reviewed resources that focus solely on infertility. We've included resources that explain the pros and cons of various "assisted reproductive technologies" (the ARTS), from "low-tech" methods to ultra "high-tech" solutions. Descriptions are given of techniques such as IUI, IVF (in vitro fertilization), GIFT, ZIFT, and more. Many of the resources we've recommended offer information and advice on the actual procedures, accompanying issues (emotional, physical), costs, and rate of success. Check out several of our recommendations before, during, and after you choose to undergo fertility assessment and treatment. Compare their respective information and feel confident you are getting the support and direction that best serve your needs.

THE COUPLE'S GUIDE TO FERTILITY
Updated With The Newest Scientific Techniques To Help You Have A Baby

★★★★

 Recommended For:
Solutions For Infertility

Description:
This 457 page directory is arranged in the following sections: What's Going On, What You Can Do, Alternatives, and Pregnancy Success. It addresses the current irony in our society of waiting to have children until one can have it all, only to discover one has waited too long. Written to directly address people in this situation, this book attempts to help the couple to understand the newest fertility treatments and techniques. Causes of infertility are explained in clear and accessible language. Social factors that have changed American lifestyle choices and affected fertility are also explained. Chapter 4—"Getting Started With A Fertility Specialist"—is designed to assist the couple with navigating the interviews, insurance, and evaluation period of getting fertility assistance. The rest of the book is a step by step explanation of current treatments and alternatives in use as of 1995. A directory of fertility specialists throughout the United States and fertility centers in Canada is provided.

Evaluation:
This book was written by two doctors and a professional medical writer who together have produced a directory that is well laid out, orderly, and easy to read and reference. Rather than focusing on infertility, this book instead presents a positive approach to the topic of fertility and all its aspects. Written for the couple to read and/or reference together, this text can be a very helpful resource for the adult trying to understand the various issues involved in fertility and the medical professionals' current approaches. Hormone treatments, surgical treatments, and microsurgical procedures are all covered in a clear and even interesting manner. In its second edition, this book is filled with current information, yet is not overwhelming or daunting. The writing is both readable and sensitive of the reader's personal issues. Thus, this book leaves one with a sense of perspective and even hope when faced with problems in conceiving a child.

Where To Find/Buy:
Bookstores and libraries.

Overall Rating
★★★★
Sensitive and well-informed advice giving guidance on issues of fertility

Design, Ease Of Use
★★★★
Easy to read, well-illustrated, well-paced

1–4 Stars

Author:
Gary S. Berger, MD, Marc Goldstein, MD, Mark Fuerst

Dr. Gary S. Berger and Dr. Marc Goldstein are specialists in male and female fertility treatment and authors of multiple books and articles. Mark Fuerst is a medical writer who has himself faced infertility.

Publisher:
Main Street Books (Bantam Doubleday Dell)

Edition:
2nd (1995)

Price:
$16.95

Pages:
457

ISBN:
0385471246

Media:
Book

Principal Subject:
Solutions For Infertility

★★★★

Overall Rating
★★★★
Comprehensive, supportive guide for the emotional and physical issues of infertility

Design, Ease Of Use
★★★★
Clear, well-referenced, with glossary, bibliography, index and resource listings

1–4 Stars

Author:
Carla Harkness

Harkness, a mother of two, spent ten years undergoing fertility tests and treatment. She has written this book to assist others with the help of more than 70 medical specialists, infertility patients, psychologists, adoptive parents, surrogate mothers, and recent parents.

Publisher:
Celestial Arts Publishing

Edition:
2nd (1992)

Price:
$16.95

Pages:
400

ISBN:
0890876649

Media:
Book

Principal Subject:
Solutions For Infertility

THE INFERTILITY BOOK
A Comprehensive Medical & Emotional Guide

 Recommended For:
Solutions For Infertility

Description:

This guidebook is more than 400 pages of information and experiences on infertility. Carla Harkness has herself experienced infertility and has used medical technology that successfully treated it. This book is part of her effort to reshape her life and, therefore, addresses the entire experience of infertility. Part One deals with the experience itself: self-image and social pressures, the emotional impact on the couple, the economics of infertility treatment, insights on the doctor-patient relationship, and ways to take care of yourself. Part Two pulls together current information on the diagnosis, causes, and treatments of infertility. It discusses various options with an eye to what it costs both financially and in terms of the personal commitment needed for various treatments. Part Three is called "Resolutions" and addresses what happens after infertility treatment, whether it works or not. Adoption, pregnancy and parenting after infertility, surrogate mothers, and child-free living are also discussed.

Evaluation:

An impressive number of experts have been consulted for the material in this book. Just looking at the numerous lists of specialists and advisors gives one a sense of the comprehensive work that went into its production. This book takes on the personal side of infertility and the emotional issues that are aroused by the unfulfilled desire for a child. Why it is so traumatic, how men and women react to the emotional rollercoaster ride, and how to deal with the emotions in a healthy way, are all compassionately addressed. This is one of the few books with tables in it that go over the diagnosis, causes, and treatments of infertility. The tables cover the procedure, its purpose, the benefits, risks and inconveniences, and the approximate costs of each, as of 1992. Other useful aids include lists of questions with check-off boxes for evaluating infertility treatment options. The sections in "Resolutions" reveal and examine options for couples who can't have a child. Adoption is supported, as is choosing to live "child-free"—an option that is not often given emotional support or validation. A well done book, and one we highly recommend.

Where To Find/Buy:

Bookstores and libraries, or order direct by calling (800) 841-BOOK.

OVERCOMING INFERTILITY
A Compassionate Resource For Getting Pregnant

 Recommended For:
Solutions For Infertility

Description:

The intent of this book is to comprehensively educate anyone with an interest in the medical aspects of infertility. There are five parts, entitled Nature, Tests, Special Treatment, Assisted Conception, and Getting What You Deserve. Each includes descriptions of where its topic is placed in the fertility matrix. The author begins by explaining the process of conception, normal fertility, and basic concepts of infertility. Included are explanations of the tests that may be used to diagnose infertility along with tests that may be given either when a miscarriage may occur or has already occurred. Explanations of many possible causes of infertility (low sperm count, blocked fallopian tubes, ectopic pregnancy, fibroids, endometriosis, etc.), options available for assisted conception, issues that may occur once pregnancy is achieved, and the role of the physician follow. In addition, the author explores the moral and ethical arguments surrounding assisted conception. A glossary and appendices ("the New Fertility and Infertility Math" and "Results of Assisted Conception") are included to supplement the main body of the book.

Evaluation:

This book is geared toward anyone seeking hard-core medical information regarding all aspects of conception and infertility. The sections are wisely divided into primary issue areas, such as testing, causes of infertility, and options available to overcome infertility. Subsections on each test, cause, and method of treatment are very detailed in their explanations, without being too overwhelming to a lay reader. Thanks to the extensive glossary, with a little time and determination a reader can achieve a clear understanding of the topic. It is not necessary to read this book cover to cover to gain the benefits of the information on a particular topic. Each is self-contained, and a reader can pick and choose the information he or she needs. Medical illustrations clarify many explanations. The author also includes sidebar articles to supplement the primary text. In the last section of the book, the author draws away from the medical, technical explanations, and offers his views on the morals and ethics of society and culture regarding infertility and assisted conception.

Where To Find/Buy:

Bookstores and libraries.

Overall Rating
★★★★
Thorough medical information that is not too technical for the lay reader

Design, Ease Of Use
★★★★
Self-contained explanations on all subjects; good use of blocked text, headings

1–4 Stars

Author:
Robert Jansen, MD
Jansen is a medical doctor at a clinic (Sydney, Australia) that treats infertility.

Publisher:
W.H. Freeman and Company

Edition:
1997

Price:
$16.95

Pages:
474

ISBN:
0716733021

Media:
Book

Principal Subject:
Solutions For Infertility

★★★★

Overall Rating
★★★★
Thorough treatment of
natural family planning

Design, Ease Of Use
★★★★
User-friendly; letter-boxed
highlights, numerous
illustrations, color

1–4 Stars

Author:
Toni Weschler, MPH

Weschler is a nationally respected
women's health educator and
speaker with a master's degree in
public health. She founded Fertility
Awareness Counseling and Training
Seminars and has lectured at
hospitals, clinics, and universities
since 1982.

Publisher:
HarperCollins Publishers
(Harper Perennial)

Edition:
1995

Price:
$22.00

Pages:
383

ISBN:
0060950536

Media:
Book

Principal Subject:
Solutions For Infertility

TAKING CHARGE OF YOUR FERTILITY
The Definitive Guide To Natural Birth Control And Pregnancy Achievement

 Recommended For:
Solutions For Infertility

Description:
The intent of this 383 book is to give you "the tools to avoid or achieve pregnancy naturally . . . (So that) information about your cycle and body will empower you with . . . self-knowledge that you rightly deserve." Part 1 explores birth control myths, offers a rationale for the Fertility Awareness Method (FAM), and compares FAM and the Rhythm Method. In Part 2, female and male reproductive anatomy is presented. The three primary fertility signs (waking temperature, cervical fluid, cervical position) are highlighted along with how to observe and chart these signs, and how to interpret variations in menstrual cycles. FAM as either a natural birth control method or a way of becoming pregnant is the topic of Parts 3 and 4. How to construct and read your FAM chart is provided along with photos, example charts, and illustrations throughout. Various related topics, such as maintaining a healthy body, your sexuality, choosing your baby's sex, PMS, menopause, and more are included in Part 5. Appendices (14, consisting of 90 pages) complete the book offering tips on FAM and breastfeeding, effectiveness of FAM, and more.

Evaluation:
This resource presents a thorough treatment of the subject of fertility. It is user-friendly but not condescending, clinical without being heavy on the medical jargon. Its explanations, detailed chart discussions, and illustrations are superior to other resources. Also, in a very informative way, the author doesn't just focus on the Fertility Awareness Method (FAM) itself but considers other areas of a woman's sexuality and her need to take charge of her fertility. For example, she points out how FAM is affected by AIDS awareness, when is the best time to schedule physical exams or surgery, how to time intercourse to increase one's chances of choosing the baby's gender, and much more. So, if there have been attempts to get pregnant which have failed or if one is looking for a resource which enables one to become pregnant without medical interventions, this book is the book.

Where To Find/Buy:
Bookstores and libraries.

WHAT TO EXPECT WHEN YOU'RE EXPERIENCING INFERTILITY
How To Cope With The Emotional Crisis And Survive

 Terrific Resource For:
The emotional aspects of dealing with infertility

 Recommended For:
Solutions For Infertility

Description:

The authors have divided this book into four sections: "Crisis," "Acceptance," "Resolution" and "Epilogue" (C.A.R.E.) to represent the emotional stages an infertile couple may go through. A fifth section, "Treating Infertility: A Guide for Professionals," is intended as a resource for medical professionals on the emotional aspects faced by those dealing with infertility. The four C.A.R.E sections are formatted as statements by men and women who have experienced infertility, followed by responses and explanations by the authors. Topics in the "Crisis" section include issues and emotional challenges a couple may face after learning of their infertility, such as dealing with the medical community, family, friends, spouse, and career. "Acceptance" deals with the issue of childlessness as a lifestyle choice and with making major life decisions based on living with infertility. "Resolution" describes the process of choosing one of three paths a couple then faces, such as continuing attempts to become pregnant, adoption, or living child-free. Lastly, "Epilogue" illustrates the effects of decisions made in the Resolution stage.

Evaluation:

This book takes a comprehensive look at the emotional side of infertility. The format is simple, presented in an easy to read way. The statements and questions posed by people who have experienced infertility problems illustrate the pain and frustration that is so much a part of everyday life for an infertile couple. Answers and explanations are clear, thoughtful, and well-reasoned. The authors address the concerns of both partners, including infertility of both the male and female. Topics include a range of concerns, such as the insensitivity of family, friends, and coworkers, how to cope with the grief of miscarriage, how to maintain faith in one's ability to conceive, and ways to deal with decision-making. The authors provide their information in a comforting, yet realistic voice. Medical information is kept to a minimum. If a couple is looking for hard medical information and options, another book would be better suited. However, those with infertility who are seeking help with emotional frustration, as well as information about how to better to cope with their situation, will find this book an excellent resource.

Where To Find/Buy:

Bookstores and libraries.

Overall Rating
★★★★
Excellent resource on how to cope emotionally with infertility

Design, Ease Of Use
★★★★
Simple, easy-to-read question and answer format

1–4 Stars

Author:
Debby Peoples and Harriette Rovner Ferguson, CSW

Peoples is a past president of Long Island RESOLVE, a freelance writer, and founder of a counseling and support center. Ferguson is a psychotherapist who counsels people with infertility. Both authors lead workshops on the emotional aspects of infertility.

Publisher:
W.W. Norton & Company

Edition:
1998

Price:
$25.00

Pages:
297

ISBN:
0393041042

Media:
Book

Principal Subject:
Solutions For Infertility

Newborn Subject:
Solutions For Infertility

Overall Rating
★★★★
Written by leading authority, this resource is easy to read, yet comprehensive

Design, Ease Of Use
★★
Progression of information somewhat confusing; photos fuzzy, indecipherable

1–4 Stars

Author:
Sherman J. Silber, MD

Silber, an internationally known pioneer in infertility treatment, is medical director of the Infertility Center of St. Louis at St. Luke's Hospital in St. Louis, Missouri. He invented or advanced many of the leading infertility treatments in use today for both men and women.

Publisher:
Warner Books (Time Warner)

Edition:
2nd (1998)

Price:
$16.99

Pages:
477

ISBN:
0446674052

Media:
Book

Principal Subject:
Solutions For Infertility

HOW TO GET PREGNANT WITH THE NEW TECHNOLOGY

 Recommended For:
Solutions For Infertility

Description:

This book is an updated version of Silber's classic, *How To Get Pregnant*. It includes an overview, based on current statistics, of the increasing problem of infertility. Silber then offers an analysis of infertility issues and discusses how technology now can overcome most fertility problems. Silber's thesis is that incorrect diagnoses and ineffective treatments have prevented many prospective parents from becoming pregnant in a timely manner. Chapters in this 477-page book range from Chapter 4, "Figuring Out What's Wrong," through Chapter 8, "Low-Tech Solutions," to Chapter 11, "Step-By-Step Details Of How 'Test-Tube' Babies Are Made," and beyond. The book's medical information is backed by the author's own research and other leading studies in the field. It focuses on the possibilities offered by the newest medical techniques, such as intra-cytoplasmic sperm injection, known as ICSI, in-vitro fertilization and Gamete Intra-Fallopian Transfer, or GIFT. The author also discusses egg and sperm donation, surrogate parenting, and the role genetics plays in the development of personality characteristics. The book includes illustrations, photos, a preface, foreword, and an index.

Evaluation:

This is a gee-whiz story comparable to those findings arising from the frontiers of quantum physics or the micro-worlds of DNA breakthroughs. Silber discusses possible reasons for increasing infertility, then proceeds to lay out technology options he says can solve even the most extreme cases. His medical approach is well-written, easily understandable, and riveting. He doesn't talk down to the reader; one seeking an overview of the problem and potential solutions will find it, another searching for in-depth explanations of pioneering science will find those, as well. Be aware that the author is not without opinions. While acknowledging—and then sidestepping—societal issues surrounding surrogate parenting and other procedures, he firmly believes that sloppy diagnoses and ineffective treatments have doomed too many treatable couples to infertility. To his credit, Silber includes discussions about how to make these treatments affordable, and how to work with insurance companies to gain coverage. The book's one drawback? Fuzzy, largely indecipherable photos. However, any reader able to get through this book without at least exclaiming, "No kidding," just isn't paying attention.

Where To Find/Buy:
Bookstores and libraries.

FERTILITY UK

Description:

The site sponsor's mission is to provide an educational service, offering instruction and counseling in fertility awareness and Natural Family Planning for women/couples. Topics covered include fertility awareness, indicators of fertility, male and female physiology, planning and avoiding pregnancy, breast-feeding, and training. Each of these topics lists links to more detailed information on related subtopics. The homepage also offers an introduction to the organization, an overview, answers to questions, and contacts; the introductory portion of the site offers a site map. "Indicators" details methods used to calculate a woman's fertile period based on a number of factors including temperature and cervix changes. "Physiology" offers details about the reproductive systems of the male and female. The newsletter index offers articles written by a number of professionals on a range of subjects. The three training sections detail seminars and courses available for more information.

Evaluation:

Fertility UK definitely is informational, not flashy. It parallels a book entitled *Fertility* by Dr. Elizabeth Clubb and Jane Knight but lacks the book's intensity, is more abbreviated and contains language that is more user-friendly. This may not be the most colorful or attention-grabbing website on the issue of fertility, but it is, however, full of information about its subject—Natural Family Planning. Couples seeking a successful pregnancy will want to first head for the "Indicators" section, where they will learn to predict fertile days, interpret fertility charts and note other indicators of fertility. There are plenty of medical illustrations, charts, graphs, and planning tools on the site. The text and discussions are arranged logically and cover the topics comprehensively. Each of the topics gives a brief initial summary, then leads to more detailed information. The introduction includes an extensive glossary of terms and a "fertility awareness quiz." This site would be useful to anyone researching Natural Family Planning or looking for nonmedical ways to predict fertility. For couples dealing with infertility problems, however, other resources would be needed.

Where To Find/Buy:

On the Internet at the URL: http://www.fertilityUK.org/

Overall Rating
★★★
Recommended for those couples and professionals exploring Natural Family Planning

Design, Ease Of Use
★★★★
Organized structure offers clear information, easy to read, with many charts

1–4 Stars

Author:
The Fertility Awareness and Natural Family Planning Service UK offers information about Natural Family Planning and other methods the organization offers for nonmedical assistance with fertility issues.

Publisher:
The Fertility Awareness and Natural Family Planning Service UK

Media:
Internet

Principal Subject:
Solutions For Infertility

★★★

Overall Rating
★★★
Proactive book describing treatments, tests, diagnoses, and more; needs some updating

Design, Ease Of Use
★★★★
User-friendly, well-organized; detailed table of contents and questionnaire

1–4 Stars

Author:
Peggy Robin

Robin is a two-time successful fertility patient, community activist, and author of several books including *Saving the Neighborhood* and *Outwitting Toddlers*.

Publisher:
William Morrow & Company

Edition:
1993

Price:
$15.00

Pages:
447

ISBN:
0688117325

Media:
Book

Principal Subject:
Solutions For Infertility

HOW TO BE A SUCCESSFUL FERTILITY PATIENT
Your Guide To Getting The Best Possible Medical Help To Have A Baby

Description:

A two-time successful fertility patient, the author claims her 447 page book is a "patient's book." The author suggests that chapter 1 be read first to determine whether or not you have a fertility problem; the other 10 chapters can be read in any order. Chapter 2 covers the topic of "smart doctor-shopping." The next 2 chapters focus on tests and what the diagnoses mean in layman's terms. Chapters 5–7 offer a questionnaire to help you decide which type of approach (conservative, moderate, aggressive) will work for you, a description of drug therapies, and an overview of assisted reproductive technologies (in vitro, etc.). The next chapter offers tips on whether or not to switch treatment methods, switch doctors, take a break, or give up when you still haven't become pregnant. The stress involved with infertility treatments is the topic of chapter 9. Chapter 10 deals with needs of non-traditional husband/wife roles (single women, gay or Lesbian couples, etc.). The last chapter offers suggestions on choosing an obstetrician should you become pregnant. A glossary, resource guide and suggested reading list are also included.

Evaluation:

Patients who find themselves feeling powerless need to become proactive to achieve their goal of having a child. To do this they need to become knowledgeable, for knowledge is power and this book empowers. As the author states, you will "find it a less daunting chore to pick the right doctor if you know how to talk with confidence to jargon-spouting specialists, how to ask the right questions, and how to decode the answers." Other useful features of this text are the extensive questionnaires (60 questions each for men and women) and follow-up analysis, advice for "non-traditional" couples, and tips on deciding when to make a switch in your fertility treatments. Its information is well-organized, follows logically within each chapter, and is up-to-date. Some recent treatments for infertility are not included, however, so other more current resources also need to be consulted along with this one. What strongly recommends this resource, however, is its lack of medical jargon (except when necessary); thus, it can be a knowledgeable and comfortable "mentor" at a time when would-be parents need a friendly hand to guide them.

Where To Find/Buy:
Bookstores and libraries.

IN PURSUIT OF FERTILITY
A Fertility Expert Tells You How To Get Pregnant

Description:
Written by a fertility specialist with contributions from other specialists, this 349-page book provides in-depth information about the human reproductive system and the evaluation and treatment of both male and female infertility. The book is divided into four main sections, Part 1 dealing exclusively with female infertility, tests, and medical treatments, including the diagnosis and treatment of endometriosis, diseases of the fallopian tubes, and hormonal imbalances. Part II discusses male infertility and treatments: risk factors, the physical exam, fertility drugs, artificial insemination and egg-sperm "micro manipulation." Part III explores issues such as unexplained infertility, repeated spontaneous abortion, and the latest medical breakthroughs in Assisted Reproduction Technology, as well as taking a look at the stress and emotions infertility can give rise to. Part IV discusses alternatives: donor insemination, surrogacy, and adoption. The book includes a glossary of medical and physiological terms.

Evaluation:
This book, as compared to others on the same subject, has a definite authorial "voice" all the way through, lending a real friendliness to much of the more technical/medical material. At the expense of absolute comprehensiveness, it focuses upon prevailing issues and treatments in infertility, leaving aside the more esoteric ones. Its writing, although medically accurate, is not overwhelmingly technical, often choosing to couch explanations of such things as endometriosis in the form of an anecdote, i.e. explaining what it is and how it is treated, then describing how a real woman handles her diagnosis and treatment. Also intriguing are the images of the reproductive system viewed through the eyes of this doctor—they are very often sensitive and even poetic (e.g. the ends of the fallopian tubes as "flowerlike tubal fingers" that "whisk the egg . . . into the oviduct."). Throughout, the book displays a real sensitivity to both men's and women's experiences of infertility (both on a practical and emotional level) and it leaves the reader with the sense of being in capable, knowledgeable hands.

Where To Find/Buy:
Bookstores and libraries.

Overall Rating
★★★
An intelligent, compassionate discussion of infertility

Design, Ease Of Use
★★★★
Writing style combines descriptiveness with medical accuracy

1–4 Stars

Author:
Robert R. Franklin, MD, and Dorothy Kay Brockman
Dr. Robert R. Franklin is a clinical professor of obstetrics and gynecology at Baylor College of Medicine in Houston, Texas, and "an acknowledged leader in his field" of infertility treatment. Dorothy Kay Brockman is a freelance writer living in Houston.

Publisher:
Owl Books (Henry Holt)

Edition:
2nd (1995)

Price:
$12.95

Pages:
349

ISBN:
0805041818

Media:
Book

Principal Subject:
Solutions For Infertility

★★★

Overall Rating
★★★
A fascinating and enlightening foray into America's "reproductive history"

Design, Ease Of Use
★★★
First-hand accounts from the colonial era onwards make this vivid and real

1–4 Stars

Author:
Elaine Tyler May

Elaine Tyler May is Professor of American Studies at the University of Minnesota.

Publisher:
Harvard University Press

Edition:
1997

Price:
$14.95

Pages:
318

ISBN:
0674061829

Media:
Book

Principal Subject:
Solutions For Infertility

BARREN IN THE PROMISED LAND
Childless Americans And The Pursuit Of Happiness

Description:

Written by a professor of American Studies at the University of Michigan, this is a 318-page study of the history of reproduction and childlessness in America from colonial times up to the present day. An introduction discusses how procreation has always been a matter of public concern in America, and it is these "intersections between the most private aspects of our lives—relationships with partners and kin, sexuality, and procreation—and the public life around us" that this book aims to study. Chapters 1–4 take us from the colonial era to the beginnings of reproductive engineering in the 19th century, "eugenics," compulsory sterilization practices, and the "baby boom" of the post-World War II era. Chapter 5 takes a close look at our growing understanding of infertility and its causes. Chapter 6 looks at the rise in voluntary childlessness after the peak of the baby boom, and the "childfree lifestyle." The last chapter focuses on the experience of infertility today, the "baby quest" through medical treatments, and modern identity and parenthood. Letters from childless individuals in response to the author's query are also used throughout this book, as are many first-hand accounts and testimonies.

Evaluation:

This book offers a fascinating glimpse into America's concern with its citizens' reproductive practices, and how the private and public attitudes towards childbearing have shifted and overlapped throughout history. It is a study of American culture: a look at ideas of motherhood and childbearing is really a look at ourselves. The author uses lots of first-hand accounts, presidents' speeches, personal letters, sermons, and diaries, to weave a vivid tapestry of both "public" and "private" values. These can often be unbearably sad (Anne Bradstreet praying for a child during the colonial era), uplifting (a 1907 woman claiming "You cannot use me to breed food for your factories"), and shocking (testimonies of women sterilized against their will). This book is not a "light" read, nor is it a "how to" book. On the other hand, it offers a fascinating cultural study of our society in its historical struggle with reproductive choices or dilemmas. As such, it can provide important background reading for American women and men who are wrestling with those same choices and dilemmas in their lives today.

Where To Find/Buy:
Bookstores and libraries.

THE FERTILITY SOURCEBOOK
Everything You Need To Know

★★★

Description:

The author addresses many issues about fertility, including causes of infertility, infertility specialists, tests, infertility drugs, Assisted Reproductive Technology (ART), same sex parenting, pregnancy loss, and alternative treatments. Chapters 1 and 3 discuss various factors that may render a couple infertile, including environmental influences. The author discusses fertility specialists, including descriptions of additional factors that may affect fertility, such as genetic disorders and sexually transmitted diseases. Tests and "work-ups" seek to determine either male factor or female factor infertility, which the author describes in two separate chapters. Fertility drugs, how to use them, and assisted conception are topics covered in Chapter 8 of this 12 chapter book. Illustrations are included to help the reader visualize the topic. Other subjects indirectly related to infertility discuss gay/lesbian fertility issues, miscarriage, and alternatives to traditional medical treatments. An appendix is included for additional support and information.

Evaluation:

There is a recurring theme in this book, one the author stresses repeatedly for the benefit of the reader—the importance of asking many questions and educating oneself about one's infertility. The author reminds a couple trying to conceive that a fertility specialist can become "God-like" in their eyes, with the result being that they will do whatever the specialist suggests in their desperation to get pregnant. The author states that it is important, and sometimes difficult, when dealing with any medical condition to remember that second opinions are available. The author also broaches an issue that too many other authors on this subject neglect as she discusses the many environmental factors that may influence a couple's infertility (stress, obesity, personal hygiene, exercise, sexual activities, and occupation). She even cites male sexual dysfunction as a source of infertility problems. This is a departure from much of the infertility literature, which more often presents infertility primarily, if not solely, as a medical dysfunction of the reproductive system.

Where To Find/Buy:

Bookstores and libraries.

Overall Rating
★★★
Clear explanations regarding testing and infertility drugs

Design, Ease Of Use
★★★
Chapters are easy to read, without being to technical

1–4 Stars

Author:
M. Sara Rosenthal

Rosenthal is a health writer and journalist who has authored other books regarding pregnancy issues. She also lectures to lay organizations about health issues and performs pro bono work for various health organizations

Publisher:
Lowell House

Edition:
2nd (1998)

Price:
$17.00

Pages:
307

ISBN:
1565658663

Media:
Book

Principal Subject:
Solutions For Infertility

★★★

Overall Rating
★★★
An accurate and clear introduction to infertility and high-risk pregnancy

Design, Ease Of Use
★★★
Readable presentation of "the facts"

1–4 Stars

Author:
Diana Raab, BS, RN

The author is a nursing consultant and medical writer, and the mother of three children after experiencing infertility and high-risk pregnancies.

Publisher:
Hunter House

Edition:
1991

Price:
$14.95

Pages:
316

ISBN:
0897930800

Media:
Book

Principal Subject:
Solutions For Infertility

GETTING PREGNANT AND STAYING PREGNANT
Overcoming Infertility And Managing Your High-Risk Pregnancy

Description:
The author, a nurse who herself experienced miscarriage, infertility, and high-risk pregnancies, wrote this book to guide both professionals in the field and women experiencing similar difficulties. The first three chapters discuss infertility: its causes, testing, and alternatives for infertile couples. Chapters 4–5 explain "high-risk factors" before and during pregnancy, including anatomical abnormalities, infections and disease, hypertension, unusual fetal positions, and ectopic pregnancies. The following three chapters discuss sexuality, nutrition, medical tests, and bed rest for high-risk pregnancies. Chapters 9–10 explain miscarriage and other losses of a fetus. Cesareans, premature births, birth defects and genetic risks are discussed next, and the last chapter focuses on special issues (single moms, teenage pregnancies) and ethics (sex selection, fetal surgery) involved in high-risk pregnancies and infertility. Appendices include a look at the female and male reproductive systems, a postnatal exercise program, an extensive list of support groups and associations (9 pages), and a glossary of terms.

Evaluation:
Information offered here about high-risk pregnancy and infertility is accurate and clear. Women experiencing these difficulties will find this a good overview of the issues involved. Including her own and other women's stories about coping with these problems adds a needed "personal" touch to the more scientific data. As the complications of high-risk pregnancy and infertility don't always occur together, this book may appeal to separate groups of readers, which has its advantages for some couples, but which may also point the way to other more detailed resources on infertility or high-risk pregnancy for readers who are experiencing one but not the other. All in all this is a useful factual resource, but people may likely find they need to refer to other books on the separate subjects of infertility (especially in light of new findings, treatments, and techniques) and dealing with a high-risk pregnancy.

Where To Find/Buy:
Bookstores and libraries, or order direct by calling (800) 266-5592.

THE LONG-AWAITED STORK
A Guide To Parenting After Infertility

Description:

Glazer, a clinical social worker specializing in the areas of infertility, pregnancy loss, adoption, and parenting after infertility, offers a look into the thoughts, feelings, and questions that arise for many parents after infertility. Her 277+ page book is broken into two parts. The first part looks at some of the feelings and concerns facing infertile couples as they first become parents and throughout the years that follow the arrival of their child (from birth through adolescence) The second half of the book focuses on special circumstances that arise for couples as a result of infertility. Chapters in this section focus on: domestic adoption, international adoption, raising biological and adopted children, donor insemination, surrogacy, new reproductive technologies (IVF, GIFT), multiple births, only children, and special needs children. Most of the experiences and observations used for the writing of this book came from the author's advertisement in a RESOLVE newsletter in which "hundreds of people" contacted her.

Evaluation:

Any parents who have wrestled with infertility will appreciate this book. In a very caring and sensitive way, the book illustrates that, unlike what most people believe, feelings of inadequacy, loss, and isolation that couples face when dealing with infertility problems do not go away once they have a child. Rather, as the narratives and anecdotes in this book show, these feelings come back to haunt couples until their child reaches the ages of 7 to 12. The catalysts for these negative feelings are others' lack of understanding, friends' subsequent pregnancies, and a sense of "feeling not quite in the club." Each chapter in the first section of the book highlights these feelings with personal stories of what others have gone through and offers emotional encouragement and suggestions on ways to deal with these feelings. This same compassionate attitude is present in the second half of the book which addresses topics from adoption to donor insemination to special needs children. In short, a basic message of this book is that pregnancy or adoption does not resolve infertility issues for couples, but instead they need sensitivity and support.

Where To Find/Buy:

Bookstores and libraries.

Overall Rating
★★★
A sensitive and informative guide to feelings arising for parents after infertility

Design, Ease Of Use
★★★
Well organized, reader friendly

1–4 Stars

Author:
Ellen Sarasohn Glazer

Glazer is a clinical social worker specializing in the areas of infertility, pregnancy loss, adoptions, and parenting after infertility. She is a former member of the national board of directors of RESOLVE, Inc.

Publisher:
Lexington Books (Macmillan)

Edition:
1990

Price:
$12.95

Pages:
277

ISBN:
002911814X

Media:
Book

Principal Subject:
Solutions For Infertility

★★★

Overall Rating
★★★
A brief but comprehensive and accurate overview of fertility

Design, Ease Of Use
★★
Somewhat dry, totally clinical presentation

1–4 Stars

Author:
Sarah Freeman, PhD, RNC, and Vern L. Bullough, PhD, RN

Sarah Freeman, Ph.D., R.N.C., is assistant professor at SUNY Buffalo's School of Nursing. Vern L. Bullough, Ph.D., R.N., is Distinguished Professor of History, also at SUNY Buffalo, and the author of other books on human sexuality.

Publisher:
Prometheus Books

Edition:
1993

Pages:
129

ISBN:
0879757981

Media:
Book

Principal Subject:
Solutions For Infertility

THE COMPLETE GUIDE TO FERTILITY & FAMILY PLANNING

Description:

Written by two professors (of Nursing and History, respectively) at SUNY Buffalo, this 129-page book offers a look at the many sides of fertility and human conception. The historical, religious, psychological and medical implications of infertility are all described, including charts and diagrams to help illustrate the human reproductive process. Chapter 1 shows us how infertility was understood throughout history and the relatively "modern-day" discoveries of how humans conceive, and current practices in artificial insemination. Chapter 2 covers the basic anatomy and physiology of men and women's reproductive systems and how they work. Chapters 3–4 discuss "What Can Go Wrong" and "Discovering What's Wrong": diagnosing causes of infertility in men and women. Chapter 5 discusses current treatments for infertility: changing sexual methods, drug therapies, surgery, in vitro fertilization, gamete transfer (GIFT), and other types of medical fertilization are discussed. The last chapter focuses on "Issues and Alternatives" to fertility treatments: surrogacy, adoption, and childlessness.

Evaluation:

This book is a little on the dry side, and its treatment of the issues is brief, but it does offer clear and accurate information about many of the issues that infertile couples may face. Although some of the psychological and religious implications of infertility are raised, focus is on the physical aspects of fertility and conception: how the reproductive system works, the causes of infertility, and medical tests and treatments. This might be a good initial resource for couples experiencing infertility. It offers short but sound "refresher courses" in human reproductive anatomy, and introduces the sometimes bewildering array of medical methods used to treat infertility, as well as looking at the alternatives for couples for whom pregnancy is ultimately not possible. Those who would like a closer look at their options as well as the more complex psychological issues at stake will find they need the help of other, more in-depth resources.

Where To Find/Buy:

Bookstores and libraries.

DR. RICHARD MARRS' FERTILITY BOOK
America's Leading Infertility Expert Tells You Everything You Need To Know About Getting Pregnant

★★★

Description:

This 506-page book pulls together an enormous amount of information pertaining to the emotional/psychological, medical, and financial aspects of infertility, written by a doctor with notable achievements in the field. Part One provides an in-depth look (with drawings) of the reproductive process in men and women. Part Two is a general introduction to infertility and its treatment, including finding the right doctor and an explanation of the basic infertility workup. Part Three looks at the current medical tests and techniques used to increase fertility, from fertility drugs to male problems and solutions; tubal, uterine, cervical and pelvic problems; and the various types of Assisted Reproductive Technologies (IVF, GIFT, ZIFT, cryopreservation). Part Four discusses the emotional response to infertility, coping techniques, as well as alternatives (surrogacy, adoption, "child-free" living). This last section ends with a discussion of the future of reproductive technology. Many chapters have their own glossary of key terms, and the book also contains a general glossary.

Evaluation:

Towards the end of this book, the author states "the emotional and medical aspects of infertility can't be addressed separately, they need to be looked at as two halves of a whole." The goal of this book, then, is to examine both the medical/technical side of infertility as well as the emotional/psychological. It accomplishes the former in a very comprehensive way, for it is an enormous book, packed with extremely valuable, although at times overly technical, information about the human reproductive system and how infertility treatments work (or don't work). It is vital for men and women to have access to this kind of accurate, specific information before launching into the world of infertility treatments. However, this kind of "techno-talk" sits somewhat uneasily with chapters focused on the personal/emotional side of things, which often feel more hurried and less convincing. As a result, although this book offers a comprehensive and knowledgeable sweep of the medical issues, it has less overall balance than other resources on the subject.

Where To Find/Buy:

Bookstores and libraries.

Overall Rating
★★★
A comprehensive, current look at the medical/technical side of infertility

Design, Ease Of Use
★★
Sheer breadth & encyclopedic scope may make this tough going

1–4 Stars

Author:
Richard Marrs, MD, Lisa Bloch, Kathy Silverman

Dr. Richard Marrs "was the second doctor in the United States to achieve the birth of a baby from in vitro fertilization; the birth of the first frozen-embryo baby in the country, as well as the world's first pregnancy using a combination of ZIFT and surrogate gestational carriers." Bloch and Silverman are a "television writing and producing team."

Publisher:
Delacorte Press
(Bantam Doubleday Dell)

Edition:
1997

Price:
$25.95

Pages:
506

ISBN:
0385314361

Media:
Book

Principal Subject:
Solutions For Infertility

★★★

Overall Rating
★★★
Best suited as a companion text to instruction on natural family planning

Design, Ease Of Use
★★
Dense text, sometimes heavy on technical jargon; detailed graphs, diagrams, charts

1–4 Stars

Author:
Dr. Elizabeth Clubb & Jane Knight

The authors are a doctor and nurse team with many years' experience teaching natural family planning methods to women, couples, and health professional. They are also extensively involved with researching, writing, and lecturing in this field.

Publisher:
David & Charles

Edition:
3rd (1997)

Price:
$14.95

Pages:
192

ISBN:
0715304240

Media:
Book

Principal Subject:
Solutions For Infertility

FERTILITY
Fertility Awareness And Natural Family Planning

Description:

A doctor and nurse team with backgrounds in the field of natural family planning (NFP) methods have developed this 192 page, 18 chapter book focusing on fertility. The book is divided into 4 parts. Part 1 is the heart of the book (roughly 65+ pages) and describes the "sympto-thermal method" (also known as the muco-thermic method or the double-check method). The male and female reproductive systems are highlighted along with first, second, and third fertility indicators (temperature, cervical mucus, and cervix). Numerous charts and graphs are offered to further explain the text. Part 2 deals with "Fertility Awareness and NFP in Special Circumstances." Here you will find information on fertility as it relates to the period after childbirth, during breast-feeding, for those who were on the Pill, and for those who are entering menopause. "Gynecology"—part 3—discusses infertility (10 pages), new technologies (saliva/cervical mucus, hormone detections, etc.), and the effect of infections, contraceptions, and more on fertility. An appendix offers a sympto-thermal chart along with instructions on how to read and use it.

Evaluation:

This book, as the authors state, is designed to complement instruction given by a qualified fertility awareness teacher. Presuming such instruction which would help the reader to digest this information which can be quite heavy and technical, there is no question that most information currently available on the sympto-thermal method and the benefits of natural family planning can be found in this guide. Without the instruction, it can only be read by couples who can concentrate on and digest such information on their own. With concomitant instruction or not, this work clearly speaks to the effectiveness of this method of natural family planning, data which many other resources ignore. Unfortunately, the writing style is dense and the margins narrow (1/2"), although these constraints are eased by the numerous charts, graphs, or diagrams found on almost every page. Medical professionals or those couples seriously interested in understanding the hows, whys and what's involved with planning for a pregnancy or avoiding a pregnancy the natural way will find this book useful.

Where To Find/Buy:

Bookstores and libraries. Their website URL is: http://www.fertilityUK.org

YOUR FERTILITY SIGNALS
Using Them To Achieve Or Avoid Pregnancy, Naturally

Description:

The author combines her backgrounds in art and biology to explore various ways to achieve or avoid pregnancy using fertility signals. The book consists of eight parts and 159 pages. In Parts 2 and 6 it presents the female's biology focusing on the three major fertility signals (cervical mucus, basal body temperature, cervix position and shape) and hormonal influences. Parts 2 and 3 detail the ovulation and the basal body temperature methods; numerous sample charts and illustrations are included. Part 4 explains how fertility changes affect energy and moods and how to achieve intimacy without intercourse. Part 5 expands on various topics such as: breast feeding, after the pill, regulating your cycle with light, choosing your baby's sex, and more. "Infertility Self-Help" in Part 7 discusses men's infertility and other infertility problems; sample mucus-temperature charts are included with lists of possibly related infertility problems. Part 8 deals with vaginal infections as related to infertility. The book ends with how to find teachers to help you use these methods along with additional resources and blank charts to record mucus-temperature readings.

Evaluation:

The author's intent in writing this book is to empower women (and couples) to "experience the marvelous power of living in harmony with" their fertility, whether they wish to become pregnant or avoid pregnancy. Through numerous sample charts and illustrations she has accomplished that intent. Her work contains very detailed and well illustrated information. Yet, as the book asserts, fertility isn't an exact science since many considerations can interfere with predicting fertile times—past surgeries, infections, stress, etc. With this as a given, the book offers an alternative and less invasive procedure than normally offered by many medical professionals, Its approach, then, has appeal for couples who, for varying philosophical, religious, or physical reasons, need alternatives to contraceptive methods or new reproductive technologies. The problems with this resource is that there is almost too much information given at times and that some sections are confusing, scattered, and repetitive.

Where To Find/Buy:

Bookstores and libraries, or order direct by writing the publisher at P.O. Box 19875, St. Louis, MO 63144 (add $2.00 for postage).

Overall Rating
★★★
Useful as an alternative to medical methods for predicting fertile periods

Design, Ease Of Use
★★
Excellent use of charts and illustrations; text sometimes rambles, repeats and confuses

1–4 Stars

Author:
Merryl Winstein

Winstein, an author, illustrator and teacher, holds a BFA with a Minor in Biology from Washington University in St. Louis.

Publisher:
Smooth Stone Press

Edition:
2nd (1997)

Price:
$13.95

Pages:
159

ISBN:
0961940107

Media:
Book

Principal Subject:
Solutions For Infertility

★★

Overall Rating
★★
Informative, but out-of-date, resource guide that deals with infertility questions

Design, Ease Of Use
★★
Question and answer format is somewhat slow and disjointed at times

1–4 Stars

Author:
Melvin J. Frisch, MD, and Gayle Rapoport

Melvin J. Frisch, M.D., is board certified by the American College of Obstetrics and Gynecology, practices in Minneapolis, and has a special interest in infertility and tubal microsurgery. Gayle Rapoport resolved her fertility problem as a patient of Dr. Frisch.

Publisher:
Berkley Publishing Group (Body Press/Perigee Books)

Edition:
1987

Price:
$14.00

Pages:
329

ISBN:
0399517111

Media:
Book

Principal Subject:
Solutions For Infertility

GETTING PREGNANT!
Over 1,000 Of The Most-Important Questions & Answers About Fertility Problems & How To Have A Baby

Description:

Getting Pregnant! is a collection of over 1,000 questions focusing on fertility problems and possible solutions available as of 1987. Written by both an OB/Gyn and a former medical secretary/ successful infertility patient, this book was written so that "people with a non-medical background could understand." It is written from a woman's point of view to make the book "personal, like a physician talking with a patient." Questions start out as simple e.g., "What happens to boys during puberty?" They then work up to complicated explanations of medical procedures e.g., "What is laparoscopy?" This book consists of 16 chapters and each chapter contains between 20 and 70 questions. Chapter topics address: infertility, the reproductive systems, how to get pregnant, causes and treatments of infertility in women and in men, endometriosis, "unexplained infertility," artificial insemination, effects of sexually transmitted diseases, medical advances, the emotional effects of infertility, and adoption.

Evaluation:

If one is new to the subject of fertility and getting pregnant, the books provides a good introduction. The writers have done a good job of starting at the beginning and working their way through the range of questions that anyone (from a sixth grader to a grandmother) might have on how to get pregnant. Explanations, such as what one has to do for a post-coital test, are clear and frank. This kind of book takes the mystery out of sitting in a cold examination room with a piece of paper thinly covering oneself, wondering what exactly the doctor is going to do next, or ask for next, or what the test is for. It examines myths and misinformation that are perpetuated by hearsay, and offers instead concise, easily understood answers to each question. A detailed glossary of terms is also included. This book may be too simplistic for some and it is certainly out-of-date, but it is uniquely informative.

Where To Find/Buy:

Bookstores and libraries.

HAVING YOUR BABY BY DONOR INSEMINATION
A Complete Resource Guide

Description:
The author, a "leader in the maternal and child health field," uses her personal experiences as a basis to address ethical, social, legal and genetic concerns arising from Donor Insemination (DI). Chapters of this 462 page book deal with male infertility, alternative routes to having children (adoption, foster parenting, child-free living), donor insemination (traditional unknown donor vs. known donor), sperm banks, and more. This book raises serious questions and Noble attempts to answer them by challenging past beliefs throughout her book: "Why does the practice of donor anonymity and secrecy remain almost universal? Why are no standard records kept of donors that can be matched to recipients? Why are parents reluctant to disclose not only the identity of the sperm donor, but even the . . . DI itself, to their children?" The intent in her book is to serve the "best interests of the child." She hopes that the direction that open adoption is taking will influence the current practice of DI and take into consideration the child's rights to know his or her paternal origins.

Evaluation:
In an era in which couples are faced with choices to make to correct fertility problems, donor insemination has become an accepted solution, especially in the areas of in vitro fertilization and surrogate motherhood. However, at the time she wrote her book ten years ago, there had been no consistent policies established to govern this practice. Although there have been some changes in this arena, parents' choices and trust concerning donor insemination are still primarily controlled by medical professionals. And these decisions are ones that literally have ramifications and consequences throughout eternity. Although this book is thick with personal opinions and criticisms, Noble's observations need to be listened to. She describes the secrecy surrounding DI as a "fetish" which confronts the child born from such a procedure with the same issues as those confronting adopted children as they search for their biological parents. Consequently, those involved with making the decisions behind DI—medical professionals, parents, family, donor—need to read the points Noble raises to make a more-informed and careful decision.

Where To Find/Buy:
Bookstores and libraries.

Overall Rating
★★
Raises serious questions concerning current practice of anonymity of donor insemination

Design, Ease Of Use
★★
Reads much like a textbook; repetitive at times; some information is dated.

1–4 Stars

Author:
Elizabeth Noble

Noble is the director of the Maternal and Child Health Center in Cambridge, Massachusetts. She is also the founder of the Obstetrics and Gynecology section of the American Physical Therapy Association.

Publisher:
Houghton Mifflin

Edition:
1987

Price:
$15.95

Pages:
462

ISBN:
039545395X

Media:
Book

Principal Subject:
Solutions For Infertility

★★

Overall Rating
★★
Strong arena for emotional support, but lacking in solid current information

Design, Ease Of Use
★★
Straightforward navigation but lack of graphics leaves the site dull and lifeless

1–4 Stars

Media:
Internet

Principal Subject:
Solutions For Infertility

RESOLVE

Description:

RESOLVE is a national non-profit organization founded in 1974 to assist people "in resolving their infertility by providing information, support, and advocacy." The homepage outlines services available: a helpline for infertility information, physician referrals, and publications for purchase (booklets, starter kits, fact sheets, newsletters); a medical helpline and infertility support groups also are available to members. The homepage also features information on topics such as: infertility myths and facts; managing family, friends and the holidays; and "How do I know if I have [an] infertility problem?" A sample fact sheet is provided focusing on "What is an infertility specialist?" (More fact sheets can be ordered). Three pages of information detail the variations between MDs, Ob/Gyns, Urologists, and Reproductive Endocrinologists, and provide information on how to select a doctor and get the most out of your care. Sample newsletter articles are also provided.

Evaluation:

If you are seeking either the latest scientific breakthroughs in the field of infertility or basic information about how to deal with infertility, you'll need to look elsewhere. The information provided here is disappointing, sometimes outdated and misleading. For example, an ovulation kit and the basal temperature method are suggested ways to determine when a woman is ovulating. However, other, more exacting techniques (that won't endanger your pocketbook) are not detailed. This site's strength lies in its emotional support for those dealing with infertility. You'll find comebacks to comments such as "So, when are you going to start a family?" or "Well, I guess we'll never be grandparents." Myths are debunked: "Why don't you relax and take a vacation?" or "If you adopt a baby, you'll get pregnant." "Coping with the Holidays" is a sensitive addition to help deal with the combined stresses of infertility, family pressures (and children), and the holiday season. Even so, we suggest other more complete references on the topic of infertility, those that provide information about the groundbreaking advances being made in this field. If you're dealing with infertility, you deserve that information.

Where To Find/Buy:

On the Internet at the URL: http://www.resolve.org/

50 ESSENTIAL THINGS TO DO WHEN THE DOCTOR SAYS IT'S INFERTILITY

Description:

An "award-winning medical and science writer," Levitt states her book's purpose is to "focus on the positive . . . and to help you take a proactive role in understanding and dealing with infertility." The 182 pages of this book are divided into seven parts. Topics include: defining infertility (includes finding infertility specialists, etc.); understanding the physiology of female infertility, male infertility, lifestyle effects on fertility (alcohol, smoking, drug, etc.); high-tech infertility solutions (AID, AIH, IVF, GIFT, and more): developing a support team: and stacking the fertility deck in your favor. These seven topics are further divided into a total of 50 "essential things to do" concerning infertility. The table of contents lists all 50 of these subtopics within each of the seven main topics. Each of these 50 subtopics amount to 2–4 pages that address the given concern, for example, "Find Out If a Genetic Disorder is Affecting Your Fertility." Each subtopic closes with a summarizing paragraph that gives you tips on "An Important Thing You Can Do."

Evaluation:

The title of this book is a catchy one and it delivers what it advertises by literally listing 50 things to do when the doctor says it's infertility. What this means in reality is that it presents a general overview of various causes and treatments concerning infertility. Its tone is friendly and provides a helpful, current introduction to the world of infertility, its causes and treatments. Consequently, the couple could find it a helpful first step in becoming familiar with this world. The main problems with this book are its organizational elements. First of all, in an introductory text which is filled with a whole new world of medical jargon, a glossary is essential. This book has none. Secondly, the Index is quite extensive, but cross-referencing is next to impossible due to the fact that all left handed pages are not numbered and many right handed pages also lack numbers. Finally, the table of contents is useful in that it lists all 50 "essentials," but they are somewhat difficult and distracting to read since they are all in capital letters. In summary, if a couple is unsure about whether or not to pursue seeing an infertility specialist or clinic, this book will give them a taste of what they are in for. But if they wish to learn about infertility in depth, they need to use other resources.

Where To Find/Buy:

Bookstores and libraries.

Overall Rating
★★
Overview of infertility causes and treatments, little in-depth treatment

Design, Ease Of Use
★
No page numbers on majority of pages; glossary would be helpful

1–4 Stars

Author:
B. Blake Levitt
Levitt is an award-winning medical and science writer, and co-author of *Before You Conceive, The Complete Pregnancy Guide*.

Edition:
1995

Price:
$10.95

Pages:
182

ISBN:
0452271193

Media:
Book

Principal Subject:
Solutions For Infertility

Overall Rating

★

Uninspired presentation focuses on high-tech approach rather than diagnostic solutions

Design, Ease Of Use

★★

Dry writing style with extensive medical jargon used; helpful analysis of option costs

1–4 Stars

Author:

Hugh D. Melnick, MD, and Nancy Intrator

Melnick, M.D., is founder and director of Advanced Fertility Services in New York City, one of the first independent, non-hospital based infertility centers. Intrator, a writer specializing in health and family topics, is a former patient, now mother of two.

Publisher:

The Josara Companies

Edition:

1998

Price:

$17.95

Pages:

184

ISBN:

0966041909

Media:

Book

Principal Subject:

Solutions For Infertility

VII. Solutions For Infertility

THE PREGNANCY PRESCRIPTION
The Success-Oriented Approach To Overcoming Infertility

Description:

This 184 page resource draws a distinction between what it calls a "diagnosis-oriented" approach to infertility and a "success-oriented" approach. According to this premise, a diagnosis approach uses any number of diagnostic procedures to discover what is preventing natural conception, then attempts to correct those problems. In contrast, the author's approach focuses early on how to achieve pregnancy moving rapidly to technology-based solutions. The result, according to the authors, is less pain and frustration for couples, lower expenses, and greater chances for a successful pregnancy. Their approach calls for use of infertility drugs with one of two types of insemination, then in-vitro fertilization if necessary. The book is divided into four parts: "Rationale For The Success-Oriented Approach," "The Pregnancy Prescription," "Other Considerations," and "The Ultimate Decision." It includes a number of comparisons and checklists, as well as a preface, photos, a glossary, and an index. Melnick's approach is based on his training and experience; patient stories are used to illustrate key points.

Evaluation:

This book presents an increasingly accepted philosophy for treating infertility—forego long and expensive tests designed to uncover the cause of a couple's infertility and move directly to the technology that offers the best chance for a successful pregnancy. The authors present that portion of their argument adequately. Where their book fails is through its overall mediocre presentation and in its discussion of options. Unfortunately, the book quickly falls into a manual of tech-speak. Medical terminology is explained, but the use of jargon throughout the text requires a dedicated reader. The writing is uninspired, and the editing will make an experienced reader wince. Some couples well-versed in infertility literature may find it comprehensible, but those new to seeking help are likely to be intimidated. An example: "Both MESA and TESE make the successful outcome of an IVF cycle even more difficult, since another variable—obtaining viable sperm—has been added." Happily for most readers, that level of information—and the approach advocated by this book—is available in other resources offering broader bases, better editing, more interesting writing, and adequate documentation.

Where To Find/Buy:

Bookstores, libraries, or order direct by calling (800) 345-6665.

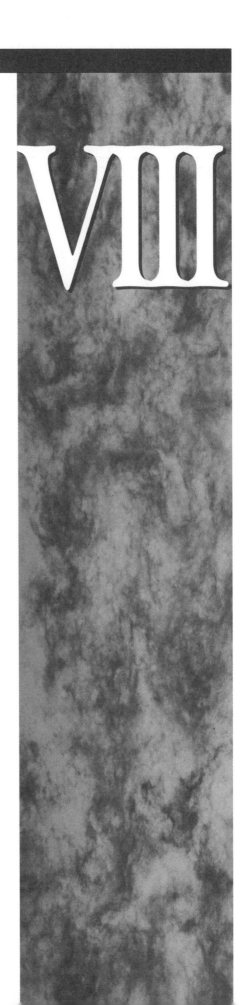

GAINING
AN OVERVIEW:
ALL-INCLUSIVE
RESOURCES

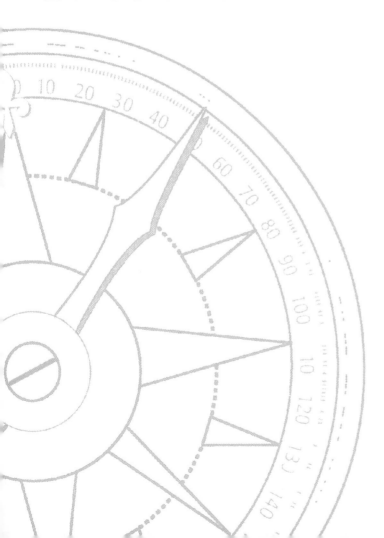

INTRODUCTION

Preparing to have a child, giving birth, and then parenting that child can be one of the most exciting and enriching parts of life. It can also be frightening—so much to learn, and so much seemingly riding on our "performance."

From the moment they hear the news that they are pregnant, parents are called upon to make important choices which will have a profound influence on the life of their unborn child. Decisions must be made during a mother's pregnancy in terms of choosing a maternal care provider, exercise, nutrition, and lifestyle choices. Childbirth also brings into focus numerous other decisions—pain management, birthing location, birthing participants, care provider, and more. And that is just the beginning of a couple's decision-making! Well before their baby is born, parents are also trying to decide how they are going to interact with and relate to this precious little person. They begin to realize the enormity of what their parenting job entails as they journey mentally down that long road toward helping this tiny, immature individual become a healthy, productive, and caring adult. They find themselves constantly asking, "How will we do this?"

With all the available childbirth choices and parenting style "labels," new parents can understandably feel overwhelmed. Most likely they will then benefit from reading a variety of suggestions and advice from professionals who have many years of experience in helping other couples make their pregnancy, childbirth, and parenting choices. By reading this book and taking advantage of the resources we have recommended earlier in this guidebook, it is clear that you want to educate yourself so you can make the right choices for you and your baby. We hope some of the resources in the previous sections will answer your specific questions about various aspects of this process of becoming a parent.

The resources in this section provide a more general overview of the process of having a baby. They are good sources to turn to for basic questions and quick answers. They may point you to topics and areas of which you want more information. As we have suggested throughout, choose a resource that fits your personal style and approach, and don't take any one source as the absolute truth.

Those of us involved with this book have found giving birth and parenting our children to be a most joyful and challenging undertaking. We wish you well as you begin your own personal adventure!

THE COMPLETE BOOK OF PREGNANCY AND CHILDBIRTH

★★★★

 Recommended For:
Gaining An Overview: All-Inclusive

Description:

This 432 page book addresses current social changes arising from "the pressure on women by a powerful medical system to surrender themselves to it as passive patients." The main focus of this book is on the experience of childbirth itself and how each step and stage feels, assisted by detailed diagrams, charts, and discussions of various birthing options available (homebirth, waterbirth, drug-free, medicated, etc.). The writer describes choices now available to women so they can decide how to have their babies, the kind of setting and care they might prefer, and how they wish to welcome their babies into the world. Information is given using the same phrases that doctors and nurses use in order to help the reader become more familiar with them and communicate more easily with these professionals. There are suggestions on what to ask the doctor and how to retain control over the experience. An overview guide is also provided to help parents understand what is happening during their pregnancy week-by-week. The first 10 days of newborn care is also explained along with breastfeeding basics, and more.

Evaluation:

This book is a comprehensive guide to pregnancy and childbirth. It focuses on many aspects of pregnancy—from the medical arena (details on the effects of various drugs, procedures, etc.) to explanations of physical and emotional changes. Although this book offers information you'd expect to find in a textbook, the book does not read like one. The writer manages her subject in a warm and friendly voice that makes it very approachable. The section of the book dealing with childbirth methods provides explanations of various options and methods in a clear and straightforward manner. The last section of the book deals with the "medical control of birth." The attitude here is that the mother is in charge, and understanding what doctors may want to do and why, will help her to make informed choices. This book is recommended, not only because it offers numerous alternatives for childbirth but because it also supports a woman's control of the childbirth experience.

Where To Find/Buy:

Bookstores and libraries.

Overall Rating
★★★★
Comprehensive treatment of women's choices and control of their childbirth

Design, Ease Of Use
★★★★
Textbook design; subheadings in table of contents & throughout; color illustrations

1–4 Stars

Author:
Sheila Kitzinger

Kitzinger is the author of twenty-two books on pregnancy, childbirth and parenting. She has an international reputation as a social anthropologist, researcher, and women's advocate on pregnancy. She lives in England with her husband and five daughters.

Publisher:
Alfred A. Knopf

Edition:
3rd (1996)

Price:
$24.00

Pages:
432

ISBN:
0679450289

Media:
Book

Principal Subject:
Gaining An Overview: All-Inclusive

★★★★

Overall Rating
★★★★
A valuable, broad-based reference written from the unusual perspective of the baby

Design, Ease Of Use
★★★★
Detailed table of contents, great visuals for reference, well-organized

1–4 Stars

Author:
Dr. Miriam Stoppard

Stoppard is the author of bestselling books on women's health, pregnancy, and baby and child care, including *The First Weeks of Life*, *The Baby and Child A to Z Medical Handbook*, *Day-by-Day Baby Care Book*, and, most recently, *The Magic of Sex*.

Publisher:
Dorling Kindersley

Edition:
1993

Price:
$29.95

Pages:
351

ISBN:
1564581829

Media:
Book

Principal Subject:
Gaining An Overview: All-Inclusive

CONCEPTION, PREGNANCY AND BIRTH

Terrific Resource For:
Understanding the prenatal, labor, and birth experiences of both baby and mother

Recommended For:
Gaining An Overview: All-Inclusive

Description:
This book begins with a general overview which describes each of the chapters of the book and what the reader will find. Then, each chapter focuses on a particular subject area: "Preparing For Pregnancy," "You and Your Developing Baby," "The Birth of Your Choice," "Food and Eating in Pregnancy," "A Fit Pregnancy," "Your Prenatal Care," "Caring For Your Unborn Baby," "Common Complaints," "Medical Emergencies," "A Sensual Pregnancy," "Getting Ready For Your Baby," "Managing Your Labor," "Your Baby is Born," "Getting to Know Your Newborn Baby," and "Adjusting to Parenthood." All of these chapters contain numerous illustrations and pictures. Also, the reader will find blocked text on nearly every page which cumulatively cover a multitude of information, such as "Empty Calories," "Will My Mood Affect My Baby?" "The Effect of Your Age," and more. "A Case Study" of different individuals appears for many topics such as "The Older Father," "An Emergency Delivery," "The Single Mother," and other special circumstances. A resource list is included for further support and information.

Evaluation:
This book is written from the unusual perspective of the baby. As the author states, "Much of what doctors encourage women to do has little real significance until we consider it in the light of the unborn child." The book begins with a helpful summary of the book, chapter by chapter. This overview encourages awareness and responsibility for making positive choices concerning pregnancy. In addition, the table of contents gives a good overview of this very detailed book. The pictures provided interestingly convey the development of the fetus and the mother. Much like an encyclopedia, there is thorough use of text formatting and pictures/illustrations, offering visual referencing of the subject matter. For example, illustrations that are coupled with the text in "Exercise For A Fit Pregnancy" enhance the book's ability to communicate clearly and concisely to the reader. This book would serve as a thorough reference for the topics contained in its title—conception, pregnancy, and birth. Both new mothers and women who have already been through a pregnancy could rely on this book as a source of abundant information.

Where To Find/Buy:
Bookstores and libraries.

HAVING TWINS

Terrific Resource For:
Parenting twins or multiples, from pregnancy through the first year

Recommended For:
Gaining An Overview: All-Inclusive

Description:

In its 19 chapters, this 430 page book is a "comprehensive resource for those giving and receiving prenatal care (in) preparation for twinbearing." This second edition of Noble's guide includes up-to-date statistics and new information focusing on prenatal communication, bonding, pregnancy experiences with twins, prenatal screening, nutrition, and what to do in the event of a loss. Other topics covered include: the biology of how twins are formed, factors contributing to having twins, how to prepare for multiple births, treatments to prolong pregnancy and prevent prematurity, labor and birth (including caesarean section and alternatives), how to take care of twins, and taking care of twins with special needs. In the book's margins are anecdotes from parents, siblings, and others illustrating their fears, reliefs, tips, and more. Three appendices list rights and responsibilities for pregnant patients, an alternative birth plan for twins in a hospital, and an action plan for parents and hospital personnel in the event of a loss. A glossary, list of resources, and bibliography are also provided.

Evaluation:

We live in a time where, as some suggest, there is an "epidemic of multiple births." The increased use of assisted reproductive technologies, treatments that enhance fertility, and women delaying childbirth until their later reproductive years all contribute to this increase. Unfortunately, most resources have yet to catch up with the demand for information made by these families of multiple births. Most of them concentrate their focus on the care, psychology and development of twins once they have been born. This book does address bonding and being with the twins once everyone arrives home, but the greater part of the book illustrates, in an easy to read and easily digested fashion, the importance of the mother's commitment to a vigilant program of nutrition, exercise, rest, and preparation prior to the births. The author does acknowledge the hazards of such pregnancies, but she offers reassurances through her strategies, tips, and up-to-date information so they are less likely to occur. Its mother-to-mother advice throughout the book, then, makes it an empowering, sensitive and recommended work.

Where To Find/Buy:

Bookstores and libraries.

Overall Rating
★★★★
An empowering book that offers sensitive & sound advice to prepare for multiple births

Design, Ease Of Use
★★★★
Short, well-organized and formatted chapters; family anecdotes in book's margins

1–4 Stars

Author:
Elizabeth Noble

Noble is the founder of the Obstetrics and Gynecology Section of the American Physical Therapy Association, and of the Maternal and Child Health Center in Cambridge, Massachusetts.

Publisher:
Houghton Mifflin

Edition:
2nd (1991)

Price:
$16.95

Pages:
430

ISBN:
0395493382

Media:
Book

Principal Subject:
Gaining An Overview: All-Inclusive

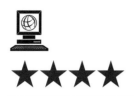

★★★★

Overall Rating
★★★★
Entertaining and informative; highly qualified expert advice, support, and fun

Design, Ease Of Use
★★★★
Expertly designed with clear pathways between topics and selections

1–4 Stars

Author:
ParentsPlace.com began three years ago as a home-based business of two parents who wanted to find a way to stay home with their newborn son. Since then, ParentsPlace.com has grown to become an award-winning site gaining recognition throughout the Internet.

Publisher:
iVillage

Media:
Internet

Principal Subject:
Gaining An Overview: All-Inclusive

PARENTSPLACE.COM
Pregnancy

 Recommended For:
Gaining An Overview: All-Inclusive

Description:
This site is a subsection of the ParentsPlace website, an iVillage parenting site. Other ParentsPlace subsections include Fertility, Health, Stages, Family, Work, Fun, Experts, Shop, Chats, Boards, and Tools. Here a visitor can choose a number of activities, including a pregnancy calendar calculator, interactive birth plan, due date calculator, and baby name finder. Informational topics include nutrition, tests, complications, gynecological concerns, information for each trimester of pregnancy, labor/birthing, postpartum recovery, newborn care, pregnancy loss, breastfeeding and bottlefeeding, maternity leave, and birth stories. The site schedules a broad array of chat room discussions and message boards on selected topics. Updated regularly are the "Today's Features" and "In the News." ParentsPlace subject experts host pages that allow visitors to submit questions. Each page lists the credentials of the subject expert and a selection of past questions and answers. The site also offers a free weekly email newsletter and a selection of email postcards.

Evaluation:
ParentsPlace.com is a joyful, colorful website engagingly presented and packed with educational, informational, and interesting topic discussions and activities. The pregnancy subsection is well integrated into the rest of the site. For those seeking information, its "Ask Our Experts" selection offers everyone from a pediatrician to a nutritionist, an attorney to a dentist. The site begs to be explored, so visitors in a hurry will be tempted to linger. ParentsPlace's goal is to serve as an Internet community, so interactivity is encouraged. An extensive community events calendar lists chats, and a daily poll offers chances to weigh in on the day's topic. The pregnancy subsection offers an interactive calendar that allows parents to create an individualized calendar timed according to the due date and stage of fetal development. The interactive birth planner is designed to help prospective parents demystify the process of labor and birth by making selections based on individual comfort levels. From the "Fertility" section to the email postcards announcing your baby's birth, ParentsPlace is a virtual community worthy of its name.

Where To Find/Buy:
On the Internet at the URL: http://www.parentsplace.com/pregnancy/

PREGNANCY, CHILDBIRTH, AND THE NEWBORN
The Complete Guide

 Recommended For:
Gaining An Overview: All-Inclusive

Description:

This book is 311 pages of tightly packed information within 15 chapters. The stated goal of this book is to "help each woman and her partner learn what they need to make good decisions, to adapt the labor techniques to suit themselves, and generally, to begin parenthood with the self-confidence that comes with understanding and active participation." Chapter titles include: "Becoming Parents," "Pregnancy," "Prenatal Care," "Nutrition in Pregnancy," "Drugs, Medications, and Environmental Hazards in Pregnancy," "Exercise, Posture, and Comfort in Pregnancy," "Preparation for Childbirth," "Labor and Birth," "Labor Variations, Complications, and Interventions," "Cesarean Birth and Vaginal Birth after a Previous Caesarean," "Medications during Labor, Birth and Postpartum," "Postpartum Period," "Caring for Baby," "Feeding Your Baby," and "Preparing Other Children for Birth and the Baby." Inserts of charts, calendars and often referenced options, like birth options, are blocked out and marked with dark borders for easy reference.

Evaluation:

Using a two column format, with large lettering to signal subject changes, this book reminds one of a good college textbook. This book is comprehensive and contains much of the information found in other books on the separate topics of pregnancy, childbirth and child care. Though last updated in 1991, the book appears to be fully up-to-date, including information on VBAC and on drugs, medications and environmental hazards during pregnancy. Throughout this book are numerous drawings and charts that provide information in a compact, useful format. If you only want to buy one book that gives a direct and clear discussion of each issue, this one could be it. Written by 2 RNs and a physical therapist with decades of experience in preparing women for childbirth and parenting, this book cuts to the heart of each issue with minimal rhetoric on methods and ideologies. This book provides the information needed to make informed decisions. It is targeted to those mothers who plan a mainstream, medically supported childbirth experience. You'll find it to be a good reference to have on your shelf.

Where To Find/Buy:

Bookstores and libraries, or order direct by calling (800) 338-2232.

★★★★

Overall Rating
★★★★
Comprehensive and up-to-date

Design, Ease Of Use
★★★★
Clear, compact and well-written

1–4 Stars

Author:
Penny Simkin, PT, Janet Whalley, RN, BSN, Ann Keppler, RN, MN

Penny Simkin, a physical therapist, has been in childbirth education since 1968. Janet Whalley, a registered nurse, has been a childbirth educator since 1975, and is a lactation specialist. Ann Keppler, a registered nurse, with a master's degree in maternal-child nursing, has taught new parent classes since 1975.

Publisher:
Meadowbrook Press
(Simon & Schuster)

Edition:
3rd (1991)

Price:
$12.00

Pages:
311

ISBN:
0671741829

Media:
Book

Principal Subject:
Gaining An Overview:
All-Inclusive

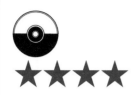

★★★★

Overall Rating
★★★★
Excellent resource combining sight and sound for first-time or prospective parents

Design, Ease Of Use
★★★★
Visually pleasing art backdrops, inspiring quotes, & video clips; navigation a breeze

1–4 Stars

Publisher:
PARENTING/Time Publishing Ventures

Edition:
1996

Price:
$34.95

Media:
CD-ROM

Principal Subject:
Gaining An Overview: All-Inclusive

YOUR PREGNANCY, YOUR NEWBORN
The Complete Guide For Expectant And New Mothers

 Recommended For:
Gaining An Overview: All-Inclusive

Description:
For Mac (3.1+, 68040/33+), Windows/DOS (3.1+,5.0+; 486/66+). Created by the editors of *PARENTING* magazine, this CD-ROM is divided into five main sections. The first three focus on pregnancy with information on how to plan for pregnancy (work, exercise, health, etc.), a month-by-month description of pregnancy (baby development, changes in the mother, doctor relations), and labor & delivery (options, pain relief). Section Four highlights the newborn. Subtopic discussions include: the newborn's appearance, warning signs, senses, reflexes, communication, bonding, breastfeeding, bottlefeeding, and more. Section Five offers parents advice for "Life With Baby." Mom's needs, dad's needs, and baby's needs (feeding, sleeping, bathing, crying, etc.) are outlined. Also provided are baby health and safety tips from immunizations to first aid to car and home safety. A discussion of childcare options and issues is also given. An interactive pregnancy calendar is available, as well as an index and gift registry (Fisher-Price items).

Evaluation:
This is a must for prospective parents. Although it comes with a pretty high price tag, it will prove valuable for calming the fears of new parents-to-be as they gain confidence in their parenting. Combining visually stunning backdrops, realtime video clips, and audio advice from experts, this CD-ROM fills a need not addressed elsewhere. Numerous experts and parents from *PARENTING* are made available to parents offering their advice about maternity leave rights, birth and delivery, the older mom's experience, exercise, breastfeeding, choosing childcare, and more. Two areas which lack depth, however, deal with how to start breastfeeding and administering first aid. For both of these areas, video clips would be an asset. More expensive than most print resources, but it will satisfy the needs of many parents.

Where To Find/Buy:
Bookstores or computer software stores.

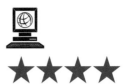

CHILDBIRTH.ORG

 Recommended For:
Gaining An Overview: All-Inclusive

Description:

Childbirth.org offers information on dozens of topics. A representative sample includes: birth plans and stories, Cesareans, complications, doulas, educators, episiotomy procedures, feeding baby, fertility, finding a childbirth class, labor, monitoring, newborns, postpartum issues, and pregnancy. Resources include: Ask the Pros, chat rooms, email, FAQs, interactive activities, and message boards. The site hosts a bookstore and an area to send and receive multimedia birth announcements and postcards. Each topic leads to selections of subcategories and offers links to other information sources. Question and answer areas offer visitors the chance to submit questions. The site includes a referral list of childbirth educators and doulas, an interactive birth planner, and a "mystic babynamer." Other interactive activities include a "baby needs calculator" which can be used to generate a shopping list, a scoring system used by doctors to determine when induction is appropriate, and a just-for-fun feature, "Will It Be A Boy Or A Girl?" Once a topic is selected, subcategories are presented and provide multiple links to other informational sources. There are several question and answer sections which a visitor would input information and then receive a report on that particular topic, specialized for them. This site is meant to provide general information for the woman or couple who are planning or expecting a baby.

Evaluation:

Childbirth, says this site, "is a natural process, not a medical procedure." From that mission statement grows a website that is attractive and full of information. It includes many of the exciting features that have become standard on pregnancy and parenting sites—an interactive birth plan program, email postcards, a bookstore and a comprehensive search function. It also includes extensive coverage of a full range of pregnancy and childbirth topics. Medical information is clear, without being too technical. Illustrations, lists, and quizzes entice a visitor to linger and explore. For example, an expectant parent can supply basic information, such as when the baby is expected along with their preferred feeding and diapering methods, and then receive a personalized shopping list. There are the usual, but useful, FAQ section, chat rooms, message boards, and archived articles on a variety of topics. One favorite of ours was "Surviving Parenthood Day by Day." The site is fairly well-designed, attractive, and professional; better organization of subtopics would be more useful to visitors rather than forcing them to wade through a lengthy list of article summaries. This site's search options, however, make this website particularly useful.

Where To Find/Buy:

On the Internet at the URL: http://www.childbirth.org/

★★★★

Overall Rating
★★★★
Informative, interactive, and extensive links to articles on the Internet

Design, Ease Of Use
★★★
Clear paths to information and activities; subtopic navigation can be confusing

1–4 Stars

Author:
Childbirth.org was founded by Robin Elise Weiss, a childbirth educator, doula and mother who went on to establish the pregnancy/childbirth website operated by The Mining Co. Contributors include subject experts, doulas, nurses, and childbirth educators.

Publisher:
Childbirth.org

Media:
Internet

Principal Subject:
Gaining An Overview: All-Inclusive

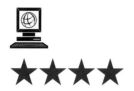

★★★★

Overall Rating
★★★★
Attractive, well-designed, unbelievably comprehensive

Design, Ease Of Use
★★★
Lots of information in an easy-to-navigate format; can get lost at times in the layers

1–4 Stars

Author:
Parent Soup is one of two parenting web sites included in the iVillage community of web sites.

Publisher:
iVillage Inc.

Media:
Internet

Principal Subject:
Gaining An Overview: All-Inclusive

PARENT SOUP

 Recommended For:
Gaining An Overview: All-Inclusive

Description:
Parent Soup, a member of the iVillage, offers many links on its website homepage. "Soup specials" include features such as child and senior care directories, chats with Random House children's authors, parental "survival kits," a children's resume maker, child development profiles, baby name finder, a book club, and a shopping service. Parent Soup offers e-communities from those considering pregnancy to those who are parents of teens. A daily parent poll seeks visitors' opinions, and the site offers a selection of daily chats and message boards. A guided tour helps a visitor learn what is available. A roster of experts offers information on early education, family counseling, child development, health and pediatrics, breastfeeding, and summer camps. Guest experts add additional voices. Other resources include Community Challenges, a community discussion of a monthly parenting challenge, iBaby, a baby needs store, a library, an online guide, and an archive of parenting news stories.

Evaluation:
Refill your tea cup, pull your chair closer to the computer screen, and prepare to spend some time at this website. Anyone with a child of any age—parent, grandparent, family member, or interested friend—will find more to do here than there is time to experience in one sitting. The decision will be where to start. The site features areas for everyone from expectant parents to parents of teens. The homepage itself offers a wealth of other informational services and entrances to discussions of individual topics. Discussion chats change daily, and special chats are scheduled with professionals in any number of fields. Information is updated continually, and topics range from the humorous which encourage the child in us all (The Whine Cellar) to the useful (Bedwetting). Site organization is energizing, attractive—and a little messy. You're sure to wander off the path, following one nugget or another, so be sure you know your way home. Program Director Susan Hahn says this is "a place to share the funny moments and everyday delights that are part of being a parent. It is a place to enrich our lives." It certainly is.

Where To Find/Buy:
On the Internet at the URL: http://www.parentsoup.com

TWINS!
Expert Advice From Two Practicing Physicians On Pregnancy, Birth, And The First Year Of Life With Twins

 Recommended For:
Gaining An Overview: All-Inclusive

Description:

The authors begin by acknowledging that twins are "miraculous . . . You're starting out on a truly epic journey." Throughout the book, readers hear both from health care professionals and other parents of twins. Introductory chapters discuss how twins are conceived, how to find the "right practitioner," and why the reader needs to take responsibility for a healthy start in their pregnancy. Fetal development is considered from several perspectives: "Your Developing Twins," "Your Pregnant Body," "Symptoms That May Be Ongoing," "The Checkup," "Transitions" (a forum for special issues and conditions), and "Roundtable Talk" in which parents and physician participants respond to an array of topics concerning the twins in their lives. Also provided are chapters on labor and delivery followed by an expanded discussion of postpartum issues which focus on the whole family. The first year of life with twins is described in a format similar to that used for fetal development—"Your Growing Twins," "Parental Questions and Concerns," "Roundtable Talk," and more. An emphasis is placed on developmental milestones, family harmony, and safety measures to consider.

Evaluation:

This book speaks both to readers who are pregnant and, more specifically, to those who are pregnant with twins. As expectations and conditions of the pregnancy are described, comparisons are often noted in relation to the "singleton mom." Similar to other books on pregnancy, the reader is told what to expect during her prenatal visits to the physician. In addition, helpful considerations for choosing a prenatal caregiver are offered. Unusual to this book are chapters that not only detail the progression of both the developing fetus and the first year of life, but also thoughtfully introduce the reader to other peers in "Roundtable Talk." Here prospective parents will find comfort in knowing their concerns are shared by others, as well as attaining advice from specialists. Throughout the book, consideration and guidance is offered to support family harmony. Thanks to its organization, bold highlights, and index, it is also easily referenced. Relevant charts and a 10 page resource guide are included to help support parents. Overall, this book can be comfortably read from cover-to-cover.

Where To Find/Buy:

Bookstores and libraries.

★★★★

Overall Rating
★★★★
Especially valuable for parents of twins; emphasizes family harmony and peer insight

Design, Ease Of Use
★★★
Excellent text, light on illustrations

1–4 Stars

Author:
Connie L. Agnew, MD, Alan H. Klein, MD, Jill Alison Ganon

All authors are parents and reside in Los Angeles, California. Agnew, a perinatologist, specializes in the care of high-risk mothers and infants. Klein, a pediatrician, specializes in high-risk infant care. Ganon is a professional writer and editor.

Publisher:
HarperPerennial (HarperCollins Publishers)

Edition:
1997

Price:
$16.00

Pages:
304

ISBN:
0062734601

Media:
Book

Principal Subject:
Gaining An Overview: All-Inclusive

★★★

Overall Rating
★★★
Broad without being overwhelming or over assuming, well-targeted information

Design, Ease Of Use
★★★★
Easily referenced, consistent format; provides in-depth and at-a-glance information

1–4 Stars

Author:
Paula Spencer with the Editors of *PARENTING* Magazine

Spencer is a contributing editor of *PARENTING* Magazine who writes about women's health, children, and family issues. A parent of three, she worked as an editorial director before becoming a freelance writer. She and her family live in Tennessee.

Publisher:
Ballantine Books
(Random House)

Edition:
1998

Price:
$12.00

Pages:
375

ISBN:
034541179X

Media:
Book

Principal Subject:
Gaining An Overview:
All-Inclusive

PARENTING GUIDE TO PREGNANCY & CHILDBIRTH

Description:

In the introduction, Spencer relates that she was pregnant during the nine months she spent researching/writing this book, and that this book "presents a total picture of pregnancy and childbirth, from the latest medical facts to enduring old wives' tales, from what's going on in your body to what's going on in your head and your heart and even your closet. You'll find explanations, advice, and ideas. But it skips the preachy lectures and scientific treatises." The book is divided into 5 chapters corresponding to the first, second, third, and fourth trimester ("Recovery & Newborn Care") of pregnancy; an additional chapter is dedicated to labor and delivery with information on pain management, "Special Situations" (VBAC, Cesarean birth, multiple births, etc.), and more. Chapters follow a similar format with subtopics, such as "What's Going on Your Body," "What's Going on in Your Head," "Checkups and Tests," "What Should I Eat?," "Work Worries," and more. A medical advisory board is included consisting of pediatric and Ob/Gyn doctors, and a childbirth educator. Black and white illustrations and photos are provided.

Evaluation:

The breadth of information offered within this book is presented in a straightforward manner. While a vast array of topics are considered, readers are wisely directed to search beyond the pages of this book for additional in-depth information on topics, such as breastfeeding, postpartum depression, and other concerns. Additionally, within the 375 pages of this book, the reader is given bridges or references to other sections of the book when further details of a topic need elaboration. Spencer's tone is casual while pertinent. Readers will find that this book really does seem to speak as "a real person's guide to having a baby." The sections on "Childbirth Basics" and "All About Pain" do a fine job of outlining pros and cons of various pain management methods, as well as other childbirth choices, encouraging women to take a proactive stance. This book contains information that is not only relevant, but also timely. For example, Spencer includes pertinent information in the "Work Worries" sections contained within each of the three chapters on pregnancy. On the whole, this book is an excellent basic resource for pregnant women.

Where To Find/Buy:

Bookstores and libraries.

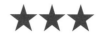

TOUCHPOINTS, VOLUME I
Pregnancy, Birth And The First Weeks Of Life

Description:

T. Berry Brazelton, "America's preeminent baby doctor," hosts this look at the changes, attitudes and worries that beset families as they await the arrival of their baby and during their babies' first few weeks of life. Six families are the focus of this 45 minute videotape: a family worried their newborn will have a similar disabling condition as the older sibling, a single mom, a couple with a very busy dad and toddler, a couple with an eventual premature baby, a couple looking to adopt a second child, and older first-time parents who previously experienced three miscarriages. Throughout the videotape, Brazelton expands upon the various "touchpoints" these families encounter. Touchpoints are "periods of time that precede a rapid growth in learning for both child and parent." As Brazelton and the camera trace the fears of these parents and their subsequent experiences during their pregnancies (or waiting period for the prospective adoptive couple), birth, and first few weeks, eight touchpoints are explained ("What kind of parent will I be like?"; "What will my delivery be like?"; "The work of attachment," etc.).

Evaluation:

Brazelton is charming in front of a camera. Many viewers will recognize him as the focal point of the popular TV series "What Every Baby Knows." The families he interviews and works with are touching; the viewer cannot help but identify with the hopes and fears of those parents as they await the magic moment of the birth. These parents are credible: they are very busy worried about giving the baby proper time, or they are older and have experienced multiple miscarriages, or they are single, or they are expecting a premature birth, or they are adopting. All this is done with excellent photography (even the home video segment is above average) which brings a dimension quite different from the printed word. However, the lack of practical information provided on those confusing first few weeks with one's newborn is disappointing. The strength of this video is found in its portrayal of these families their emotional and attitudinal changes; it could be an effective tool for prenatal couples to use in their own home.

Where To Find/Buy:

Bookstores and libraries, or order direct by calling (800) 756-8792.

Overall Rating
★★★
Brazelton's charming, the families endearing; practical information is sparse

Design, Ease Of Use
★★★★
Touchpoints are progressive, delineated by title blocks introduced by Brazelton

---

1–4 Stars

Author:
T. Berry Brazelton, MD

Publisher:
Pipher Films

Edition:
1991

Price:
$29.99

ISBN:
1878983091

Media:
Videotape

Principal Subject:
Gaining An Overview:
All-Inclusive

★★★

Overall Rating
★★★
Thorough, practical treatment of subject without being overwhelming

Design, Ease Of Use
★★★★
Information is concise and well organized, visuals/layout provide clear presentation

1–4 Stars

Author:
George E. Verrilli, MD, FACOG, Anne Marie Mueser, EdD

Eighteen years ago, Verrilli delivered the daughter of Mueser, an author of children's books and educational materials. Now a Chief of Obstetrics, Verrilli has delivered over 14,000 babies and pioneered new approaches to family-centered childbirth.

Publisher:
St. Martin's Griffin

Edition:
2nd (1998)

Price:
$7.95

Pages:
168

ISBN:
0312187750

Media:
Book

Principal Subject:
Gaining An Overview: All-Inclusive

WHILE WAITING

Description:

This 168 page guide consists of six sections. Section One, "Working With Your Care Provider," details what to expect on your first visit to a prenatal caregiver. Also included is a month-by-month drawing and description of pregnancy. Possible topics and questions for discussion are provided along with full-page charts entitled "Appointment Record" and "Questions and Notes." Section Two, "Coping With Bodily Changes," describes when and why changes occur, offering advice in sections entitled "Try This." Section Three, "Keeping Healthy and Fit," provides nutritional information to encourage healthful nutrition; illustrations, dietary examples, and record-keeping worksheets are given. Also provided in this section are fitness and relaxation suggestions specific to the needs of pregnancy. Section Four presents alphabetical descriptions of situations which may affect pregnant women from acne and Caesarean delivery to ultrasound and x-rays. The last section addresses "Labor and Delivery" and "Postpartum Care." The author's intent throughout is to encourage the reader to have dialog with her physician.

Evaluation:

Curtis describes this as a companion book for taking to physician visits, and the reader is continually encouraged to work together with her prenatal care provider. Information provided is both precise and effectively organized. Section topics are arranged alphabetically, where applicable, making this guide quite convenient for busy women wanting quick answers. Throughout the book, the author helps bridge understanding between the reader's possible lack of knowledge and the author's professional experience through numerous cross-references to more detailed information in the book. "Hints For Helping" during stages of labor offer clear and comforting insight for birthing partners who will be present during the mother's labor. Although most of the book pertains to all women who are pregnant, Section Four also addresses some more specific situations, such as "Vegetarianism," "Teenagers," and more. Thanks to the 1998 revision, current topics, such as "Olestra Alert" in Section Three, are also aptly addressed. After reading this book, a pregnant woman should be well-prepared to take an active, responsible role in the birth process.

Where To Find/Buy:
Bookstores and libraries.

25 THINGS EVERY NEW MOTHER SHOULD KNOW

★★★

Description:

Written by two experts in the field of parenting and child care, this slim guide seeks to encompass the key elements of motherhood for first-time mothers. With conciseness as its goal, this book does not cover the practicalities of baby care, but chooses to focus on the transition into motherhood and effective parenting. The authors speak from both professional and personal experience as the parents of eight children in writing this book. The book's philosophical foundation is what the authors call "attachment parenting," which "includes closeness right from birth, responding sensitively to cries, babywearing, sharing sleep, and breastfeeding." It is the authors' belief that such parenting leads to the greatest closeness between mother and child as well as healthy, stable children. There are 25 separate sections to this book, each of which focuses on a separate parenting issue, such as breast/bottle-feeding, how to respond to the baby's crying, how to address baby's needs during the day and during the night, making the decision to stay home with the baby, learning to trust intuition and become the best "expert" on the baby's care, and more.

Evaluation:

For mothers without much time to wade through the sheer volume of baby books out there, this little volume includes much sage advice about mothering. It wisely leaves the practicalities to other books in order to focus exclusively on the elements of successful mothering. This book represents a shift in parenting styles away from a model of strict, authoritarian parenting towards a style of parenting that believes a mother can interpret and respond to a baby's needs without fear of "spoiling" or "ruining" the child. The authors believe the closest attachment of an infant to her mother occurs through exclusive breastfeeding, immediately responding to a baby's cries, sharing sleeping arrangements in the early months, and being a full-time mother. Even if these ideas feel conflicting for some, this book can enrich every mother's perspective without dominating her own style of mothering.

Where To Find/Buy:

Bookstores and libraries.

Overall Rating
★★★
An insightful guide to ways mothers can bond with their infants

Design, Ease Of Use
★★★
Quite readable and concise

1–4 Stars

Author:
Martha Sears, RN, with William Sears, MD

Martha Sears, R.N., is a certified childbirth educator, breastfeeding consultant, and labor support expert. Together with her husband, William Sears, M.D., a pediatrician, they have authored several books on parenting, including *The Birth Book* and *The Baby Book*.

Publisher:
Harvard Common Press

Edition:
1995

Price:
$7.95

Pages:
117

ISBN:
1558320695

Media:
Book

Principal Subject:
Gaining An Overview: All-Inclusive

★★★

Overall Rating
★★★
Thorough, basic information on hundreds of health topics

Design, Ease Of Use
★★★
Search engine and clear subtitles make finding topics easy

1–4 Stars

Author:
This site is sponsored by the American Academy of Family Physicians, one of the largest medical associations in the U.S.

Media:
Internet

Principal Subject:
Gaining An Overview: All-Inclusive

AMERICAN ACADEMY OF FAMILY PHYSICIANS

Description:

This site is provided by the American Academy of Family Physicians, one of the largest medical associations in the U.S. It includes information about a broad range of medical issues handled by family physicians. The group's mission is to promote and maintain "high standards for family physicians—the doctors who specialize in you," according to the site's homepage. Four major headings can be accessed on the site's homepage: "Healthy Living," "Common Conditions/ Diseases/Disorders," "Treatments," and "The Body." A search engine helps viewers locate specific health information, or visitors can quickly click through subcategories to reach topics such as "Newborns, Infants and Children's Health," "Pregnancy," "Women's Health" (all located under the heading "Healthy Living"), and "Female Reproductive System" (located under the heading "The Body").

Evaluation:

The extensive bank of information presented here is compiled and maintained by the American Academy of Family Physicians. Sections offer information about every imaginable health topic, and a search engine and clear site layout makes information easy to find. The information presented is parent-friendly, void of unnecessary medical jargon, and the explanations are clear, complete, and easy to understand. The "Newborns, Infants and Children's Health" section lists dozens of topics, from "Runny Nose in Children" (which provides an interesting explanation of runny noses) and "Pets and Parasites" to "Checking Your Child's Hearing" and "Taking Care of Twins." The information provided is mainstream medical advice, well-grounded in tradition. This isn't the site to investigate the latest medical or alternative treatments, but it is a comforting place for parents who just need to know what to do about pinworms or earaches or runny noses.

Where To Find/Buy:

On the Internet at http://www.aafp.org/patientinfo/

CHECKLIST FOR YOUR FIRST BABY

Description:
This book is designed to help new mothers-to-be organize and prepare for the arrival of a new baby. Focusing on pregnancy, birth, and the first six postpartum weeks, this book offers "checklists" for vital needs, helpful tips and information on a variety of topics. Section One discusses the first, second, and third trimesters, and changes you can expect through the months. Section Two contains information and checklists for health, nutrition, and exercise for the first trimester. Section Three looks at second trimester topics: how (and when) to announce the news, health insurance, equipping the nursery, purchasing maternity and baby clothes, childbirth classes, and bottle- vs. breast-feeding. Section Four includes a checklist of questions for one's pediatrician, choosing child care, and packing for the hospital during the third trimester. Section Five contains important tips for the weeks following the baby's birth: general care, the 6-week check-up, birth control choices, and traveling and playing with the baby. The last section is a "pregnancy calendar" to note appointments and stay organized until the birth.

Evaluation:
The key to this little book's usefulness is in its design. It gives the absolute basic information for such things as nutrition and baby care (more comprehensively covered in other books) but contains reminders and checklists for little everyday necessities that bigger books may overlook. For example, how to choose maternity and baby wear while keeping costs down, nursery needs, what to pack for the hospital, and useful, practical baby care tips. Also helpful are the lists of suggested questions for one's health-care provider before and after birth that may easily be forgotten in the thick of things (e.g. "What is your attitude about pain relief during labor?" "What type of breast-feeding tips can you provide me?" "When can I start exercising?"). Although the information offered here is very simple and basic, this book points the way towards getting the in-depth information one needs from the appropriate sources, while staying on top of the overall planning process for the baby's arrival.

Where To Find/Buy:
Bookstores and libraries.

Overall Rating
★★★
A useful planning tool for baby's arrival; includes small, easily-overlooked necessities

Design, Ease Of Use
★★★
Helpful "checklist" format; monthly pregnancy calendars provided to track to-do list

---

1–4 Stars

Author:
Susan Kagen Podell, MS, RD

Susan Kagen Podell, M.S., R.D. is a Registered Dietitian and Certified Diabetes Educator, and the author of other books on nutrition.

Publisher:
Main Street Books
(Bantam Doubleday Dell)

Edition:
1997

Price:
$6.99

Pages:
212

ISBN:
038547797X

Media:
Book

Principal Subject:
Gaining An Overview: All-Inclusive

★★★

Overall Rating
★★★
A moving and powerful visual account of pregnancy and birth, some info needs updating

Design, Ease Of Use
★★★
Stunning photographs and clear, unobtrusive text

1–4 Stars

Author:
Lennart Nilsson, MD (Hon.); text by Lars Hamberger, MD

Lennart Nilsson is an internationally renowned medical and scientific photographer. His books, including this one, have been translated into 18 languages. Lars Hamberger, M.D., is Professor and Chairman of Obstetrics and Gynecology at a Gothenburg University in Sweden.

Publisher:
Dell Publishing
(Bantam Doubleday Dell)

Edition:
2nd (1990)

Price:
$18.95

Pages:
216

ISBN:
0440506913

Media:
Book

Principal Subject:
Gaining An Overview:
All-Inclusive

A CHILD IS BORN

Description:

This book chronicles the miracle of reproduction and childbirth through color photographs and explanatory text, from ovulation to conception, and through the stages of pregnancy to birth. In its 2nd edition, this book, originally published in Sweden, was written by an internationally recognized medical/scientific photographer and an expert in human reproduction. The first 5 of 15 chapters take us from the origins of life through human sexual development, ovulation, fertilization, and the beginning of the "long journey" of the fertilized ovum through the fallopian tubes and implantation in the uterus. The next 6 chapters describe the extraordinary changes of the embryo during the first weeks, the emotions and concerns of early pregnancy, medical tests, and the development of the fetus up until birth. The actual labor and delivery are depicted in the next chapter, as well as births requiring special care. The last 2 chapters discuss the role genes play, and issues in infertility and its treatment.

Evaluation:

The photographs in this book are almost as much of a miracle as childbirth itself. Using sophisticated photographic equipment, Nilsson shows us—clearly, in color—how life takes hold and grows inside a woman's body. The photographs are awe-inspiring, and, oddly, humbling; upon viewing these photos, we feel ignorant of the complexities of a process that can sometimes be taken for granted. The photographs, especially, of the developing fetus are stunning. The pictures of childbirth are also powerful, although additional resources on pain management and childbirth alternatives are advised. Most of the accompanying text is clear and well-written, complementing, but never overpowering the photos themselves. A disappointment for some readers may be that most of the pictures here show only people of a certain ethnicity (Swedish) who appear to represent a certain class and age group. Also, some topics need updating, namely in the discussions regarding infertility treatment. However, overlooking these flaws, "A Child is Born" is an enthralling visual testimony to pregnancy and birth.

Where To Find/Buy:

Bookstores and libraries.

FAMILY.COM
Disney.Com

Description:

Coordinated with Disney, this site covers a range of family related information including activities, education, parenting, shopping, and cooking. Options available at the homepage allow a visitor to choose one of those categories or select an article from "current feature," which, at this visit, discussed healthy snacks, whining, parenting an only child and activities, such as making puppets and snowmen. There are more than a few search engines included at this website: one to search any topic, one to search meals and recipes by ingredient, and one to search a visitor's geographic area for local information on family activities. In the "Activities" section, a visitor can choose from several feature articles or search for an activity by indicating a topic and an age group. In "Education," one can again choose from a number of articles or search through the archives using the same criteria. Other sections of the website that use that format include the food and parenting sections. Bulletin boards are available on many topics, which are categorized into sections such as "All About You," "Family Ties," and many more.

Evaluation:

This site looks just like a slick magazine cover, overwhelming the senses and with abundant commercialism. However, unusual to this site are the vast number of customized searches available and the reprints from respected authorities' books. Whether parents require a check-off list for evaluating preschools, need support for their parenting decisions, or want a quick activity for their three year old on a snowy day, they will find it here. Parents looking for others to share ideas and tips with will find the "Boards" to be a well-organized feature. Topics are arranged under the same headings as the site's homepage, with multiple subtopics found under each, and age ranges can be chosen. A novel feature to this segment is that visitors can specify that they want to read only the most current postings or include those more than a year old. This saves busy parents from wasted time and effort responding to chats that are no longer current. One won't find a lot of technical advice about heavy parenting issues or how to take care of a newborn at this site. This site, while comprehensive, is better suited for parents of toddlers, preschoolers, and older children.

Where To Find/Buy:

On the Internet at the URL: http://family.go.com

Overall Rating
★★★
Comprehensive, but best for parents of older kids; customized searches, active "Boards"

Design, Ease Of Use
★★★
Commercialism abounds; easily navigated, well-organized site; book reprinted online

1–4 Stars

Media:
Internet

Principal Subject:
Gaining An Overview: All-Inclusive

★★★

Overall Rating
★★★
Unique approach invites parents to develop their own style while relaying others' tips

Design, Ease Of Use
★★★
Use the table of contents and index to guide you; could use bolder headings and graphics

1–4 Stars

Author:
Linda Albi, Deborah Johnson, Debra Catlin, Donna Florien Deurloo, and Sheryll Greatwood

Linda Albi, Deborah Johnson, Debra Catlin, Donna Florien Deurloo, and Sheryll Greatwood are mothers of twins and members of the same support group.

Publisher:
Fireside (Simon & Schuster)

Edition:
1993

Price:
$14.00

Pages:
414

ISBN:
067172357X

Media:
Book

Principal Subject:
Gaining An Overview: All-Inclusive

MOTHERING TWINS
From Hearing The News To Beyond The Terrible Twos

Description:
This guide's 15 chapters focus on having and caring for twins. Chapter 1 begins with parents' revelation when they find out they are carrying twins and continues with what to expect. Chapter 2 through 4 take parents through the birthing experience including information on what to expect and focusing on the possibility of having premature twins. Chapters 6 through 9 show parents how to establish a support system, locate childcare, and help older siblings adjust. Chapters 11 and 12 speak to the "couple relationship" and how to find time to regenerate oneself. Chapters 5, 10, 13, and 14 discuss the development of twins from the first six months through preschool. Chapter 15 is dedicated to the father's perspective of life with twins. An epilogue of the authors' final thoughts and reflections follows this final chapter. A resource directory is given supplying contact information for organizations, support groups, and more. A suggested reading list and a 9 page index are also provided.

Evaluation:
Offering a variety of personal narratives and "it worked for me" solutions, this 414 page guide is a unique approach to the caring for twins. Emphasizing individuality and adaptability, the authors seek to encourage mothers to develop their own parenting approach based on what's best for themselves and their children. This is a wonderful book full of insight and practical tips. A special chapter is Chapter 15: five fathers of twins (the authors' husbands) give their touching and sensitive perspectives on what it's like to have twins. Parents of twins will find this to be a well-written guide—relaxed, but comprehensive. Neither dictating nor forcing solutions, the authors merely express suggestions and advice from their own experiences. Parents of twins will find this very thoughtful book to be both interesting and informative from all five points of view. This resource has managed to cover a lot of ground, while being careful not to omit the essentials.

Where To Find/Buy:
Bookstores and libraries.

PLANNING FOR PREGNANCY, BIRTH, & BEYOND

★★★

Description:

Planning For Pregnancy, Birth & Beyond contains 3 sections and 17 chapters. Section I, "Preconceptional Care," covers "Planning Your Pregnancy" and "How Reproduction Occurs." Topics included focus on family and medical history, later childbearing, detecting ovulation, and more. Section II, "Pregnancy," discusses signs and diagnosis of pregnancy, growth and development of mother and fetus, childbirth preparation, prenatal care, genetic disorders and birth defects, nutrition, exercise, work, sex, special situations (high blood pressure, heart disease, thyroid disease, etc.), complications (vaginal bleeding, breech, preterm labor, etc.), and infections (STD, hepatitis, urinary tract infections, etc.) during pregnancy. Section III covers labor, delivery, and postpartum care. Topics include how labor begins, monitoring, delivery, vaginal birth after Cesarean, the newborn, and more. Also in Section III is a chapter on dealing with loss. Each chapter concludes with "Questions to Consider," which are designed to reinforce key concepts and present questions the patient may want to ask her doctor. This book contains some illustrations, tables, and charts. A "Personal Pregnancy Diary," baby growth charts, glossary, and index are also provided.

Evaluation:

This is a comprehensive book on pregnancy and birth. It fills in much of the A through Z of preconception through postpartum care. The book generally gives a chronological layout of the events and concerns during and after pregnancy, and much more. Surprises (as these topics may not be expected in a book on pregnancy and birth) include infant car safety seat, battered women, and an entire chapter on dealing with loss. The illustrations, tables, and charts, although not abundant for such a comprehensive book as this, are well placed and effective visual aids. The glossary is short, but the index is rather comprehensive, which helps make this book a good reference book if one does not want to read it in its entirety. The members of The American College of Obstetricians and Gynecologists who wrote this book have made a tremendous contribution to expectant parents by packing in as much information as they have in this book. The breadth of coverage makes this definitely a good one for expectant parents to consult. Its design is awkward (compact, pocket-size) but its handiness in being carried in purse or bag might make it well-used.

Where To Find/Buy:

Bookstores and libraries.

Overall Rating
★★★
Comprehensive information on pregnancy and childbirth—all the basics and much more

Design, Ease Of Use
★★★
Jam-packed, overwhelming at first, but easier once the reader gets used to the format

1–4 Stars

Author:
The American College of Obstetricians and Gynecologists
This book was created by members of the American College of Obstetricians and Gynecologists—the most respected authority on preconception, pregnancy, and postpartum health care.

Publisher:
Signet (Penguin Group/ Penguin Books)

Edition:
2nd (1995)

Price:
$6.99

Pages:
338

ISBN:
0451191757

Media:
Book

Principal Subject:
Gaining An Overview: All-Inclusive

Overall Rating
★★★
Vast amount of concise information on topics from pregnancy to baby's first year

Design, Ease Of Use
★★
Cumbersome subtopic list (often 100+) can be difficult to access, but worth the search

1–4 Stars

Media:
Internet

Principal Subject:
Gaining An Overview: All-Inclusive

BABYCENTER
Complete Pregnancy & Baby Information

Description:

Launched in November 1997, this site offers many areas of parenting information from "preconception" to "baby." Other options available at the homepage include daily "Features" that address issues such as infertility, eating during pregnancy, nannies, and spanking. Another option includes "Popular Areas" with subtopics such as "The Dads Page," "Ask the Experts," "Pregnancy Calendar," "Find a Health Provider," and more. Experts in "Ask the Experts" include 19 different professionals and their biographies, from pediatricians (Brazelton and Dixon) and lactation consultants to clinical psychiatrists and midwives. Previously asked questions are summarized, along with the particular expert that responded, in a list format. There are numerous polls throughout the site on various topics regarding pregnancy and childcare. "BabyCenter Community" offers a visitor opportunities to participate in the website through its bulletin boards, chats, "Great Debates" and "Community Update." Online shopping is available as well.

Evaluation:

At first (and second and third) glance, this site is an assault on the senses. The numerous commercial advertisements and disorganized layout make an initial visit seem daunting. The homepage merits a quick glance for interesting, daily updated features, but if one is looking for specific information, skip the homepage and go directly to the Site Index or the Table of Contents. Once one learns to navigate the maze, valuable and concise information can be found. For example, a parent seeking information on a baby's development also will be given links to related topics, other sources (websites and print references) and other parents. Some subtopics ("baby sleeping through the night") also reference bulletin boards on the same topic ("babies and sleep") and "great debates" ("baby sleeps alone vs. the family bed"), offering pros and cons on an issue, experts' advice, and more. The only area needing some help is in the access of these articles. Parents will need to read through a rather unwieldy list of titles (often 100+), although a search can be conducted. The sheer volume of information can take a significant amount of time, but it is well worth it.

Where To Find/Buy:

On the Internet at the URL: http://www.babycenter.com

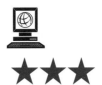

PARENTTIME

Description:

Access to this site's features can begin with either selecting a child's age range or a topic-driven department for specific information. Age range choices include pregnancy, baby, toddler, preschool, and school-age. "Departments" feature many articles and sub-articles focusing on a child's growth and health concerns, issues for parents, finances, "Parenting A to Z," a "Pregnancy Primer," celebrity parents, fun and games, and more. The age range selection takes a visitor to age-appropriate features, "This Week's Feature," "Expert," and "Boards and Chats." The Table of Contents lists all of the site's articles and information, organized into topics: Parent Time Specials, Travel, Fun & Games, Health Guide (which includes a medical encyclopedia and a first aid resource), Parenting A to Z, Parent Talk, Pregnancy Primer, and Expert Advice. This site is owned by Time Inc. and Proctor & Gamble Productions, with references including links to other publications such as *Money*, *Time* and *People* magazines, Dr. Ruth Westheimer, and *Parenting* and *BabyTalk* magazines.

Evaluation:

Once a visitor finds his or her way through the maze of commercialism and product and company advertisements to arrive at the Table of Contents, a wealth of information is available to answer most questions and address most concerns. The pages specialized for particular age ranges offer helpful, if limited, tips and advice. Boards and chat rooms discuss topics pertaining to that age range. "Ask an Expert," the question and answer section, and experts' perspectives on topical parenting issues are features not be missed. The Health Guide's encyclopedia of medical terms and first aid (help in treating emergencies) are especially useful resources to have readily available. The site's archived articles—primarily reprints from Parenting magazine—cover a wide variety of parenting topics, from the technical to the supportive to the whimsical (sending an e-card in the Fun and Games department). This website even covers financial situations that parents (or others) may face, such as buying a home; some of this information is actually in the format of links to other websites. Another particular plus—a project planner that offers easy craft projects for each month. Once one learns the route, time spent at this site will definitely be worthwhile.

Where To Find/Buy:

On the Internet at the URL: http://www.pathfinder.com/ParentTime/homepage/homepage.all.html

---

Overall Rating
★★★
Access to abundant info, discussions on selected topics

Design, Ease Of Use
★★
Most info is buried deep, but fairly well-categorized, graphics slow down the process

1–4 Stars

Media:
Internet

Principal Subject:
Gaining An Overview: All-Inclusive

★★★

Overall Rating
★★★
Interactive, immediate, colorful

Design, Ease Of Use
★
Search engine, thoughtful site design, but much difficulty returning to main menus

1–4 Stars

Publisher:
Parent Garden.com

Media:
Internet

Principal Subject:
Gaining An Overview:
All-Inclusive

BABYSOON.COM

Description:

Babysoon.com features include "Week By Week," information about fetal development; "Pregnancy Guide," more than 200 articles on key pregnancy-related topics; "Baby Bulletin," the opportunity to sign up for weekly pregnancy updates sent via email; "The First Time," a new mother's journey; "Baby Blueprints," which provides illustrations from conception to birth; and a due date calculator. The site is updated daily; interactive features include a daily poll, an "In The News" section, a question of the day, and a topic of the day. Visitors may review archived results of earlier polls and questions. A search function makes finding information on a particular topic easier.

Evaluation:

Babysoon.com, a Parent Garden.com site, is an attractive, interactive site for parents and parents-to-be. Updated daily, its immediacy is one of its most attractive features. Many of its offerings have become common to parenting websites, but that does not lessen their value. Each site's "Today's Poll" or "Topic of the Day" offers parents new chances to be heard and to join with others to influence a site's content and direction. Each list of links and topics increases the chances that the one bit of information a new parent needs to feel comfortable and confident will be available to them. As the Internet continues to evolve, expectations for sophisticated and complicated sites increase. Yet there will always be a demand for clear, colorful, interesting sites, ones that present basic information needed by large numbers of today's parents. Babysoon.com is one of those sites. The primary problem visitors will find with this site lies in accessing the site's content. Although the site is well-organized and well-thought out, once a visitor finds articles via text links, there is considerable difficulty returning to the main menus. Hopefully, future plans for this site will include restructuring its organizational elements.

Where To Find/Buy:

On the Internet at http://www.expecting.net

MULTIPLE BLESSINGS
From Pregnancy Through Childhood, A Guide For Parents Of Twins, Triplets, Or More

★★

Description:

This guidebook is divided into four sections. The first section is about pregnancy and includes such topics as the delivery, planning for your multiples' births, premature babies and coping with the loss of a child. Section Two's focus is on "Life with Multiples," dealing with the parent partnership and expectations, naming your babies, breastfeeding, and the logistics of caring for multiples. It also includes advice on how to select a pediatrician and helping siblings to adjust. Section Three offers advice on enlisting help and support, finding babysitters, and a discussion of Mothers of Twins Clubs and a listing of other resources. The final section speaks to the parenting challenges and joys. One-on-one time, overcoming favoritism, bonding, handling stress, and making comparisons are just a few of the subtopics in this section. The appendices include a glossary of terms, additional resources, a bibliography, and a listing of books for children about twins and triplets. An index is also included.

Evaluation:

Using quotes from interviews with the family of multiples, this 383-page book offers advice and suggestions on raising twins, triplets, and more. A large section of the book deals, in general, with the birthing/delivery aspect, followed by broad-based blanketed advice on what parents might expect life to be with multiples. One valuable section in Part Two is "Multiple Feats: The Logistics of Caring for Multiples." Some of the subtopics in this section include how to bathe babies; deal with mealtime, scheduling and routines; toilet training; and record keeping. "Parenting Challenges and Joys," Section Four, contains good material (handling stress, giving equal love, avoiding typecasting, etc.), but otherwise seems a rather random array of issues. The resource section includes periodicals, organizations, and mail-order buying information for parents of multiples. There are, however, more comprehensive books on multiples than this one.

Where To Find/Buy:

Bookstores and libraries.

Overall Rating
★★
Lots of info and resources given to cover topics of pregnancy through early child care

Design, Ease Of Use
★★★★
Numerous quotes from families of multiples; detailed table of contents and index

1–4 Stars

Author:
Betty Rothbart, MSW

Betty Rothbart is a psychiatric social worker. She is currently a science and health writer, educator, and trainer of teachers for the New York City Board of Education. She is also an adjunct professor at the Bank Street College of Education.

Publisher:
Hearst Books
(William Morrow)

Edition:
1994

Price:
$12.00

Pages:
383

ISBN:
0688116426

Media:
Book

Principal Subject:
Gaining An Overview:
All-Inclusive

★★

Overall Rating
★★
Information and advice from "authorities" rather succinct; shopping and chats good

Design, Ease Of Use
★★★★
Good graphics in their "mall," easily navigated, well-organized headings

1–4 Stars

Media:
Internet

Principal Subject:
Gaining An Overview: All-Inclusive

THE NATIONAL PARENTING CENTER

Description:

Programmed and hosted by ParentsPlace.com, The National Parenting Center (TNPC) was founded in July 1989 to provide parents "with comprehensive and responsible guidance from nine of the world's most renowned child-rearing authorities. . . ." Features at the homepage include articles, a mall, chat facilities, and a daily feature. Articles, presented through the "ParentTalk Newsletter," are written by the panel of parenting authorities (bios include a psychologist, pediatrician, parenting authors, and more). Information is grouped by the following categories: pregnancy, newborns, infancy, toddler, preschool, preteens, and adolescence; various subcategories then are presented, along with the respective author. Articles typically range from half a page to one page in length. "Chat" leads a visitor to ParentsPlace.com's discussion rooms with 100+ topics that are divided into categories. TNPC's "Mall/Shopping Center" houses award-winning products from the group's Seal of Approval program. Products are organized by age groups and can be purchased online.

Evaluation:

Visitors to this site will be initially impressed by the discussion forums available here. The topics are more numerous than most other sites, they're clearly labeled for access, and the participants are active. At the "Mall," the lists of toys, books, music, furniture, and other child-related products are, of course, limited to those that were tested by the group's volunteers. It would be helpful to know what products overall were evaluated. For example, is a particular product not a "quality" product or has it simply not been tested by the parent judges? The articles were adequate, but just that and nothing more. The advice given is succinct, albeit a bit too brief to be of any real help to a struggling parent. In one instance, helpful hints for "Terrible Twos" invite the parent to remember the authors five rules to "escape toddlerhood in one piece." Such directions are rather negative and simplistic. Visitors are likely to miss the Q & A information archives available at other sites. Other sites, as well, provide more in-depth follow-through and situational help than this one.

Where To Find/Buy:

On the Internet at the URL: http://www.tnpc.com/ or by calling (800) 753-6667

PREGNANCY & CHILDBIRTH
The Basic Illustrated Guide

Description:

Pregnancy & Childbirth is a 126 page book containing 18 unnumbered "chapters" or "sections." Topics include "A Woman's Body," "How the Baby Grows," "What Happens Inside the Woman's Body as the Baby Grows?" "A Good Diet Is Important," "Birth: Labor—What Is It?" "The First Week" (baby and mother), "What's Good About Breastfeeding," and more. The first, second, and third stages of labor are also discussed. Many illustrations accompany the text. Actual size drawings of the baby's in utero growth from 1 month through 9 months are included in the section titled "How the Baby Grows." Also provided are actual size drawings of cervical dilation during labor. Two appendix-type sections are provided at the back of the book on "Childbirth Classes" and "A Guide to Healthy Eating." The "Healthy Eating" section contains tips on healthy eating, lists of food groups and servings, and a diet worksheet.

Evaluation:

This is about as basic a book on pregnancy and childbirth as it gets. The book will appeal to expectant parents of all backgrounds, with its simple, unencumbered language and illustrations. The book's design itself is simple yet attractive: the type is extra large and the numerous illustrations are a little reminiscent of drawings in a preschooler's book. That is, the drawings are done with heavy black lines and details are often sparse. However, the contents of this quaint book is nonetheless very informative and highly readable. *Pregnancy & Childbirth* is a good choice for expectant parents who have little time to read, who want an overview of what will basically occur during pregnancy and childbirth, or for those who otherwise would not read any other book on these topics. It also can be a fun primer before heading into resources offering more details. However, for those readers wanting to take a proactive role in their pregnancy, deal effectively with childbirth and pain management, or seeking other specific how-tos on topics such as breastfeeding, this resource won't suit their purposes.

Where To Find/Buy:

Bookstores and libraries.

Overall Rating
★★
The basics on what occurs during pregnancy and childbirth are clearly presented

Design, Ease Of Use
★★★★
Simple language and illustrations make this an easy book to read

1–4 Stars

Author:
Margaret Martin, MPH

Martin has taught thousands of expectant parents how to prepare for childbirth. She is the founder of the Pregnancy and Natural Childbirth Education Center in Los Angeles, California.

Publisher:
Fisher Books

Edition:
2nd (1997)

Price:
$9.95

Pages:
126

ISBN:
1555611141

Media:
Book

Principal Subject:
Gaining An Overview: All-Inclusive

★★

Overall Rating
★★
Fun treatment of old wives' tales using fact (and opinion); good for shower present

Design, Ease Of Use
★★★
Layout and design attractive

1–4 Stars

Author:
Colleen Davis Gardephe & Steve Ettlinger

Gardephe is a writer and editor specializing in parenting topics. Her articles have appeared in many magazines (*Woman's Day, Parenting, American Baby, Healthy Kids*). Ettlinger is an author specializing in popular reference books.

Publisher:
Chronicle Books

Edition:
1993

Price:
$9.95

Pages:
95

ISBN:
0811802426

Media:
Book

Principal Subject:
Gaining An Overview: All-Inclusive

DON'T PICK UP THE BABY OR YOU'LL SPOIL THE CHILD
And Other Old Wives' Tales About Pregnancy And Parenting

Description:

As mentioned in the foreword, the advice expectant mothers are given is well-meant, but certain sayings have passed from generation to generation and can "mislead a woman at a time when she is trying to be . . . careful about everything she does." This book is intended for those times when "everyone starts telling you what to do . . . what to expect . . . spewing out old superstitions and homespun wisdom with the certainty of a prophet." This little (7" x 7") 95 page book is broken into two parts that list myths and sayings about pregnancy and parenting. Each part is further divided into common threads. Part 1—about pregnancy—includes myths about determining your baby's sex, labor and delivery, health or looks of the mother and baby-to-be, and "myths that need no response" ("If you conceived in the morning, you'll have a boy"). The second part—about parenting—includes myths about feeding, sleeping, discipline, development, breast-feeding, bottle-feeding, and more. Each "old wives' tale" is highlighted and then a paragraph follows which debunks, explains, or extends the myth using input from the authors and a "panel of physicians."

Evaluation:

Exaggerations and superstitions abound in this little book. It's fun and it's easy to read; its format is friendly and its illustrations lend an informal, sweet touch. Much of the authors' advice accompanying the "old wives' tales" is sound, based upon facts. Some, however, is based on opinion with little basis in facts, e.g. "around seven months, however, babies can start to manipulate their parents." New parents need to be careful using this little book as a source of real information to help get through pregnancy or to obtain suggestions about parenting. Rather, it should be used in a fun way by a newly pregnant couple or passed around at a baby shower or given to those who constantly offer well-intended, but misinformed, advice. On the other hand, if a couple were to use this as their principal reference point, they would have a source that does have some solid facts, but also contains opinions that taint its solidarity. And if they heed ALL the advice contained within, they will find themselves swimming in yet another sea of tales.

Where To Find/Buy:

Bookstores and libraries.

JANE'S BREASTFEEDING AND CHILDBIRTH RESOURCES

★ ★

Description:

A British "mum" of three daughters and her husband host this site. She trained with the National Childbirth Trust to become a breastfeeding counselor and worked as a breastfeeding supporter with the Breastfeeding Network. She supports the idea that all parents should be offered sound, factual information about feeding their babies so that they may make an informed choice about their method of feeding. The options available at this website include a video store, book list, links to specific organizations, a support option, and links to "the largest collection of breastfeeding and childbirth-related sites available anywhere." There are also options to contact the site author's organization—the Breastfeeding Network—as well as information regarding the training available through the National Childbirth Trust. An option to post a message to the bulletin board also is provided. Links new to the web page are added to "What's New," then transferred to the relevant section on the site. Links new to the site at this visit include "UK Mums," "Birthingway Place," "Dawson & Son," "Definition for Healthy Breasts," and others. The directory currently includes only UK based organizations, although there are plans to expand to a worldwide directory.

Evaluation:

"Although breastfeeding is natural, it is not necessarily instinctive or easy, and a certain amount of perseverance and determination may be necessary," states this website's author. Unfortunately, the site is not equipped to follow up on this comment. The resource lists that it offers include a video list, book list, a very small list of organizations in the United Kingdom (although there are plans to expand worldwide), and the "largest collection of related sites available anywhere." However, even though the link list is impressive—nine pages long under the Pregnancy and Childbirth section—and listed alphabetically, it is a generous claim. Links are organized into categories of "What's New," "Breastfeeding & Nutrition," "Pregnancy and Birth Info," "Commercial Sites," "Newsgroups," and more. A description of the categories would be helpful, but in lieu of that, descriptions are provided for each link. The only two areas of support are the bulletin board (the most inactive we've seen, with less than a handful of postings) and the support area where one can email a question to one of the site's volunteers. This site is almost exclusively a resource list in itself with no original material to support anyone interested in breastfeeding.

Where To Find/Buy:

On the Internet at the URL: http://www.breastfeeding.co.uk/

Overall Rating
★★
No original information, this site instead hosts extensive links to other resources

Design, Ease Of Use
★★★
Simple, effective layout

1–4 Stars

Media:
Internet

Principal Subject:
Gaining An Overview: All-Inclusive

Overall Rating
★★
Offers Christian parenting perspectives without being fanatical

Design, Ease Of Use
★★★
Straightforward, succinct; numerous links to get more information

1–4 Stars

Media:
Internet

Principal Subject:
Gaining An Overview: All-Inclusive

THE KIDZ ARE PEOPLE TOO PAGE

Description:

Pregnancy, childbirth, breastfeeding, and infant care are some of the major topics at this website created by a Christian mother. Her site's focus is that "children should be treated with respect, too." The homepage to this site includes a Table of Contents to the entire site. Each topic includes links to other sites offering further information. Pregnancy links include those offering general overviews, nutrition, low tech ways to conceive, etc. Also included are essays and brochures detailing an unborn child's right to life and sites offering alternatives to abortions. "Childbirth" offers birth stories and invites users of the site to submit their own stories. Links at this topic include Advice on Childbirth, Birth Stories, Siblings at Birth, Birth Links, and more. Areas linked under "Infant Care" include diapering, weaning your baby, understanding your baby's cries, the family bed, and more. "Breastfeeding" offers highlights of "why breast is best," along with links to articles supporting that choice; also included are tips on starting solids, nursing toddlers, etc. Excerpts from the Bible are offered to support the site's focus and beliefs.

Evaluation:

Two distinctive approaches to parenting have evolved and steer current parenting practices. One approach, "attachment parenting," believes in heeding the baby's every cry, sharing sleep with one's baby, breastfeeding, etc. The second approach (termed by some "detachment parenting") believes that a baby needs to be taught to be independent, cry it out, learn to sleep by himself/herself, etc. This site takes both elements into account. In doing so, it uses quotes from the Bible, couples this guidance with the author's own experiences and attitudes, and supplies additional informational sources. The tone of the website is loving and joyful. The author offers her Christian background as a basis for her parenting methods, without being preachy. The best part of this site is that the homepage is a table of contents for the entire site. There are not many graphics, which can make a website boring and dry. However, with this site, the lack of graphics makes it easy to read and navigate. The site is positive, well-organized, and straightforward in its approach. Visitors wishing forums or chats will need to go elsewhere.

Where To Find/Buy:

On the Internet at the URL: http://www.geocities.com/Heartland/8148

YOUR PREGNANCY QUESTIONS & ANSWERS

★ ★

Description:

This book was written to "provide patients with many types of information about gynecological and obstetrical conditions they may have, problems they may encounter and procedures they may undergo." Teachings are conveyed in a question and answer format throughout this book's 4 main parts which include discussions of "Before Pregnancy," "Your Pregnancy," "The Birth of Your Baby," and "After Your Baby Is Born." Further clarification is provided in tables that are frequently used to summarize a collection of answers. Also included to further reinforce and clarify the author's responses are pencil sketches, a glossary, and an index. The questions contained within this 403 page book originate from Curtis' patients and those of other physicians he knows. This book attempts to not only convey an overview of pregnancy, but to also answer questions about special problems patients have had historically. For example, the author provides a list of questions pertaining to possible legal concerns; Curtis leaves these questions unanswered, instead advising the reader to consult a family law attorney.

Evaluation:

Using the question and answer format to present information flows much like a conversation between doctor and patient. As each question is asked, the answer offered nearly leads to the next question. Strings of questions (printed in bold type) build upon one another in this manner which makes for easy referencing, while still providing broad coverage. The Q/A text, which requires an abundance of words, is contrasted by the many tables found throughout the book that summarize information at a glance. A glossary and index further highlight information and terminology. Some of the illustrations contained throughout the book serve to provide detail, while others serve more as a visual reference point. The book is arranged in sections, yet the divisions are not rigid and there is some overlap of information. Given the broad coverage of information beginning with basic terminology ("What is the purpose of the menstrual cycle?"), this book could best serve first-time mothers as a source of explanation and reassurance for minor concerns. For more critical concerns, the reader is clearly directed to her physician.

Where To Find/Buy:

Bookstores and libraries.

Overall Rating
★★
Q/A format seems to put a focus on problems rather than solutions or joys

Design, Ease Of Use
★★★
Information easily found and cross-referenced

1–4 Stars

Author:
Glade B. Curtis, MD

Curtis is a practicing physician who has written two other books on pregnancy (*Your Pregnancy Week by Week* and *Your Pregnancy After 30*), and co-authored a book on female surgeries.

Publisher:
Fisher Books

Edition:
1995

Price:
$12.95

Pages:
403

ISBN:
1555611508

Media:
Book

Principal Subject:
Gaining An Overview: All-Inclusive

★ ★

Overall Rating
★★
Comprehensive, emphasis on medically-based model of childbirth

Design, Ease Of Use
★★
Easy to read; conversational style of writing; no graphics to lighten the text or educate

1–4 Stars

Author:
Shari E. Brasner, MD

Publisher:
Hyperion

Edition:
1998

Price:
$12.95

Pages:
250

ISBN:
0786883391

Media:
Book

Principal Subject:
Gaining An Overview: All-Inclusive

ADVICE FROM A PREGNANT OBSTETRICIAN
An Insider's Guide

Description:

This 250 page, 11 chapter book was written by a woman obstetrician who gave birth to twins at 32-1/2 weeks by Cesarean section. The book is divided into three parts: First Trimester, Second Trimester, and Third Trimester. The "First Trimester" section contains information about changes in the woman's body, fears and problems during the first trimester, genetic testing, multiple fetuses, diet and exercise, sex, and more. The "Second Trimester" section discusses the relatively "calm" period between the first and third trimesters, tests, and changes during this period. The "Third Trimester" section covers changes in the woman, fetal growth, hypertension and preeclampsia, prelabor, labor, and various intervention methods (epidural, forceps, etc.). Cesarean delivery is discussed in a chapter of its own. The last chapter contains postpartum information: breastfeeding or bottlefeeding, circumcision, depression, sex, exercise, and more. An index is provided at the back of the book.

Evaluation:

This book on pregnancy and childbirth is unique in its design. It is journal-like, chronicling some of Brasner's own experiences during her pregnancy and childbearing. It is also casual in the presentation of facts and advice. Brasner often uses a conversational writing style, with many "Is" and "yous." Some of her advice may be controversial to readers. For example, she is not shy about suggesting numerous obstetrical interventions (fetal monitoring, pain management medications, epidurals, etc.) and she "routinely suggests . . . half a glass of wine when [the expectant mother] gets home from her amnio[centesis], if she wants"; this is not to say, however, that she advocates regular consumption of alcohol during pregnancy. Brasner recognizes that her approach and methods may not be embraced by those who are set on a "natural" delivery. However, for those interested in knowing what modern medical technology has to offer, this book will help educate and inform. It is well-rounded, taking the reader from conception through delivery and postpartum. Brasner makes a true effort to give the reader a one-on-one book "from both sides of the stirrups."

Where To Find/Buy:

Bookstores and libraries.

BABY BAG
The In-Site To Parenting: Prenatal To Preschool

Description:

The creators of this website have divided it into two separate parts—"Our Departments" and "Interactive." Within the first section, visitors may select various options ranging from pregnancy information to parenting tips. Articles included about pregnancy range from birth stories, baby shower games and baby shopping lists to overcoming infertility, exercise, and doulas. Information returned generally amounts to several pages of dense text (sometimes tempered with graphics) written by a variety of professionals; for "overcoming infertility," five pages were provided by a writer for the FDA Consumer. The site's "Interactive" section contains various means for parents to communicate with one another. Bulletin boards are provided and are organized into a general category with nine specific categories ("parents over 30," "single parents," "feeding," etc.). Birth announcements, birth stories, shopping opportunities, and more are also provided. Within this segment, one also may "Ask the Professional" (a pharmacist, a childbirth educator, a midwife, a home-based employment specialist).

Evaluation:

Parents-to-be and new parents want information and advice, and this site attempts to provide it. The information provided tends to be no-nonsense and to the point. The site's creators collaborate with many professionals and agencies, who submit articles at this site. For example, "Healthy Eating During Pregnancy" is co-sponsored by the March of Dimes, with information provided by the National Academy of Science and U.S. Department of Agriculture. Most parenting websites offer chat rooms and bulletin boards; at first glance, we were thrilled to note that this site's bulletin board area was sub-categorized, making it easier for parents interested in a particular topic to find one another. Unfortunately, the conversational summaries given were vague and difficult to decipher. Overall, the range of "professionals" offer interesting choices; a pediatrician or child care provider's voice would be a welcome addition. The information found here is adequate, and the bulletin boards are active. In all, the site's creators have pulled together a myriad of sources on many topics to make a website that is useful and easy to understand and navigate.

Where To Find/Buy:

On the Internet at the URL: http://www.babybag.com/

Overall Rating
★★
Includes information about specific concerns of pregnancy, childbirth, etc.

Design, Ease Of Use
★★
Site design has improved; bulletin board forums need better summaries

---

1–4 Stars

Media:
Internet

Principal Subject:
Gaining An Overview: All-Inclusive

★★

Overall Rating
★★
Those who like lists will love this; otherwise, too many lists, too much time involved

Design, Ease Of Use
★★
Two separate table of contents organize information by topic and by trimester; no index

1–4 Stars

Author:
Maureen Bard

Bard is a wife, a mother of two, and a career woman who lives in Indianapolis and is a faculty member at Indiana State University.

Publisher:
Meadowbrook Press

Edition:
2nd (1995)

Price:
$9.00

Pages:
175

ISBN:
0881662429

Media:
Book

Principal Subject:
Gaining An Overview: All-Inclusive

GETTING ORGANIZED FOR YOUR NEW BABY
A Checklist And Planner For Busy Parents-To-Be

Description:
A wife and mother of two has compiled numerous check-off lists, fill-in-the-blank forms, outlines, graphs, charts, and more to "make your pregnancy preparations as simple and convenient as possible." Her 175 page planner is organized in two ways—information given by topic and then subsequently by trimester. The ten topic chapters consist of the following: planning for a baby (plotting menstrual cycles, basal body temps), prenatal planning (selecting caregiver and birthsite, morning sickness, etc.), mother's needs (clothing, meds, manicures, etc.), baby's needs, (breast vs. bottle feeding), family members and household needs (siblings, duties, shopping, menus, etc.), financial planning (budgets, insurance, investments), celebrations (showers, religious ceremonies), day care and babysitters, final countdown (labor, going home), and postpartum considerations (support systems). A second and separate table of contents lists organizers based upon trimester with pages listed for cross-referencing. Each page within the text is also labeled by trimester to establish a reference point.

Evaluation:
The reader of this resource will find list upon list, chart upon chart, and more organizer tools than she/he ever dreamed of. Due to the wide number and variety of topics, one list or another is bound to be a helpful tool to "getting organized" during pregnancy. A disclaimer: "each pregnancy is unique and the lists presented in this book are offered only as guidelines to help one organized." Consequently, the reader must think through the purpose and value of each particular list as he/she uses it. In this way the reader will not fall prey to ONLY relying on the author's list. Also, some lists appear to be superfluous and/or intimidating to most first-time parents. Truly, there is a need to get organized for the delightful, traumatic entry to a new person into one's life. But there is also the learning by living through the experience of this entry which too many lists and organization can so overly anticipate, that the event becomes more a project than a mystery to be experienced. The book's central image is a very busy mother orchestrating all, but such an emphasis seems to ignore the evolving role of fathers both before and following the birth. If one lives for checking off lists and filling in charts, this resource will be a help.

Where To Find/Buy:
Bookstores and libraries, or order direct by calling (800) 338-2232.

BIRTH OVER THIRTY-FIVE
The Practical, Reassuring Guide To The Joys And Challenges

★★

Description:

As the author states in her introduction, "this is not a how-to book, packed with dos and don'ts." Using her background as a social anthropologist, she explores the emotional aspects of birth and raising children from the viewpoint of women over the "safest age range"—women in their thirties and early forties. Most of the information in this 9 chapter, 180 page book was obtained through Kitzinger's advertisement in a British national newspaper. The concerns and realities of the 289 women that responded is coupled with those obtained through the author's own childbirth classes and from 28 women in South Africa replying to a different newspaper article. The book centers on the decision to have a baby. Numerous narratives from women are featured on various subjects, such as: planning for pregnancy (mother's nutrition, lifestyle, etc.); prenatal care (what to expect at doctor's office visits); risk factors (amniocentesis, genetic tests, ultrasounds, etc.); "life after the baby comes"; roles of parents, siblings, and other family members; and single motherhood.

Evaluation:

The facts are there—more and more women are having children in their late thirties and early forties whether by choice or "surprise." Obviously, these women will have concerns and be in search of advice that may differ from women in other age groups. Knowing others share the same doubts, fears, frustrations, and thrills may help some mothers, but mothers will most likely feel shortchanged as they look for answers in this book. Some subjects are neglected, such as dealing with multiple births, adoption, or having an only child; others are treated superficially (social isolation, career decisions). Keep in mind that opinions of women in a different culture—European—form the basis of this book, and that the author's sample size is small. The targeted audience for this book is "older mothers," however, we find the audience that would most benefit from this book will be those involved in counseling and medical fields. For those who counsel others, there is a store of "realities" in this book that may shed some light on what mothers over 35 years of age may experience emotionally, physically, and socially.

Where To Find/Buy:

Bookstores and libraries.

Overall Rating
★★
"Not a how-to" for "older mothers"; best used by counselors

Design, Ease Of Use
★
Poorly organized; based on British survey of 289 women

1–4 Stars

Author:
Sheila Kitzinger

Kitzinger, "an internationally respected educator and writer on birth and motherhood," was educated as a social anthropologist at Oxford. She has done field research on sex, pregnancy, and childbirth among women in diverse settings.

Publisher:
Penguin Books
(Penguin Group)

Edition:
3rd (1994)

Price:
$9.95

Pages:
180

ISBN:
0140241418

Media:
Book

Principal Subject:
Gaining An Overview:
All-Inclusive

★★

Overall Rating
★★
Excellent graphics, much opportunity for visitor participation

Design, Ease Of Use
★
Horribly disorganized, information not worth the effort needed to find it

1–4 Stars

Media:
Internet

Principal Subject:
Gaining An Overview: All-Inclusive

PARENTHOODWEB

Description:

Various options are available at this website's homepage. Visitors can gain quick access to spotlighted topical questions, participate in a quick poll to express an opinion on a given subject, review "facts and figures" (news abstracts) and note the latest product recall notices. Also available are birth announcements, greeting cards, and links to other parenting sites. The visitor to this site can offer her/his opinion on pregnancy and parenting issues. Articles focusing on pregnancy, labor, childcare, and parenting issues are available throughout the website. Many articles are linked to other websites. Additional resources are listed and a weekly newsletter is available through email. Various areas allow you to either ask questions of experts (their bios are given) or read their responses to others' questions. Links to topics include shopping, pregnancy, recipes, sleep, names, safety, chat rooms, and boards. Graphics, photos, and illustrations of particular issues are woven throughout.

Evaluation:

Good luck to any visitor trying to find a way around this navigational nightmare. This site is so disorganized that it distracts, even discourages, a visitor from taking the time to unearth valuable information. Much of this site offers parents chances to be heard and to hear others; this certainly will fill a need for parents at home looking for others' feedback. The homepage offers many links to articles and information, none of it organized in any recognizable manner. The information available needs to be categorized in age groups or main issues. On the positive side, this site offers good opportunities for a visitor to participate in polls, chat areas, and message boards. The graphics are excellent. For example, in the Pregnancy section, photographs of fetal ultrasounds are better than those found in most doctors' offices. Also available in the same section are a series of charts that detail fetal growth in each month of pregnancy, supplemented by detailed illustrations. Overall, however, this site offers nothing that one can't find elsewhere with much less effort and confusion.

Where To Find/Buy:

On the Internet at the URL: http://www.parenthoodweb.com/

GETTING READY FOR BABY

Description:

"Getting Ready For Baby" is one of three videos in the Video Parents' series. Others include "Your Baby's First Six Months" and "Your Baby's First Steps." This 52 minute video is divided into clearly marked "chapters" to allow viewers to easily return to particular portions for review. The 12 segments include physical and psychological changes, proper nutrition, job and household work, outings and trips, the benefits of proper exercise, intimacy and sex during pregnancy, fathering, preparing the home for baby's arrival, preparing for childbirth, labor and childbirth (including Cesarean sections), the postpartum period, and bonding with a baby. The information offered focuses exclusively on those who choose birth in a hospital setting. Voice-overs include both male and female narrators, who refer to the pregnant woman in the third person.

Evaluation:

While this video presents very basic information in an overall pleasant manner, it is hard to imagine many prospective parents who will want to view it more than once. "Getting Ready For Baby" covers general topics, from lifestyle changes that are suggested before attempting conception to necessary baby supplies. It seems strictly geared toward couples who are planning hospital births. It makes no mention of some of the most important trends emerging in birthing practices, nor of some of the newest information on what is best for baby and mother. For example, there is no mention of birthing locations other than in a hospital, such as a home birth or birthing center. A mother is shown first bottlefeeding her infant—even as the narrator says breastfeeding is best for baby—and breastfeeding is shown later in the video. And judgmental statements abound throughout. One example: lying down is said to be the preferred position for labor. Another: the narrator says it is "common to experience some difficulty breastfeeding," then proceeds to give suggestions "to avoid despair." With the wealth of insightful material available on pregnancy and labor, one is hard pressed to see the need for this particular offering.

Where To Find/Buy:

Bookstores, libraries, videotape dealers, or order direct by calling Library Video Company at (800) 843-3620, through FAX at (610) 645-4040, or online at libraryvideo.com.

Overall Rating
★
Very general, very basic information, presented in an often judgmental fashion

Design, Ease Of Use
★★★
Topics tabbed for easy review

1–4 Stars

Publisher:
Ceres International
(BMG Entertainment)

Edition:
1994

Price:
$14.95

ISBN:
1568120559

Media:
Videotape

Principal Subject:
Gaining An Overview:
All-Inclusive

Overall Rating
★
Watch for hidden commercials; subtly encourages use of Enfamil® baby formula

Design, Ease Of Use
★★
Easy to navigate

1–4 Stars

Media:
Internet

Principal Subject:
Gaining An Overview: All-Inclusive

MOMNESS CENTER

Description:

The Momness Center web site is sponsored by Mead Johnson, makers of the Enfamil® family of baby formulas. Its goal is to be "the place for information and inspiration for moms and moms-to-be." The homepage offers a number of selections, including "Baby Care," a collection of guides for the new mother, from breastfeeding to daycare; "As Your Baby Grows," a month by month account of fetal development from conception to the first few weeks after birth; "Chronicle of a New Mom," the personal story of one new mother; and "Beautiful Mom . . . and Mom-to-be," which offers information on the physiological changes during pregnancy, wardrobe tips for pregnant women, and "thoughts from the online community on what makes motherhood beautiful." A fifth selection, "Baby 123" invites visitors to join the site's online club and receive special product offers and discounts. The site also offers archived informational material on everything from a list of what to pack for the hospital to "Help! My Baby is Turning Into a Toddler," FAQs, and links.

Evaluation:

This is an attractive and well-designed site full of helpful basic information. It also is a website that requires a strong caution. It is sponsored by Mead Johnson, the makers of the Enfamil® family of baby formulas. While the site includes sections that discuss why breastfeeding is best for baby and mother with tips on successful breastfeeding, breast care, and expressing and storing mother's milk, it includes many other references that suggest, incorrectly, that most breastfeeding women will want to rely to some extent on commercial infant formulas. The wording is subtle and, while it may be unintentional, it also is obvious. Example: a large subheading is entitled "When You Need to Supplement," instead of "If You Need to Supplement." That section then proceeds to say that "almost every nursing mother will need (ed: not choose) to supplement her baby with bottled breast milk or an infant formula." Another section contains wording that suggests Enfamil® formulas are almost identical to breast milk. Inaccuracies such as these mar an otherwise enjoyable site and lend worry that inexperienced parents will accept these statements as fact, when more accurate and supportive information about breastfeeding and its benefits is available elsewhere.

Where To Find/Buy:

On the Internet at http://www.womenslink.com/momness/index.htm

DAILY PARENT

Description:

This site offers a list of articles regarding many subjects pertinent to parenting. At the homepage, a visitor must choose a topic that is listed under one of four "channels," which include "Family," "Pregnancy," "Health," and "Education and Development." That chosen topic leads to a list of articles which discuss various related parenting issues. The articles are written by various authors with the Scripps Howard News Service, and all topics and issues are organized alphabetically. A visitor also can submit comments, and read others' comments and responses regarding that issue. Topics listed under the "Family Channel" include auto safety, family finances, nutrition, summer camps, and more. "Health Channel" topics include allergies, exercise, menopause, and stress. Bedwetting, childcare, back to school, self-esteem, and other issues are listed under the "Education and Development Channel." Finally, the "Pregnancy Channel" covers issues such as premature babies, birth, and postpartum depression.

Evaluation:

The visitor to this site can only be amazed when accessing its lengthy topic list. The information offered in the articles provides good, direct advice, along with examples of real-life situations and suggested ways of using that advice. But that's where the excitement ends. First of all, the list of topics is cumbersome and awkward. It needs to be better organized into smaller distinct categories (such as "Child Health Concerns," "Discipline Problems," etc.). Also, the discussion forums seem nicely laid-out at first glance, but upon further research one discovers that the chats are relatively inactive compared to other sites. One must also question the source of the information. Little information is given regarding the expertise of the authors of these articles. Some information doesn't pertain to parenting. For example, information in the "Health Channel" includes discussions of menopause and breast cancer. Also, some areas pertinent to new moms' needs are minimal. For example, "breastfeeding" contain two articles both of which address how to breastfeed upon returning to work. In short, this site's problem can be summed up with one word: scattered. One can certainly find clearer routes to information at other sites.

Where To Find/Buy:

On the Internet at the URL: http://www.dailyparent.com/

Overall Rating

★

A variety of info is available but not easily accessed

Design, Ease Of Use

★

Topics arranged alphabetically in cumbersome list, no graphics, inactive discussions

1–4 Stars

Media:
Internet

Principal Subject:
Gaining An Overview: All-Inclusive

Overall Rating

★

This site lacks substance and direction

Design, Ease Of Use

★

Must register to use site's features; past Q & A topics can't be easily accessed/ retrieved

1–4 Stars

Media:
Internet

Principal Subject:
Gaining An Overview: All-Inclusive

THE MOMMY TIMES
Dedicated To Preserving The Sanity Of Moms Everywhere

Description:

The Mommy Times website, also billed as "The Mom to Mom Support Community on the Web," established itself first as a publication in 1992 and as a website in 1995. Registration is required to access the site's features, which include the following: "Mommy e-mail," "Mommy-to-Mommy," and back issues of "The Mommy Times." The site hosts articles, and questions and answers "written for moms by moms . . . everything from pregnancy and puberty and many topics in between." Through "Mommye-mail," moms may quickly post messages to one another. "Mommy-to-Mommy" offers a chance for moms to create new topics, post a question and read others' responses, or read archives of past questions and answers. Past issues of "The Mommy Times" may be accessed either through the website (from the October/November 1996 issue forward). The current online issue of "The Mommy Times" (November/December 1998) includes 12 articles on topics such as the holidays, life with twins, toys for less, and consumer product tips.

Evaluation:

Many websites have been developed to support the needs of busy moms who want to communicate with others in a convenient manner with no time constraints. This site, however, lacks substance, has no direction, and is more frustrating than it is supportive. Question and answer forums are inviting, but without a helpful structure. For example, if one wants to read others' concerns and feedback regarding bedtime rituals, she needs to scroll through endless pages of posted topic headings to find the appropriate ones. What would be extremely helpful here is some categorization, e.g. "Bedtime Rituals." Also, if a mother wants to respond to a question or topic posted in the "Mommy-to-Mommy" archive, she must create a topic in the new section (since the archive is closed to responses), recap the question, and then add her response. It would be helpful to have an index of topics from past issues, so that a visitor looking for specific information could find it easily. If a mom has the time, this site is a mildly amusing place to check into routinely, but all in all, busy moms could well be spending their precious time elsewhere.

Where To Find/Buy:

On the Internet at the URL: http://www.mommytimes.com/

ONLINE BIRTH CENTER
Information On Midwifery, Pregnancy, Birth And Breastfeeding

Description:
Several options are available at this website's homepage including information on midwifery, pregnancy, and breastfeeding. Other areas include "The Parents Page," a media center, newsgroups and mailing lists for parents, an organization list for anyone involved with childbirth, and information on nutrition during pregnancy, high risk situations, and complications in pregnancy, labor, and birth. The Parents Page focuses on resources for prospective parents as well as parents of infants and small children; most of the information is obtained through links to other sites and includes topics such as "birth alternatives," "finding a practitioner," "adoption, family planning, infertility, grief and loss," and more. The Media Center lists magazines, journals, books, videos, and other media centering on pregnancy, birth, and midwifery. Various groups may be contacted through "Newsgroups and Mailing Lists"; lists include Bradley® Method teachers, doulas, a homebirth mailing list, nursing moms, and more; these lists are intended for both professionals and parents.

Evaluation:
Pregnancy, childbirth, midwifery, breastfeeding, and more? If it sounds as if this site is shooting for the moon, they are. Venture into their site, though, and you'll find yourself hurled into outer space. It's confusing, it's exhausting to wade through, and at best case you'll come away with information you probably already knew or could more easily have found in a different site or resource. Most of the original material at this site is pretty basic, without graphics and without inspiration. One problem at this site was the lack of a unifying theme or emphasis. The information here appears lifeless and unimpressive. Many sites deal with the topics of pregnancy, childbirth (and midwifery), and breastfeeding. We've also found that only some sites can credibly stand on their linked information to other sites, not so with this one. Abandon this ship and check into other sites we have recommended instead.

Where To Find/Buy:
On the Internet at the URL: http://www.efn.org/~djz/birth/birthindex.html

---

Overall Rating

★

Meek potpourri of linked and original info dealing with pregnancy, childbirth, etc.

Design, Ease Of Use

★

Navigation slow, layout haphazard, graphics noticeably absent

---

1–4 Stars

Media:
Internet

Principal Subject:
Gaining An Overview: All-Inclusive

Overall Rating

★

Very basic information; access to overall information limited based on registration data

Design, Ease Of Use

★

Navigation frustrating at times; must register to use the site

1–4 Stars

Publisher:
women.com Network

Media:
Internet

Principal Subject:
Gaining An Overview:
All-Inclusive

STORKSITE
The Premier Pregnancy And New Parenting Website

Description:

StorkSite's goal is to "provide emotional and informational support in an interactive, community-based environment." A visitor must register to gain access to the site's free features, which include "The Front Porch," the "Stork Site Library," "The Storkzine," and "The Picket Fence." The Front Porch offers a personal due date ticker, suggested baby names, email notices, access to a reference library, chat rooms, Baby Grams and more. Baby Grams are one page monthly descriptions of a baby's growth and development from early pregnancy to about 2 years of age. The Storkzine, the online magazine, offers various articles (typically one page) on pregnancy, childbirth, and the first year; recent articles dealt with postpartum blues, hot spots to raise children, and myths regarding birth control pills. "Ask Tori R.N." is a Q & A forum for issues concerning pregnancy and childbirth. Users can access a glossary, name database, medical references, and more through The Stork Site Library. The Picket Fence, "the heart and soul of Stork Site's community," offers chat rooms, "Best Friends Forums," and other features.

Evaluation:

This website offers little information on pregnancy, childbirth or baby care. Once a visitor has registered, information provided at various points is specific only to the biographical information submitted through the registration process. This limits the user to finding information that may be current to his or her situation, but doesn't allow a visitor to explore ideas or problems in general. The user is unable to access Baby Grams on older children (just those under 2 years old). Reference materials available through both The Storkzine and The Stork Site Library may be useful for some. Many of these references, however, are either too unwieldy (medical abstracts) or too brief to be relevant to many parents' needs. The Picket Fence may provide some emotional support; the Q & A forum provides interesting feedback, but it's one person's viewpoint, not a team that might offer varying points of view to consider. In short, a parent can look elsewhere for more comprehensive and user-friendly information.

Where To Find/Buy:

On the Internet at the URL: http://www. storksite.com/index2.html

TERRIFIC
RESOURCES FOR
SELECTED TOPICS

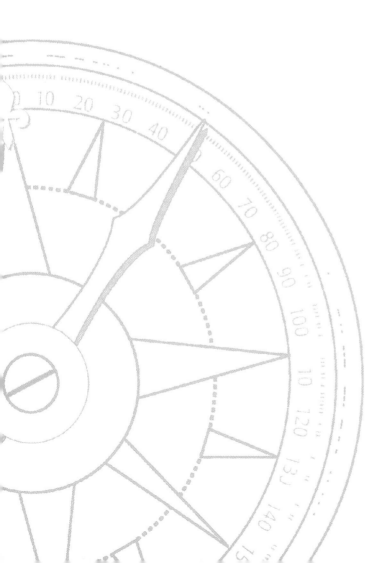

INTRODUCTION

During the course of our ongoing research, we've determined several other "views" of the resources we've reviewed. The sixteen resources listed in this section uniquely meet specific purposes as you become a parent. We've placed a short description of each here so you get a foretaste, and we've cross-referenced the full page review on each so you can follow up.

These specific resources focus on:

- An exercise program to help prepare for a fit pregnancy, easier labor, and fast recovery

- Pregnant teenagers considering their options for handling an unplanned teenage pregnancy

- Parenting twins or multiples, from pregnancy through the first year

- Birth partners offering support and coaching during childbirth

- An overview of the various childbirth options available to women

- Alternative childbirth practices and philosophies

- Understanding the prenatal, labor, and birth experiences of both baby and mother

- Couples seeking a childbirth experience that encompasses inward and outer guidance

- Nursing mothers who want to continue breastfeeding when they return to work

- The how-tos of infant care and development (through a videotape)

- Choosing a nanny as caregiver of your baby

- Describing the pros and cons of various child care options

- Raising and taking care of twins or multiples

- Advice and support for new moms through Internet dialogs with other moms

- Advice and support for new moms through online dialogs with other moms

- The emotional aspects of dealing with infertility

Take some time to read the full descriptions and evaluations for each recommended resource carefully. We're certain that you will discover the right resources to best serve your needs.

An exercise program to help prepare for a fit pregnancy, easier labor, and fast recovery

Title:	**Maternal Fitness**
Subtitle:	Preparing For A Healthy Pregnancy, An Easier Labor, And A Quick Recovery
Author:	Julie Tupler, RN (with Andrea Thompson)
Overall Rating:	★★★★
Media Type:	Book
Short Description:	The author, a personal trainer and fitness instructor, explains the rationale and methodology for her exercise program called "Maternal Fitness." Her routine is based upon three goals: prevention, preparation, and restoration. Her program also includes the "BAKS Basics" which strengthens your body for Maternal Fitness. Numerous illustrations and detailed narrative describe each exercise.

■ **Read The Full Review Of This Resource On Page 31.**

Pregnant teenagers considering their options for handling an unplanned teenage pregnancy

Title:	**I'm Pregnant, Now What Do I Do?**
Author:	Dr. Robert W. Buckingham, PH & Mary P. Derby, RN, MPH
Overall Rating:	★★★★
Media Type:	Book
Short Description:	This book presents the decision-making process for unplanned teenage pregnancies. Three options are presented for what to do: giving the child up for adoption, terminating the pregnancy through abortion, and continuing with the pregnancy. Three specific case studies are provided which outline three teenagers' decision-making thoughts regarding each of these three options. Numerous teenagers' anecdotes are also included throughout.

■ **Read The Full Review Of This Resource On Page 19.**

Parenting twins or multiples, from pregnancy through the first year

Title:	**Having Twins**
Author:	Elizabeth Noble
Overall Rating:	★★★★
Media Type:	Book
Short Description:	The second edition of Noble's guide is a "comprehensive resource for those giving and receiving prenatal care (in) preparation for twinbearing." Topics covered include: prenatal communication, bonding, pregnancy, ways to prolong pregnancy and prevent prematurity, labor and birth, taking care of twins, dealing with loss, and more. Anecdotes are given in the book's margins illustrating fears, reliefs, and tips from those that have had multiples.

■ **Read The Full Review Of This Resource On Page 223.**

Birth partners offering support and coaching during childbirth

Title:	**The Birth Partner**
Subtitle:	Everything You Need To Know To Help A Woman Through Childbirth
Author:	Penny Simkin, PT
Overall Rating:	★★★★
Media Type:	Book
Short Description:	This book is written specifically for the person who will be coaching or assisting a woman during her labor and childbirth. Written from the perspective of an advocate and a teacher, it is designed to be a tool to be referenced before and during the experience. Unique to this book is the "Take-Charge Routine" which points out ways in which the birth partner can be most supportive and effective during labor and childbirth.

■ **Read The Full Review Of This Resource On Page 55.**

An overview of the various childbirth choices available to women

Title:	**The Birth Book**
Subtitle:	Everything You Need To Know To Have A Safe And Satisfying Birth
Author:	William Sears, MD & Martha Sears, RN
Overall Rating:	★★★★
Media Type:	Book
Short Description:	This is the Sears' perspective on preparing for birth, what to do while in labor, and the experience of giving birth. Their premise throughout is to offer you enough information, medically and otherwise, so you can determine the birth you want and find out how to get it. Fourteen chapters of this 269 page book focus on past birthing practices, current choices, pain management, labor and delivery, writing birth plans, VBACs, C-sections, and more.

■ **Read The Full Review Of This Resource On Page 49.**

Alternative childbirth practices and philosophies

Title:	**Gentle Birth Choices**
Subtitle:	A Guide To Making Informed Decisions About Birthing Centers, Birth Attendants, Water Birth, Home Birth, Hospital Birth
Author:	Barbara Harper, RN
Overall Rating:	★★★★
Media Type:	Book
Short Description:	This book is written to support the choice of natural childbirth. It includes observations made all over the world on alternative childbirth options. The author's perspective on medical technology vs. natural childbirth is detailed in eight chapters. From history to myths to midwives, this book attempts to familiarize the reader with the concept of choice and power over the childbirth process.

■ **Read The Full Review Of This Resource On Page 57.**

Understanding the prenatal, labor, and birth experiences of both baby and mother

Title:	**Conception, Pregnancy And Birth**
Author:	Dr. Miriam Stoppard
Overall Rating:	★★★★
Media Type:	Book

Short Description:

■ **Read The Full Review Of This Resource On Page 222.**

This book covers its titled subject matter in 351 pages, 15 chapters. An overview summarizes the book from "Preparing for Pregnancy" to "Adjusting to Parenthood." Additionally, two pages of "Useful Addresses" are included at the back of the book. Sidebars, tables, illustrations, photographs, and bulleted highlights are used to present the book's information in addition to narrative text. Case studies of specific situations are also given.

Couples seeking a childbirth experience that encompasses inward and outer guidance

Title:	**Birthing From Within**
Subtitle:	An Extra-Ordinary Guide To Childbirth Preparation
Author:	Pam England, CNM, MA, and Rob Horowitz, PhD
Overall Rating:	★★★★
Media Type:	Book

Short Description:

■ **Read The Full Review Of This Resource On Page 56.**

This book is based on pregnancy classes developed by author Pam England. Her vision: "parents learning through interactive, creative participation, in a spirit of fun and curiosity." The book is divided into seven sections, from "Beginning Your Journey" and "Preparing Your Birth Place" to "Being Powerful in Birth" and "Fathers and Birth Companions." The book includes many illustrations, "birthing art," and other drawings.

Nursing mothers who want to continue breastfeeding when they return to work

Title:	**Nursing Mother, Working Mother**
Subtitle:	The Essential Guide For Breastfeeding And Staying Close To Your Baby After You Return To Work
Author:	Gale Pryor
Overall Rating:	★★★★
Media Type:	Book

Short Description:

■ **Read The Full Review Of This Resource On Page 153.**

Extending a section of her other book, *Nursing Your Baby*, Pryor discusses how to combine work and breastfeeding. Within its 184 pages, this seven chapter book highlights the whys and hows of breastfeeding along with a plea to change workplace attitudes toward motherhood. Three chapters specifically focus on the transition from new motherhood to work including maternity leave, getting ready (supplies, finding care, etc.), and returning.

The how-tos of infant care and development (through a videotape)

Title:	**Baby Basics (Videotape)**
Subtitle:	The Complete Video Guide For New And Expectant Parents
Overall Rating:	★★★★
Media Type:	Videotape
Short Description:	Divided into eight "chapters," this 110 minute videotape focuses on the care and development of newborns and infants. Topics discussed include: the newborn's appearances, postpartum care of the mother, the adjustment during the first days at home, daily care (bathing, diapering, dressing, and more), feeding (breastfeeding, bottlefeeding), health and safety, babies' cries, sleep patterns, and infants' growth and development.

■ **Read The Full Review Of This Resource On Page 118.**

Choosing a nanny as caregiver of your baby

Title:	**The Complete Nanny Guide**
Subtitle:	Solutions To Parents' Questions About Hiring And Keeping An In-Home Caregiver
Author:	Cora Hilton Thomas
Overall Rating:	★★★★
Media Type:	Book
Short Description:	This book contains information on finding and choosing appropriate in-home care. Chapter topics in this 154 guide include finding the right person, costs, interviewing, screening, keeping a nanny, filing government forms, using a placement agency, and more. One chapter focuses on finding care for children that have special needs. Appendices contain numerous forms and checklists (criminal background release forms, tax and government forms, etc.).

■ **Read The Full Review Of This Resource On Page 168.**

Describing the pros and cons of various childcare options

Title:	**Child Care That Works**
Subtitle:	A Parent's Guide To Finding Quality Child Care
Author:	Eva Cochran and Mon Cochran
Overall Rating:	★★★★
Media Type:	Book
Short Description:	How to find quality child care is the focus of this 355 page book. The six parts of this guide deal separately with the various options that are available, the possible emotional reactions children and parents may have to child care, ways to build a partnership with a caregiver, how much to pay, and how to become an advocate for quality care. Checklists, forms, and organization contact information are given in the appendices.

■ **Read The Full Review Of This Resource On Page 167.**

Raising and taking care of twins or multiples

Title:	**The Joy Of Twins And Other Multiple Births**
Subtitle:	Having, Raising, And Loving Babies Who Arrive In Groups
Author:	Pamela Patrick Novotny
Overall Rating:	★★★★
Media Type:	Book
Short Description:	The author strives to offer "an upbeat, practical guide to raising and loving babies that arrive in groups of two or more." This 324 page book contains medical, psychological, and sociological findings on all aspects of caring for two or more children simultaneously. Chapter topics include: the logistics of caring for multiples after birth, to their first year, and beyond; mothercare; family adjustments; premature births; and more.

■ **Read The Full Review Of This Resource On Page 123.**

Advice and support for new moms through Internet dialogs with other moms

Title:	**Moms Online (Internet)**
Subtitle:	A Home For Moms In Cyberspace
Overall Rating:	★★★★
Media Type:	Internet
Short Description:	Billing themselves as "a home for Moms in cyberspace," Moms Online offers the following at their website: a daily journal detailing life with a 4-year old boy and a baby girl; "hot tips"; contributions, essays, and advice from other moms; and a "mom of the week" and her perspectives. An online newsletter, Mother News, is available, as well as a virtual spa for moms, a recipe index, and advice from professionals.

■ **Read The Full Review Of This Resource On Page 126.**

Advice and support for new moms through dialogs with other moms on AOL

Title:	**Moms Online (AOL)**
Subtitle:	A Home For Moms In Cyberspace
Overall Rating:	★★★★
Media Type:	Online Service
Short Description:	Billing themselves as "a home for Moms in cyberspace," Moms Online offers the following at their website: a daily journal detailing life with a 4-year old boy and a baby girl; "hot tips"; contributions, essays, and advice from other moms; and a "mom of the week" and her perspectives. An online newsletter, Mother News, is available, as well as a virtual spa for moms, a recipe index, Teen Center, Homeschooling Center, and advice from professionals.

■ **Read The Full Review Of This Resource On Page 125.**

The emotional aspects of dealing with infertility

Title:	**What To Expect When You're Experiencing Infertility**
Subtitle:	How To Cope With The Emotional Crisis And Survive
Author:	Debby Peoples and Harriette Rovner Ferguson, CSW
Overall Rating:	★★★★
Media Type:	Book
Short Description:	The authors have divided this book into four sections—"Crisis," "Acceptance," "Resolution,"

■ **Read The Full Review Of This Resource On Page 201.**

The authors have divided this book into four sections—"Crisis," "Acceptance," "Resolution," and "Epilogue" (C.A.R.E.)—to deal strictly with the emotional effects a couple experiencing infertility may expect. The authors respond to statements and questions from people who have gone through this experience. Little medical information is given; the focus deals solely with the daily pain and frustration of those dealing with infertility.

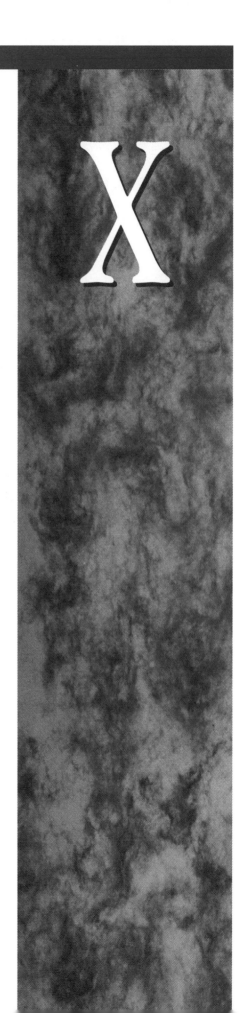

SUPPORT ORGANIZATIONS & OTHER HELPFUL RESOURCES

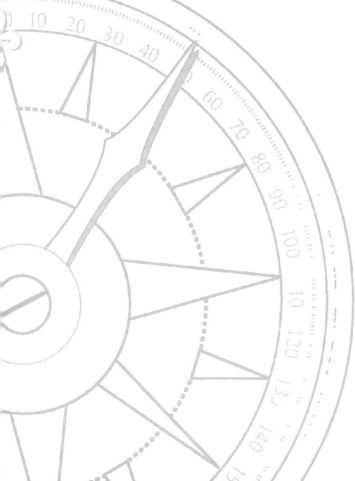

INTRODUCTION

Many of the resources we've reviewed include contact information on support groups, associations, and other organizations. On the pages that follow, we've listed a number of these organizations. They are grouped by the principal focus of their work using the major subject classifications we've used for this guidebook. You'll find that many of these organizations can further refer you to other local, regional, or national organizations that may offer you additional benefits or aspects of support that meet your needs.

The support groups, associations, and other organizations which follow are listed alphabetically within the following topics and subtopics:

SUPPORT ORGANIZATIONS

General Overview

American College Of Obstetricians And Gynecologists Resource Center

409 Twelfth Street, S.W.
Washington, DC 20024
(202) 638-5577;
publication order line (800) 762-2264

Professional organization of OB/GYNs which provides publications for doctors and patients on variety of subjects, including infertility.

American Foundation For Maternal And Child Health

439 East 51st Street
New York, NY 10022
(212) 759-5510

Global Maternal/Child Health Association, Inc. (GMCHA)

P.O. Box 140
Wilsonville, OR 97070
(503) 682-3600
Fax: (503) 682-3434
URL: http://www.geocities.com/
HotSprings/2840/about.htm

This association was incorporated in 1989 in order to facilitate maternity care reform. Their stated purpose is to preserve, protect and enhance the well-being of women and children during pregnancy, birth, infancy, and early childhood. GMCHA is working to alter the "current technological dependency, excessive drug use and rising caesarean rate by educating medical professionals and the public on the benefits of family-centered, natural childbirth, midwifery as the model for maternity care, and the use of warm-water immersion during labor and birth."

Mothers Of Supertwins (MOST)

P.O. Box 951
Brentwood, NY 11717
(516) 434-MOST

This national support network is for families who are expecting, or who are already the parents of, triplets or more. One of the organization's goals is to help families make informed decisions regarding their pregnancy and their children's development.

National Perinatal Information Center

1 State Street, Suite 102
Providence, RI 02908
(401) 274-0650

Provides perinatal information.

National Women's Health Network

1325 G Street NW, Lower Level
Washington, DC 20005
(202) 347-1140

This advocacy group focuses on women's health issues and strives to educate people about women's health rights.

Twin Services

P.O. Box 10066
Berkeley, CA 94709
(415) 524-0863

This group offer free over-the-phone counseling for parents, educators, and other professionals on issues such as pregnancy, parenting, and child development of multiple-birth children. They also offer their members a quarterly newsletter and an annual conference geared toward both parents and professionals.

Pregnancy & Fetal Development

American Diabetes Association

12660 Duke Street
Alexandria, VA 22314
(703) 549-1500

This organization offers advice and information for pregnant women with diabetes. They provide support through publications and an informational hot-line.

Birthright

3424 Hardee Ave
Chamblee, GA 30359
(800) 550-4900, or (206) 789-5676
email: info@birthright.org
URL: http://www.birthright.org/

Birthright provides free, confidential support to women who are facing an unplanned pregnancy. They offer a toll free hotline, abortion alternatives, emotional support, free pregnancy tests, and several other services. Birthright branches are spread throughout the United States.

March Of Dimes Birth Defects Foundation

1275 Mamaroneck Avenue
White Plains, NY 10605
(914) 428-7100

This nonprofit organization fights birth defects by offering informational pamphlets.

National Abortion Federation

1436 U Street NW, Suite 103
Washington, DC 20009
Hotline: (800) 772-9100, or (202) 667-5881
email: naf@prochoice.org
URL: http://www.prochoice.org/

The National Abortion Federation was founded in 1977 as a professional association of abortion providers throughout the US and Canada. They wish to preserve and enhance the quality of and access to abortion services. The NAF provides educational information and referrals to quality providers.

Sidelines

P.O. Box 1808
Laguna Beach, CA 92651
(949) 497-2265
URL: http://www.sidelines.org

This group provides support, education, and advocacy to women with high-risk pregnancies and their families. They have community-based chapters throughout the U.S., publish Left Sidelines for women with complicated pregnancies (particularly those who are confined to bed), provide pamphlets and books, and aim to be sensitive to the issues surrounding pregnancy following infertility.

The American College Of Obstetricians And Gynecologists (ACOG)

409-12th St. SW
P.O. Box 96920
Washington, DC 20004-2188
(202) 638-5577
URL: http://www.acog.com

Membership organization for obstetricians and gynecologists. This organization also provides the general public with informational pamphlets and keeps its members informed about care standards based on the most recent scientific research.

Childbirth

American Academy Of Husband-Coached Childbirth (AAHCC-Bradley)

P.O. Box 5224
Sherman Oaks, CA 91413
(818) 788-6662; (800) 423-2397;
or (800) 4-A-BIRTH (Pregnancy Hotline)

Offers information on the Bradley® method of natural childbirth offering referrals to classes in your area. When you call, leave a message along with your address since all responses are handled by mail.

American College Of Home Obstetrics

P.O. Box 508
Oak Park, IL 60303
(708) 388-1461

American College Of Nurse-Midwives (ACNM)

818 Connecticut Ave., NW, Suite 900
Washington, DC 20006
(202) 728-9860
Email: info@acnm.org
URL: http://www.midwife.org

This is a membership organization for nurse-midwives. They also provide guidelines for standards and practices, and can make referrals to certified nurse-midwives in your area.

Association For Childbirth At Home International

P.O. Box 430
Glendale, CA 91209
(213) 667-0839

Organization offers advice to pregnant women who desire to give birth at home.

Association Of Childbirth Educators And Labor Assistants

P.O. Box 382724
Cambridge, MA 02238-2724
(617) 441-2500
Fax: (617) 441-3167

This organization's goal is to help empower women and families throughout the process of childbirth. They provide childbirth training and offer referrals to parents.

California Association Of Midwives (CAM)

P.O. Box 460606
San Francisco, CA 94146
(800) 829-5791
Email: midwives@wenet.net
URL: http://www.wenet.net/~midwives/index.html

CAM started in 1978 as a professional organization representing midwives throughout California. Their goals are to increase recognition of midwives as primary caregivers and childbirth experts. They want women to have access to midwives in their homes as well as birthing centers and hospitals.

Cesarean Support, Education And Concern (C/SEC, Inc.)

22 Forest Road
Framingham, MA 01701
(508) 877-8266

Organization offers information and pamphlets regarding Cesarean section births. Also makes referrals to local listings of Cesarean support groups in your area.

Childbirth & Family Education, Inc. (CFE)

287 Whiteface Mountain Dr.
Johnson, VT 05656
(802) 635-2142
URL: http://www.childbirth.org/CFE.html

This organization provides information on labor assistants, labor support, doula training, and referrals.

Doulas Of North America (DONA)/Pennypress Inc.

1100 23rd Avenue East
Seattle, WA 98112
Pennypress (206) 325-1419
DONA (206) 324-5440
Fax: DONA (206) 325-0472

Founded by Penny Simkin in 1992, this association provides certification for individual labor doulas, provide a network for individual women and families seeking a labor doula, and trains women who wish to become a doula. They are the sister organization to NAPCS.

Informed Homebirth/Informed Birth And Parenting

P.O. Box 3675
Ann Arbor, MI 48106
(313) 662-6857

Organization offers information on alternative birth methods, and provides training for childbirth educators and childbirth assistants.

International Cesarean Awareness Network (ICAN)

1304 Kingsdale Ave.
Redondo Beach, CA 90278
(310) 542-6400
Email: ICANinc@aol.com
URL: http://www.childbirth.org/section/ican

This organization provides information and education with the aim to lower the number of repeat and unnecessary Cesarean sections. They also offer a newsletter, conferences, and nationwide support groups for Cesarean prevention and vaginal birth after Cesarean.

International Childbirth Education Association (ICEA)

P.O. Box 20048
Minneapolis, MN 55420
(612) 854-8660
Email: info@icea.org
URL: http://www.icea.org

This interdisciplinary organization trains childbirth educators, and provides books, pamphlets, and other materials on childbirth and maternity care.

Lamaze International

1200 19th Street, N.W., Suite 300
Washington, DC 20036-2422
(800) 368-4404
URL: http://www.lamaze-childbirth.com

This childbirth education program provides referrals to local certified Lamaze instructors. Videos, books, and pamphlets on pregnancy, labor, and childbirth are also available by mail order.

Maternity Center Association

48 E. 92nd Street
New York, NY 10128
(212) 369-7300

Midwives' Alliance Of North America (MANA)

600 Fifth Street
Monett, MO 65708
(888) 923-6262
Email: manainfo@aol.com
URL: http://www.mana.org

This organization provides information on midwifery and referrals to midwives in your area.

National Association Of Childbearing Centers

2123 Gottschall Road
Perkiomenville, PA 18074
(215) 234-8068

Provides pamphlets to parents about birthing centers in their area along with information on how to choose one.

National Association Of Childbirth Assistants (NACA)

205 Copco Lane
San Jose, CA 95123

259 Meridian Ave.
San Jose, CA 95126
(408) 225-9167

Founded in 1985, NACA's members are persons who are specially trained to provide labor support and educational counseling.

National Association Of Parents And Professionals For Safe Alternatives In Childbirth (NAPSAC)

Route 1, Box 646
Marble Hill, MO 63764
(573) 238-2010
Email: stewartdl@compuserve.com

This umbrella organization for the alternative birth movement provides information, a quarterly newsletter, a mail-order book service, and an international directory of alternative birth services.

Read Natural Childbirth Foundation, Inc.

P.O. Box 150956
San Rafael, CA 94915
(415) 456-8462

This foundation is based on the work of Dick Grantly-Read.

Water Birth International,
A project of Global Maternal/Child Health Association

P.O. Box 1400
Wilsonville, OR 97070
(503) 682-3600
Email: waterbirth@aol.com
URL: http://www.geocities.com/
hotsprings/2840

Directed by Barbara Harper, this organization provides information on natural childbirth, including birth in water. They also sell books and videotapes by mail order, and rent and sell portable, inflatable birthing tubs which can be shipped anywhere within the U.S.

Postpartum Care Issues

Depression After Delivery (DAD)

P.O. Box 1282
Morrisville, PA 19067
(800) 944-4PPD (4773), or (215) 295-3994

This national, nonprofit organization was the first group of its kind to offer information and support to women who suffer from postpartum depression. They also provide referrals and a quarterly newsletter called "Heart Strings" to its members.

Marcé Society

Department of Psychology
University of Iowa
Iowa City, IA 52242
(319) 335-2452

This society was founded in England in 1980, and was named for Dr. Louis Victor Marce who in 1858 published a study of postpartum psychosis in France. The society is committed to improving the understanding, treatment, and prevention of postpartum disorders.

National Association Of Postpartum Care Services (NAPCS)

General Information:
P.O. Box 1020
Edmonds, WA 98020

Membership Information:
326 Shields Street
San Francisco, CA 94132
(800) 45-DOULA (453-6852)

Founded in 1989, this is the first national organization of doula postpartum caregivers. NAPCS acts as a referral source for women looking for local

service and for those women who wish to start a service. The organization provides a free list of consultants who will work on a for-fee basis with a new service.

National Depressive And Manic Depressive Association

730 N. Franklin, Suite 501
Chicago, IL 60610
(312) 642-0049
URL: http://www.ndmda.org/

This organization's goal is to educate families, patients, mental health professionals, and the general public concerning depressive and manic-depressive illness as treatable medical diseases. They hope to eliminate patient discrimination, bring about self-help for families and patients, and improve access to care.

National Institute Of Mental Health, Depression Awareness, Recognition And Treatment (DART)

Public Inquiries:
5600 Fishers Lane, Rm. 15-C-05
Rockville, MD 20857
(800) 421-4211, or (301) 443-2403
URL: http://nimh.nih.gov/publicat/
eduprogs/dart.htm

The Depression Awareness, Recognition, and Treatment Program (DART,) a branch of the NIMH, is a public and professional education service intended to reduce the prevalence of depressive disorders by encouraging early identification and treatments. They offer information brochures through their toll free line.

Postpartum Adjustment Support Services (PASS-CAN)

P.O. Box 7282
Oakville, Ontario L6J 6C6 CANADA
(905) 844-9009, or (905) 897-MAMA (6262)

Links Canadian support services to ensure families gets up-to-date information, education, support, and services regarding postpartum issues. They also can provide a packet on postpartum adjustment disorders.

Postpartum Stress Center (The)

1062 Lancaster Ave., Suite 18-D
Rosemont, PA 19010
(610) 525-7527

Started in 1987, this support and counseling service offers couples therapy, referrals to local support groups, and a pregnancy support program to identify and support those women at risk for PPD or stress.

Postpartum Support International (PSI)

927 N. Kellogg Avenue
Santa Barbara, CA 93111
(805) 967-7636
Email: thonikman@compuserve.com
URL: http://www.iup.edu/an/postpartum

International network of individuals and groups which is dedicated to increasing awareness about the emotional health of pregnant and postpartum women and their families.

Pregnancy and Postpartum Treatment Program (The)

Department of Psychiatry
University of Illinois at Chicago
912 South Wood Street
Chicago, IL 60612
(312) 996-7362, or (312) 996-2972

This outpatient treatment program offers parent-centered treatment and support for postpartum women. Services include mental health services, pregnancy planning for women who have experienced PPD before, consultation for breastfeeding mothers, risk assessment, family and marital therapy, support for new fathers, and more. They also make referrals to community self-help programs, pediatric care, and parenting skills training.

Loss Of A Pregnancy Or Child

Abiding Hearts

P.O. Box 5245
Bozeman, MT 59717
(406) 587-7421
Fax: (406) 587-7197
URL: http://asfhelp.com/asf/sgi/ah/ahtoc.htm

Abiding Hearts gives information and support to parents who chose to continue their pregnancies after prenatal tests have shown fatal or non-fatal birth defects. They wish to connect parents with similar problems and provide support and information. They are a not-for-profit organization that relies on donations.

AMEND (Aiding A Mother & Father Experiencing Neonatal Death)

4324 Berrywick Terrace
St. Louis, MO 63128
(314) 487-7582

This organization provides support for parents whose babies die through stillbirth, miscarriage, or other means. They typically get referrals through hospitals. The organization provides one-on-one contact and support for parents.

Bereaved Parents of the USA (BPUSA)

P.O. Box 95
Park Forest, IL 60466
(708) 748-7672
Fax: (708) 748-9184

This is a nationwide support group for bereaved parents. The organization provides support through local chapters, listing of groups worldwide, program materials, and educational services.

Center For Loss In Multiple Birth (CLIMB)

P.O. Box 1064
Palmer, AK 99645
(907) 746-6123
Email: climb@ pobox.alaska.net
URL: http://www.climb-support.org/

This organization is devoted to parents throughout the US, Canada, and beyond who have experienced the death of one or more of their children. It is aimed at parents who have lost their children through twin, triplet, or other multiple pregnancies, or in early childhood. CLIMB publishes a quarterly newsletter and a contact list for parents who have lost one or more babies. They also can provide samples of birth and memorial announcements.

Compassionate Friends

National Office
P.O. Box 3696
Oak Brook, IL 60522-3696
(630) 990-0010
Fax: (630) 990-0246

This international self-help organization offers friendship and understanding to bereaved families who have lost a child of any age or any cause of death. They provide a free newsletter and brochures as well as referrals to local groups to help parents and siblings reach a positive resolution to their grief.

Elisabeth Kubler-Ross Center

South Route 616
Head Waters, VA 24442
(703) 396-3441

This center provides a network for grieving families of a child who is sick or has died. They offer a quarterly newsletter and can refer you to workshops in your area.

Helping Other Parents In Normal Grieving (HOPING)

Sparrow Hospital
1215 E. Michigan Ave.
P.O. Box 30480
Lansing, MI 48909
(517) 483-3873

Infertility And Pregnancy Loss (INCIID Links And Online Resources)

P.O. Box 3863
Arlington, VA 22206
(703) 379-9178, or (520) 544-9548
Fax: (214) 509-5251
Email: nancy@inciid.org
URL: http://www.inciid.org

This nonprofit, consumer-oriented organization provides links to current information on the Internet about the many types of infertility. They take care to provide links only to those websites and articles that offer accurate, medically responsible points of view as reviewed by qualified physicians or therapists. They also provide fact sheets on specific subjects, as well as a directory of professionals in a given area.

National SIDS Resource Center

2070 Chain Bridge Road
Vienna, VA 22182
(703) 821-8955
Fax: (703) 821-2098
Email: info@circsol.com
URL: http://www.circsol.com/SIDS/index.HTM

The National SIDS Resource Center provides assistance and information on Sudden Infant Death Syndrome (SIDS). The organization's goal is to promote understanding of SIDS and provide support and comfort to those who have lost a child.

Pen-Parents, Inc.

P.O. Box 8738
Reno, NV 89507-8738
(702) 826-7332
Fax: (702) 323-2489
Email: PenParents@prodigy.com or
URL: PenParents@aol.com

This international support network
for grieving parents offers a quarterly
newsletter and additional items for
memorials. A group for grandparents
is also available (Pen-Grandparents).

Pregnancy And Infant Loss Center (PILC)

1421 East Wayzata Boulevard, Suite 30
Wayzata, MN 55391
(612) 473-9372
Fax: (612) 473-8978

This nonprofit organization offers support,
resources, and education to parents and
families who have experienced pregnancy
and infant loss. They also provide cards,
memory albums, certificates of birth/
baptism or blessing, and burial gowns.

Pregnancy Loss Support Program For Miscarriage, Stillbirth, And Newborn Death

9 East 69th Street
New York, NY 10021
(212) 535-5900

This is a nonsectarian project of the
National Council of Jewish Women.

Resolve Through Sharing / RTS LaCrosse-Lutheran Hospital

Gundersen Lutheran Medical Center
1910 South Avenue
LaCrosse, WI 54601
(608) 791-4747, or (800) 362-9567 x4747
Fax: 608-791-5137
Email: berservs@gundluth.org
URL: www.gundluth.org/bereave

RTS is an international perinatal
bereavement program formerly known
as Resolve Through Sharing. They provide
training and support materials to
professionals working with parents who
have lost a baby through miscarriage,
stillbirth, ectopic pregnancy, or newborn
death. Their goal is to present a
compassionate staff that listens to the
needs of individual parents. They also
have an RTS training program for
professionals.

SHARE (A Source Of Help In Airing And Resolving Experiences) St. Joseph Health Center

St. Joseph Health Center
300 First Capitol Drive
St. Charles, MO 63301
(314) 947-6164
Fax: (314) 947-7486
URL: http://www.nationalshareoffice.com

This national organization provides
support, counseling, assistance, and
resources for bereaved families who
have lost infants and newborns due to
miscarriage, stillbirth, or other neonatal
death. They also offer publications.

SIDS Alliance

1314 Bedford Avenue, Suite 210
Baltimore, MD 21208

10500 Little Patuxent Parkway, Suite 420
Columbia, MD 21044
(800) 221-SIDS, or (800) 638-SIDS
Email: sidshq@charm.net

This organization offers referrals to local
support groups, counseling services, and
literature for parents who have lost a
baby to sudden infant death syndrome.
Their national toll-free hotline is staffed
24 hours with a counselor.

Baby Care—General

American Academy Of Pediatrics

141 Northwest Point Blvd.
Elk Grove Village, IL 60009-0927
(847) 228-5005
URL: http://www.aap.org

Provides information and publishes free
brochures on children's health issues.

Association For Retarded Citizens Of The United States (ARC)

National Headquarters
P.O. Box 6109
Arlington, TX 76005
(817) 640-0204

This organization makes referrals to local
chapters throughout the U.S. It provides
parents with early intervention services
for babies and toddlers in an effort to
give them a head start through
developing their motor skills, coordination,
and recognition. This organization also
offers free and low-cost brochures,
booklets, and videos.

Center For Study Of Multiple Birth

339 East Superior Street
Chicago, IL 60611
(312) 266-9093
Fax: (312) 280-8500
Email: lgk395@nwu.edu
URL: http://multiplebirth.com/

The CSMB's goal is to promote and
advance the health of women and
children, especially multiple birth children,
through public service, education, and
research. Their future goals are to reduce
the medical and social costs of multiple
births, encourage medical research, and
conduct research of their own.

National Association Of Mothers Centers

64 Division Avenue
Levittown, NY 11756
(800) 645-3828

This national network of support and
resource groups for new parents can
help connect you with a local support
center or help you start your own.

National Down's Syndrome Association

141 5th Avenue
New York, NY 10018
(212) 460-9330

National organization that promotes
research and public awareness of Down's
syndrome. Also provides free printed
information packets, video cassettes, and
a directory and early intervention and
parent support groups.

National Organization Of Mothers Of Twins Clubs, Inc.

P.O. Box 23188
Albuquerque, NM 87192-1188

Rockville, MD 20853
(800) 243-2276
URL: http://www.NOMOTC.org

This organization offers a complimentary
brochure of helpful hints. They also offer
referrals to local support groups.

Parent Care, Inc.

101-1/2 South Union Street
Alexandria, VA 22314-3323

9041 Colgate Street
Indianapolis, IN 46268
(in IN) (317) 872-9913

This coalition aims to support parents of
premature babies by connecting them

with their local support groups. They provide information, resources, and support, a quarterly newsletter, and issues papers which outline the concerns faced by parents of premature and high-risk infants. They also provide a handbook to help parents care for the preterm baby.

Parents of Premature And High-Risk Infants, International, Inc.

c/o National Self-Help Clearinghouse
24 West 43 Street, Room 620
New York, NY 10036
(212) 642-2944

Parents Of Prematures (POP)

P.O. Box 3046
Kirkland, WA 98033

This nonprofit organization is run by parents who have experienced the birth of a premature child. They offer emotional support, a national newsletters, a baby book and clothing patterns geared toward the premature infant.

Baby Care—Breastfeeding

Breastfeeding National Network (BNN) Medela, Inc.

P.O. Box 660
4610 Prime Parkway
McHenry, IL 60050-0660
(800) TELL-YOU (835-5968)
URL: http://www.medela.com

This manufacturer of breast pumps and breastfeeding support materials also offers a list of local lactation consultants. You can leave an email message at their website, and receive a personal email message reply.

Center For Breastfeeding Information

(847) 519-7730 x241

This center handles inquiries from health professionals, breastfeeding counselors, and researchers (a fee is charged).

Centers For Disease Control And Prevention Office Of Public Inquiries

1600 Clifton Road
NE Atlanta, GA 30333
(800) 311-3435

This center offers advice regarding infectious diseases and breastfeeding.

Denver Mothers' Milk Bank

Presbyterian/St. Luke's Medical Center
1719 East 19th Ave.
Denver, CO 80218
(303) 869-1888

This organization is the largest distributing milk bank in North America, providing screened and processed donor breast milk.

Human Milk Banking Association Of North America

8 Han Sebastian Way, #13
Sandwich, MA 02563
(508) 888-4041, or (888) 232-8809

This is an organization of distributing donor milk banks in North America. They provide information on milk banking and the location of milk banks.

International Lactation Consultants Association (ILCA)

4101 Lake Boone Trail, Suite 201
Raleigh, NC 27607-6518
(919) 787-5181

This association can help you find a lactation consultant in your area.

La Leche League International, Inc.

91400 N. Meacham Rd.
P.O. Box 4079
Schaumberg, IL 60168-4079
(847) 519-7730, or (800) LALECHE

Provides information, support, and materials to women about breastfeeding their baby. Their 800 number is paid for by Motherwear, staffed buy a volunteer La Leche League leader, and offers referrals to a local La Leche League support group.

Mother's Help Line

(800) 824-6351

This is sponsored by White River Concepts and offers free basic breastfeeding advice and care plans in English and in Spanish.

National Alliance For Breastfeeding Advocacy Office Of Educational Services

254 Conant Road
Weston, MA 02193
(617) 893-3553
Fax: (617) 893-8608
Email: MarshaLact@aol.com

This is an education and lobbying organization for breastfeeding reform in the US. They do not provide materials for parenting issues.

Nursing Mothers Council, Inc.

2509 NE Thompson
Portland, OR 97212

P.O. Box 50063
Palo Alto, CA 94303
(503) 293-0661, (650) 599-3669,
(415) 591-6688, or (408) 272-1448
URL: http://www.nursingmothers.org

Nonprofit, nonaffiliated organization that aims to "help mothers enjoy a relaxed and happy feeding relationship with their baby" by providing breastfeeding information and support through chapters in various cities in California, and in Denver, Fort Wayne, and Atlanta.

Baby Care—Choosing A Caregiver

American Council Of Nanny Schools

A-74 Delta College University Center,
Michigan 48740
(517) 686-9417

An information packet can be sent to families upon request.

Au Pair Care/European Nanny Service

1 Post Street, Suite 700
San Francisco, CA 94104
(800) 428-7247, or (415) 434-8788

This service provides au pair referrals and connections for families. Their 12 month childcare and cultural exchange program matches families with screened foreign students 18–26 years of age. There is typically a six to eight week waiting period for families upon applying. Au pairs may work up to 45 hours a week with a maximum limit of 10 hours a day. Families provide a stipend and room and board. The service's au pairs are not professional childcare professionals, but are trained in first aid and child development.

Au Pair In America American Institute For Foreign Study

102 Greenwich Ave.
Greenwich, Connecticut 06830
(800) 727-2437

This "largest and oldest au pair agency" offers opportunities for foreign students to work in American family homes. They also offer an international companion program during the summer months.

Au Pair Programme USA

6965 Union Park Center, Suite 100
Salt Lake City, 84047
(800) 937-6264
Fax: (801) 255-7782
Email: jacque@app/childcrest.com

This agency was originally established as a nanny referral organization and served families for 15 years. Since 1989, they became one of six authorized agencies which bring au pairs into the US. There is a $280 application fee and a $4180 placement fee for their services, which includes the au pair's airfare, medical insurance, a counselor, visa work, and 32 hours of training. Students commit to one year of au pair service.

Au Pair Exchange

161 - 6th Ave.
New York, NY, 10013
(800) 287-2477

This cultural exchange program matches families with foreign students. Cost for hosting an au pair is $230 per week, and includes up to 45 hours flexible live-in child care.

Child Care Action Campaign

330 Seventh Ave., 17th Floor
New York, NY 10001
(212) 239-0138
Fax: (212) 268-6515
Email: hn5746@handsnet.org
URL: http://www.ccac.org

The Child Care Action Campaign is a national childcare advocacy organization which serves the general public, parents, government agencies, and the media. The organization sponsors an electronic discussion group called "Children, Youth and Families Forum" which provides information on childcare advocacy and current legislation. The discussion list email address is: HN0003@handsnet.org

Child Care Aware

1319 F St. NW, Suite 810
Washington, DC 20004
(800) 424-2246
Fax: (202) 393-1109
Email: hn6125@handsnet.org

Offering a "connection to good quality care sponsored by Cheerios," this organization's nationwide 1-800 number can refer parents to phone numbers of local childcare resources and referrals. Parents may also call Child Care Aware

and request their free packet ($10 for pack of 100) of tip sheets for choosing quality child care. This includes checklists to use for interviewing careproviders, advice on how to find quality childcare, information on accreditation of childcare centers and homes, and more. A list of their national non-profit partners and corporate sponsors is also available through their phone number.

International Nanny Association (The)

900 Haddon Ave., Suite 438
Collingswood, NJ 08108
(609) 858-0808
Fax: (609) 858-2519
Email: ina@nanny.org
URL: http://www.nanny.org/

Since 1986, the INA (a non-profit association) has served as a clearinghouse for information on the in-home child care industry. The INA serves over 700 members who are committed to professional in-home childcare. Their membership is made up of nannies, nanny educators, nanny referral agency owners and personnel, and individuals who support the in-home childcare industry. Those members who join agree to abide by the association's recommended practices.

National Association For Family Child Care (NAFCC)

206-6th Ave., Suite 900
Des Moines, Iowa 50309-4018
(515) 282-8192
Fax: (515) 282-9117
Email: nafcc@nafcc.org
URL: http://www.nafcc.org

A nationwide study of family daycare in 1978 recommended formation of the National Association for Family Day Care (NAFDC) in 1982. This was later reestablished in 1994 as the National Association for Family Child Care. This "national voice for family child care" provides technical assistance to family childcare associations. This assistance is provided through developing leadership and professionalism, addressing issues of diversity, and by promoting quality and professionalism through NAFCC's Family Child Care Accreditation.

National Child Care Information Center

243 Church Street NW, 2nd floor
Vienna, VA 22180
(800) 616-2242
Fax: (800) 716-2242
Email: agoldste@nccic.org
URL: http://www.nccic.org

This is a clearinghouse for information on childcare. They disseminate information to anyone interested in finding out how to choose childcare—parents, national or local organizations, state agencies, employers, schools, media, journalists, etc. The center was established about five years ago, and offers no endorsement of information they offer. If information is not available through the center, they will refer you to other organizations that might have that information.

Solutions To Infertility

American Society For Reproductive Medicine (ASRM)

1209 Montgomery Highway
Birmingham, AL 35216-2809
(205) 978-5000
Email: asrm@asrm.com
URL: http://www.asrm.com

Formerly known as the American Fertility Society (formed in 1944), this professional organization is dedicated to advancing knowledge and expertise in reproductive medicine and biology. It is comprised of ob/gyns, reproductive endocrinologists, nurses, urologists, andrologists, psychologists, social workers, research scientists, and other health-care professionals. They provide patients with referrals to the organization's members along with numerous patient information fact sheets and pamphlets. Their publications include a monthly medical journal, guidelines for practicing clinicians, and ethics reports.

Endometriosis Association

8585 N. 76th Place
Milwaukee, WI 53233
(800) 992-3636

This international self-help nonprofit organization, which performs research on the disease, provides support and education for patients with endometriosis and their families.

**Institute For Reproductive Health
Georgetown University School Of
Medicine**

2115 Wisconsin Avenue NW, Suite 602
Washington, DC 20007

Georgetown University Medical Center
3 PHC, Room 3004
3800 Reservoir Rd, NW
Washington, DC 20007
(202) 687-1392
Fax: (202) 687-6846
Email: irhinfo@gunet.georgetown.edu
URL: http://www.dml.georgetown.edu/depts/irh/

This organization provides policy support
for Fertility Awareness and Natural Family
Planning. The institute conducts research
and advances scientific information. It is
meant to be a resource for policy
planners, non-governmental organizations,
researchers, educators, governmental
agencies, and community-based program
managers.

RESOLVE, Inc.

1310 Broadway, Dept. GM
Somerville, MA 02144-1731
(617) 623-0744
Fax: (617) 623-0252
Email: resolveinc@aol.com
URL: http://www.resolve.org

This national organization's mission is to
provide timely, compassionate support,
and information to people experiencing
infertility. They work to increase
awareness of fertility issues through
advocacy and public education. Offering
referrals to local chapters and support
groups, this organization also provides
their membership with a national
newsletter, discounts on literature, and
access to medical information.

The Barren Foundation

60 East Monroe Street
Chicago, IL 60603

**The InterNational Council On
Fertility Information Dissemination,
Inc. (INCIID)**

P.O. Box 6836
Arlington, VA 22206
(703) 379-9178
Fax: (703) 379-1593
Email: INCIIDinfo@inciid.org
URL: http://www.inciid.org/

INCIID is a nonprofit organization that
provides up to date information regarding
the diagnosis, treatment, and prevention
of pregnancy loss and infertility. They
provide resource referrals including
doctor, therapist, and attorney listings, as
well as providing information on other
non-profit and fertility sites.

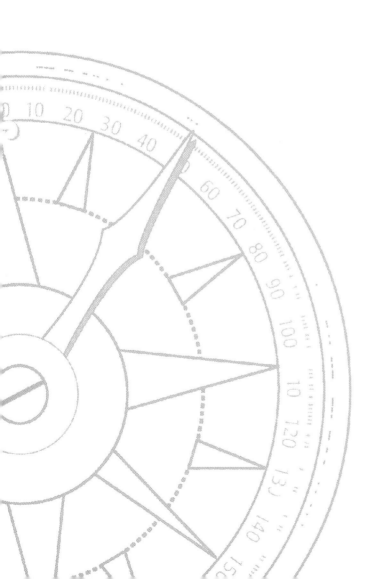

INDICES

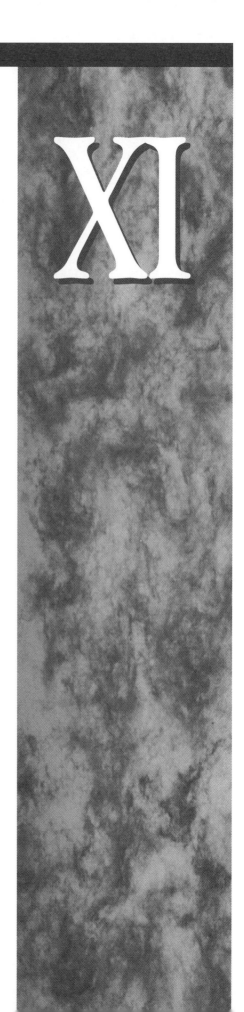

TITLE INDEX

AUTHOR INDEX

XI. Indices

PUBLISHER INDEX

MEDIA INDEX

Internet Websites

CD-ROMs

On-Line Service

Videotapes

SUBJECT INDEX
1–4 Stars (4 = Best)

XI. Indices

APPENDICES

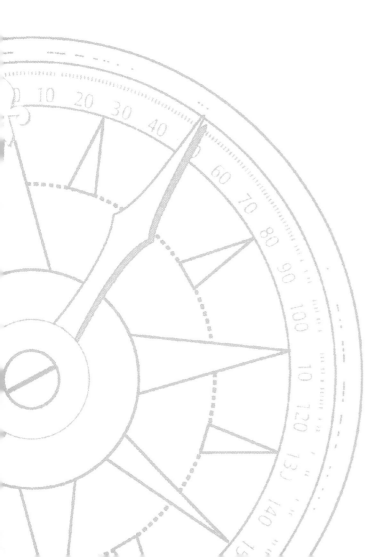

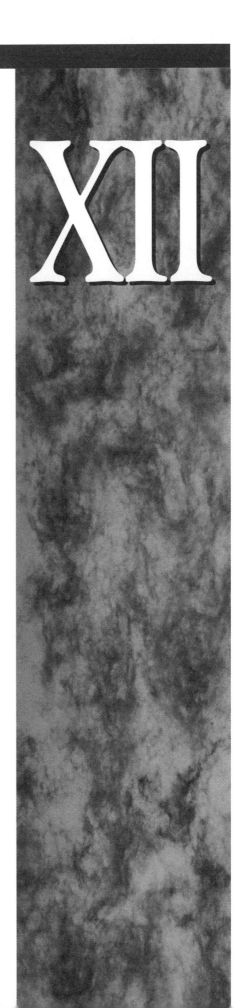

ABOUT THE EDITOR

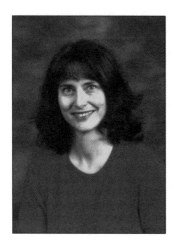

Anne Montgomery, MD, IBCLC, FAAFP, is a Board Certified Family Physician, an International Board Certified Lactation Consultant, and Clinical Associate Professor of Family Medicine at the University of Washington. Since 1994, she has served on the faculty of the Providence St. Peter Hospital Family Practice Residency Program where she serves as Chair of the Obstetrics/ Gynecology/Pediatrics Curriculum work group and serves on the Educational Management Team. At St. Peter Hospital, she has chaired the Primary Care Department Committee, and served on the Family Birth Center Council. Having graduated from Mayo Medical School and after doing her residency at the St. John's Unit of the University of Minnesota Family Practice training program, Anne practiced for five years in southern Minnesota before moving west. Her past appointments also include Clinical Assistant Professor at the Department of Family Practice and Community Health at the University of Minnesota Medical School. Anne was recently elected to the Board of Directors of the Academy of Breastfeeding Medicine, a multi-specialty international association of physicians dedicated to breastfeeding promotion and physician education. She is an active member of the American Academy of Family Physicians (AAFP) in which she has served on numerous committees, as well as representing Residents and Women Physicians in the Congress of Delegates. She also served on the Minnesota Academy of Family Physicians Board of Directors. Her practice and teaching emphasize maternal health, birth, and breastfeeding. At present, she is involved with the South Sound Breastfeeding Network, the Washington Healthy Mothers Healthy Babies Coalition, and La Leche League. Anne has also been a presenter at numerous conferences concerned with maternal health and breastfeeding, and has written professional articles on these subjects. She has attended hundreds of births and still finds each one a unique miracle. As a family physician, she feels especially blessed to be able to care for moms and babies before, during, and after birth—and to care for dads and grandparents, too! In addition to her professional experience, her knowledge in this field has been greatly enhanced by her own personal experience of pregnancy, birth, and breastfeeding. She lives in Olympia, Washington with her husband and eight-year-old son.

OUR ADVISORY COUNCIL FOR THIS EDITION

Resource Pathways would like to thank our Advisory Council for their contributions to this revised edition! Our Advisory Council includes professionals (who are in most cases parents too) that are involved with maternal and family health concerns, and familiar with decisions prospective parents face. While each Council member has made suggestions and provided input incorporated into this edition, their support does not imply their endorsement of individual resource ratings and recommendations—those decisions are the sole responsibility of our editors and researchers.

Janice Anderson, MD, Family Physician, Monroeville, PA

Dr. Anderson is a graduate of the University of Pittsburgh Medical School and Shadyside Hospital Family Practice Program. She spent five years in rural West Virginia under the National Health Service Scholarship Program. She now devotes her professional time to Forbes Family Practice Residency Program where she is Coordinator of the Ob/Gyn Curriculum. Dr. Anderson also is a member of the Ob/Gyn Subcommittee for HighMark Blue Cross and Blue Shield in Western Pennsylvania. As a member of the Advisory Council, she worked collaboratively with Anita MacDonald, MD, Rachel Gilman, MD, Joan Price, RNC, PNP, and Michael Yao, MD.

Anne Barash, MSW, MD, Assistant Professor, State University of New York Health Science Center, Syracuse, NY

Dr. Barash is an Assistant Professor in the Department of Family Medicine at the State University of New York Health Science Center at Syracuse, NY. She is responsible for the women's health, adolescent, and communications curriculum for medical students. She also serves on the Executive Committee of the Onondaga County Healthy Start Project and the Adolescent Work Group of the New York State Department of Health. Dr. Barash has also served as Director of Maternal Child Health at the Mid-Hudson Rural Family Practice Residency of New York Medical College, and has been a member of the Department of Family Practice at Mid-Hudson Family Health Institute, Kingston, New York. She holds memberships in the American Academy of Family Practice, National Association of Social Workers, the Medical Society of the State of New York, Central New York Council on Adolescent Pregnancy, and the Family Ties Network.

Joyce Blangiardo, RN, BS, LCCE, FACCE, IBCLC, Faculty member for the Lamaze™ Teacher Certification Program, Long Island, NY, and Director of Childbirth Education, North Shore Woman's Health Pavilion, Long Island, NY

In practice for over 32 years as a Registered Nurse in Obstetrics and specializing in Childbirth Education, Joyce Blangiardo is a Lamaze™ Certified Childbirth Educator, a Fellow in the American College of Childbirth Educators, and for the past 20 years a member of the national faculty for Lamaze™ International's Childbirth Educator Certification Program. Ms. Blangiardo has also been a breastfeeding educator and consultant for 28 years, and an International Board Certified Lactation Consultant for 12 years. She is currently Director of Childbirth Education at the North Shore Woman's Health Pavilion in Nassau, and the Woman's Health Pavilion in Queens. She has held these positions for the last twenty years. Ms. Blangiardo is active in a number of Internet professional discussion groups as well as a number of professional associations—Lamaze™ International, International Childbirth Education Association, International Lactation Consultants Association, and the Association of Women's Health, Obstetrical and Neonatal Nursing. She currently offers Lamaze™ and lactation classes in three counties on Long Island. Her private practice, Lamaze™ with Joy, reflects her sincere commitment to present comprehensive childbirth classes in a caring, enjoyable learning climate.

Andrea Eastman, MA, CCE, IBCLC, Certified Childbirth Educator, International Board Certified Lactation Consultant, Granville, OH

Andrea Eastman lives in Granville, Ohio with her husband and two daughters. She received a Bachelor of Arts degree in Biology from Denison University, and a Master of Arts degree in Environmental Conservation Education from New York University. She is a Certified Childbirth Educator and an International Board Certified Lactation Consultant in private practice. Ms. Eastman maintains her own informational website under the name of her business and self-designed childbirth classes—Gentle Birth Alternatives (www.geocities.com/HotSprings/8978). Volunteering for several organizations, she is the Breastfeeding & Childbirth Education Pro for "Moms Online" (www.momsonline.com), and the Research Committee Chairperson and Professional Advisory Board Coordinator & Member for Promotion of Mother's Milk, Inc., also known as "ProMoM" (www.promom.org). Ms. Eastman has been working with families in the fields of childbirth and breastfeeding since 1993.

Misty L. Gersley, CCE, Certified Perinatal and Childbirth Educator, San Diego, CA

A graduate from the University of San Diego Extension program, Misty Gersley is a Certified Perinatal and Childbirth Educator. She works at a local clinic serving as a prenatal outreach specialist as well as a childbirth educator. Her professional work aims to assure and facilitate the meeting of her clients' needs, as well as renewing each client's faith in her own body and her ability to birth. Married to a United States Marine, Ms. Gersley has been extremely active in the military community, it being the main focus of her outreach, and has volunteered to teach and speak at various military-related functions. She is pursing a degree in Social Work, and plans to continue her path to aid in pregnancy and childbirth related matters.

Molly Pessl, BSN, IBCLC, Registered Nurse, Lamaze™ Certified Childbirth Educator, Certified Lactation Consultant, Kirkland, WA

Since 1985, Molly Pessl has worked at the Family Maternity Center of Evergreen Hospital in Kirkland, WA. She coordinated the Baby Friendly Hospital Initiative at Evergreen, culminating in Evergreen becoming the first "Baby Friendly" hospital in the US. Ms. Pessl is a registered nurse, a Lamaze™ Certified Childbirth Educator, and a Certified Lactation Consultant with over 35 years of experience. She has developed preconception, prenatal, and postpartum education programs, created the regional Breastfeeding Center, and coordinates the Family Maternity Center's Professional Education Program. Ms. Pessl's current faculty appointments include Board Member, International Board of Lactation Consultant Examiners and UNICEF Breastfeeding Trainer. Her past appointments have included Academic Staff at the University of Washington and Clinical Nurse Faculty at Seattle Pacific University. Ms. Pessl is a popular speaker and lecturer, appearing at conferences, lectures, and workshops throughout the US. Her major concerns deal with the difficulties of parenting in today's society and the roles of health care providers in today's parenting issues. She is the mother of five children.

Milisa K. Rizer, MD, MPH, Family Practice Physician, Medical Director Georgetown University Medical Center

In private practice and academic practice for over 12 years, Milisa Rizer is a Family Practice Physician and a Fellow in the American Academy of Family Practice. She is presently Medical Director of the Student Primary Care Clinic at Georgetown University Medical Center in Washington, DC. Dr. Rizer is also currently an Associate Professor at Georgetown University in the Department of Family Medicine, the Department of Pediatrics, and the Department of Internal Medicine. Recipient of numerous awards for her excellence as a teacher, Dr. Rizer has also lectured at various conferences. She is also the proud mother of 28 month old Kaylin Rizer Allshouse.

Joseph Shaeffer, ARNP/CNM, Certified Ob/Gyn Nurse Practitioner, Certified Nurse Midwife, Spokane, WA

Joseph Shaeffer is a Women's Health Care Nurse Practitioner/ Certified Nurse Midwife (CNM) currently in an HMO practice with three other CNMs providing complete Women's Health Care and Obstetric services. He is affiliated with the American College of Nurse Midwives, the Nurse Practitioner Group of Spokane, and the American College of Obstetricians and Gynecologists. A guest faculty member at several nursing schools, Mr. Shaeffer has also lectured at various conferences on topics such as nurse midwifery, nurse practitioner, family nurse practitioner, and reproductive health. His previous appointments also include teaching childbirth education classes at the YWCA and at a family birth center. Mr. Shaeffer is the father of five children and grandfather to two with 25 years of experience in women's health care, many of those as a Labor and Delivery Nurse, Childbirth Educator, and for the past six years as a Nurse Midwife.

Karen Stern, OTR/ICCE-CPE, Registered Occupational Therapist, ICEA Certified Childbirth Educator, ICEA Certified Postnatal Educator, Philadelphia, PA

Karen Stern is a Registered Occupational Therapist and an ICEA (International Childbirth Education Association) Certified Childbirth Educator with over ten years teaching experience. She is also an ICEA Certified Postnatal Educator, and the founder and owner of Apres Baby Doula Services, Inc. which provides postpartum support to new families. Ms. Stern's professional memberships include DONA (Doulas of North America), NAPCS (National Association of Postpartum Care Services), ICEA, and AOTA (American Occupational Therapy Association). She resides with her husband and three children in Philadelphia.

Deborah Wage, MSN, FNP, CNM, Certified Family Nurse Practitioner, Certified Nurse Midwife, Nashville, TN

Deborah Wage is Director of Nashville Women's Health Associates in Nashville, Tennessee, a private midwifery practice. She delivers babies at Centennial Women's Hospital and Baptist Hospital in Nashville. Ms. Wage received her Master's degree from Vanderbilt University School of Nursing, and is dual board-certified as a Family Nurse Practitioner and a Nurse Midwife. She has been providing health care to the Nashville community for eight years. Ms. Wage is co-president of Middle Tennessee Advance Practice Nurses, and a member of the American College of Nurse Midwives and the American Academy of Nurse Practitioners. She is active at the local, state, and national levels in various activities to improve the quality of maternity services.

Shirley Wingate, RNC, CD, Childbirth Educator, Certified Doula, Urbana, IL

Shirley Wingate has been an Ob/Gyn Nurse for the past 12 years and is certified in women's health. She is an experienced labor and postpartum doula in private practice for the past three years. Ms. Wingate is the founder and Director of Birth Matters, Inc., a prenatal and parenting resource and support center offering classes for prepared childbirth, teen pregnancy, new fathers, adoptive parenting, and other parenting topics. Throughout her career, Ms. Wingate has been involved in developing, teaching, and expanding services in the community to educate families and support them as they face the changes, challenges, and choices that childbearing brings. She has been quoted in *Midwifery Today* and her article, "Full Circle," was published in *The International Journal of Childbirth Education*. Recently, Ms. Wingate has joined "Childbirth.org" as their "Ask a Nurse Pro."

She is a Childbirth Educator and a member of the International Childbirth Education Association (ICEA) and Doulas of North America (DONA). She is also a Certified Doula through DONA and has completed the requirements as a Doula Trainer.

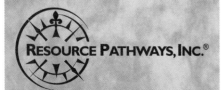

GUIDEBOOKS FOR LIFE'S BIG DECISIONS

For every important issue we face, there are resources available that offer suggestions and help. Unfortunately, we don't always know much about the issue we've enountered. Thus, we don't know:

- Where to find these sources of information
- Much about their quality, value, or relevance

Resource Pathways guidebooks help those facing an important decision or challenging life-event, by directing them to the information they need to understand the issues they face and make decisions with confidence. Every Resource Pathways guidebook includes these important values:

- We **describe and evaluate virtually all quality resources** available in any media (books, the Internet, CD-ROMs, videotape, audiotape, and more).

- We **explain the issues** that are typically encountered in dealing with each subject, and **classify each resource** we review according to its primary focus.

- We **make a reasoned judgment** about the quality of each resource, give it a **rating**, and decide whether or not a resource should be **recommended**. We select only the best as "Recommended" (roughly 1 in 4).

- We **provide information on where to buy or how to access** each resource, including ISBN numbers for books and URL "addresses" for Internet websites.

- We **publish a new edition of each guidebook frequently**, with updated reviews and recommendations.

Those who turn to Resource Pathways guidebooks will be able to locate the resource they need, saving time, money, and frustration as they begin their research and learning process.

LIFECYCLES SERIES

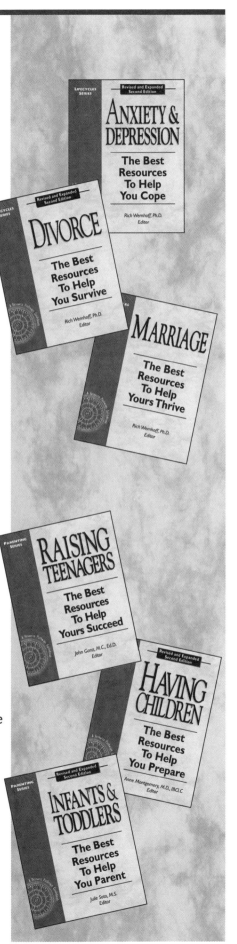

■ *". . . a calm and hope-filled guide . . ."*

Anxiety & Depression:
The Best Resources To Help You Cope

Editor: Rich Wemhoff, PhD
ISBN: 1-892148-09-9 (2nd Ed)
256 Pages (Available July, 1999)

■ *". . . an invaluable guide that will save time,*
emotional energy, and money . . ."

Divorce: The Best Resources To Help You Survive

Editor: Rich Wemhoff, PhD
ISBN: 1-892148-00-5 (2nd Ed)
324 Pages

■ *". . . valuable and remarkable directory . . ."*

Marriage: The Best Resources To Help Yours Thrive

Editor: Rich Wemhoff, PhD
ISBN: 1-892148-05-6
256 Pages (Available April, 1999)

PARENTING SERIES

■ *". . . an incredible resource guide . . ."*

Raising Teenagers:
The Best Resources To Help Yours Succeed

Editor: John Ganz, MC, EdD
ISBN: 1-892148-04-8
268 Pages

■ *"A comprehensive gem of a resource*
guide! . . . a great time-saver . . ."

Having Children: The Best Resources To Help You Prepare

Editor: Anne Montgomery, MD, IBCLC, FAAFP
ISBN: 1-892148-06-4 (2nd Ed)
312 Pages (Available May, 1999)

■ *". . . exciting, comprehensive, and hands-on*
practical . . ."

Infants & Toddlers:
The Best Resources To Help You Parent

Editor: Julie Soto, MS
ISBN: 1-892148-10-2 (2nd Ed)
390 Pages (Available August, 1999)

HIGHER EDUCATION
& CAREERS SERIES

■ *"... quintessential guide to the guides ..."*

College Choice & Admissions:
The Best Resources To Help You Get In

Editor: Dodge Johnson, PhD
ISBN: 0-9653424-9-2 (3rd Ed)
336 Pages

■ *"... comprehensive ... a real time and money saver ..."*

College Financial Aid:
The Best Resources To Help You Find The Money

Editor: David Hoy
ISBN: 1-892148-01-3 (3rd Ed)
278 Pages

■ *"... thorough, honest, and complete ..."*

Graduate School:
The Best Resources To Help You Choose, Get In, & Pay

Editor: Jane Finkle, MS
ISBN: 0-9653424-7-6
278 Pages

■ **Career Transitions:**
The Best Resources To Help You Advance

Editor: Resource Pathways Editors
ISBN: 1-892148-08-0
256 Pages (Available June, 1999)

■ *"... a clear and concise roadmap ..."*

Starting Your Career:
The Best Resources To Help You Find The Right Job

Editor: Laura Praglin, PhD
ISBN: 1-892148-03-X
248 Pages

Your favorite bookstore or library may order any of these guidebooks for you, or you can order direct, using the pre-paid postcards on the following pages.

ORDERING INFORMATION

Order by phone: 888-702-8882 (Toll-free 24/7)
Order by fax: 425-557-4366
Order by mail: Resource Pathways, Inc.
22525 SE 64th Place, Suite 253
Issaquah, WA 98027-5387

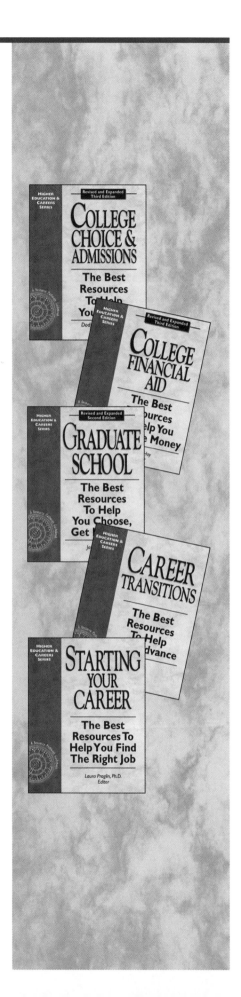

ORDER FORM

Order by phone: 888-702-8882 (Toll-free 24/7)
Order by fax: 425-557-4366

Order by mail: Resource Pathways, Inc.
22525 SE 64th Place, Suite 253
Issaquah, WA 98027-5387

☐ *Anxiety & Depression:*
The Best Resources To Help You Cope

☐ *Divorce:* The Best Resources To Help You Survive

☐ *Marriage:* The Best Resources To Help Yours Thrive

☐ *Raising Teenagers:*
The Best Resources To Help Yours Succeed

☐ *Having Children:* The Best Resources To Help You Prepare

☐ *Infants & Toddlers:* The Best Resources To Help You Parent

☐ *College Choice & Admissions:*
The Best Resources To Help You Get In

☐ *College Financial Aid:*
The Best Resources To Help You Find The Money

☐ *Graduate School:*
The Best Resources To Help You Choose, Get In, & Pay

☐ *Career Transitions:* The Best Resources To Help You Advance

☐ *Starting Your Career:*
The Best Resources To Help You Find The Right Job

_____ copies at $24.95 = _____

Shipping (USPS Priority Mail): $3.95 for first copy; $2.00/copy for additional copies

\+ Shipping & Handling = _____

We will include an invoice with your shipment

Total = _____

Name (please print) _____

Organization _____ Title _____

Address _____

City _____ State _____ Zip _____

Phone _____ Email _____

ORDER FORM

Order by phone: 888-702-8882 (Toll-free 24/7)
Order by fax: 425-557-4366

Order by mail: Resource Pathways, Inc.
22525 SE 64th Place, Suite 253
Issaquah, WA 98027-5387

☐ *Anxiety & Depression:*
The Best Resources To Help You Cope

☐ *Divorce:* The Best Resources To Help You Survive

☐ *Marriage:* The Best Resources To Help Yours Thrive

☐ *Raising Teenagers:*
The Best Resources To Help Yours Succeed

☐ *Having Children:* The Best Resources To Help You Prepare

☐ *Infants & Toddlers:* The Best Resources To Help You Parent

☐ *College Choice & Admissions:*
The Best Resources To Help You Get In

☐ *College Financial Aid:*
The Best Resources To Help You Find The Money

☐ *Graduate School:*
The Best Resources To Help You Choose, Get In, & Pay

☐ *Career Transitions:* The Best Resources To Help You Advance

☐ *Starting Your Career:*
The Best Resources To Help You Find The Right Job

_____ copies at $24.95 = _____

Shipping (USPS Priority Mail): $3.95 for first copy; $2.00/copy for additional copies

\+ Shipping & Handling = _____

We will include an invoice with your shipment

Total = _____

Name (please print) _____

Organization _____ Title _____

Address _____

City _____ State _____ Zip _____

Phone _____ Email _____

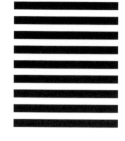

BUSINESS REPLY MAIL
FIRST-CLASS MAIL   PERMIT NO. 176   ISSAQUAH, WA

POSTAGE WILL BE PAID BY ADDRESSEE

RESOURCE PATHWAYS INC.

22525 SE 64TH PL STE 253

ISSAQUAH WA 98027-9939

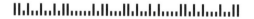

BUSINESS REPLY MAIL
FIRST-CLASS MAIL   PERMIT NO. 176   ISSAQUAH, WA

POSTAGE WILL BE PAID BY ADDRESSEE

RESOURCE PATHWAYS INC.

22525 SE 64TH PL STE 253

ISSAQUAH WA 98027-9939

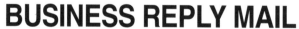

DISCOUNTS AND SUBSCRIPTIONS FOR PROFESSIONALS

Do you provide professional services to couples or families experiencing these life-events?

If so, you should know that Resource Pathways offers very attractive discounts to professionals for subscriptions to current and new editions of any title.

To obtain additional information or place an order, complete and return this postcard, or call 425-557-4382 (8-6 PST), or 888-702-8882 (Toll-free 24/7).

Name (please print) _____

Organization _____ Title _____

Address _____

City _____ State _____ Zip _____

Phone _____ Email _____

DISCOUNTS AND STANDING ORDERS FOR LIBRARIES

Resource Pathways' titles are distributed to libraries throughout North America by the National Book Network, through Ingram, Baker & Taylor, and many other regional wholesalers.

You can order any of our titles through your usual wholesaler or distributor, or direct from the National Book Network:

National Book Network, Inc., 15200 NBN Way, Blue Ridge Summit, PA 17214
800-462-6420 / 800-338-4550 (fax)

You can order directly from Resource Pathways at very attractive discounts, for both individual and standing orders.

To obtain additional information or place an order, complete and return this postcard, or call 425-557-4382 (8-6 PST), or 888-702-8882 (Toll-free 24/7).

Name (please print) _____

Organization _____ Title _____

Address _____

City _____ State _____ Zip _____

Phone _____ Email _____

BUSINESS REPLY MAIL

FIRST-CLASS MAIL   PERMIT NO. 176   ISSAQUAH, WA

POSTAGE WILL BE PAID BY ADDRESSEE

RESOURCE PATHWAYS INC.

22525 SE 64TH PL STE 253

ISSAQUAH WA 98027-9811

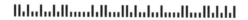

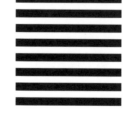

BUSINESS REPLY MAIL

FIRST-CLASS MAIL   PERMIT NO. 176   ISSAQUAH, WA

POSTAGE WILL BE PAID BY ADDRESSEE

RESOURCE PATHWAYS INC.

22525 SE 64TH PL STE 253

ISSAQUAH WA 98027-9811